Sarcoma

Peter F. M. Choong
Editor

Sarcoma

A Practical Guide to Multidisciplinary Management

Springer

Editor
Peter F. M. Choong
St. Vincent's Hospital Melbourne, Peter MacCallum Cancer Centre and
University of Melbourne Department of Surgery
Victoria, VIC
Australia

ISBN 978-981-15-9416-8 ISBN 978-981-15-9414-4 (eBook)
https://doi.org/10.1007/978-981-15-9414-4

This Springer imprint is published by the registered company Springer Nature Singapore Pte Ltd.
The registered company address is: 152 Beach Road, #21-01/04 Gateway East, Singapore 189721, Singapore

Preface

Sarcoma is a heterogeneous group of tumours that arise from mesenchymal tissue. Unlike the more common carcinoma, sarcoma is rare, and whose behaviour is characterised by substantial growth, a propensity to metastasise and aggressive recurrence if managed sub-optimally. The rarity of this tumour also means that for the majority of clinicians, diagnosis and treatment of such a tumour is typically confined to exceedingly low numbers over a lifetime. With this low level of exposure comes an inexperience which underpins earlier reported rates of treatment failure. For the patient, life and limb loss has been the sequel to a diagnosis of sarcoma in the past.

Modern sarcoma care is now characterised by a multidisciplinary, centre-based approach which capitalises on advances in diagnostics, radiotherapy, chemotherapy and surgery. Limb preservation surgery is now the norm for many who in the past faced amputation. For a condition with a near fatal outcome only 50 years ago, patients may now expect 5-year survival rates over 70%, one of the most substantial survival improvements amongst all solid cancers.

Appropriate management from the beginning underpins good treatment outcomes. This requires a systematic understanding and approach to care. This book brings together the expertise of a major sarcoma centre and highlights the multidisciplinary nature of the "team". The kernel of the multidisciplinary approach is the regular multidisciplinary meeting, so-called MDM. In this meeting, cases are discussed and the distilled wisdom of experts in imaging, pathology, genetics, radiotherapy, chemotherapy and surgery is collected to inform care paths and the ultimate patient journey. The opportunity that this provides to both patients and clinicians is the chance to model through debate and evidence the best care for each individual patient.

This book provides a pragmatism born from over a quarter of a century as one of Australia's leading sarcoma centres. The regimes discussed in this book are those that have evolved from global evidence that has been shaped by local context. For each recommended treatment path, we acknowledge that there will be others in the literature that will differ. This book discusses the principles and foundations upon which the sarcoma care provided by the partners of the Victorian Comprehensive Cancer Centre is based.

This book will be an excellent resource for residents, trainees, consultants and those interested in a centre-based multidisciplinary approach to sarcoma care.

Victoria, VIC, Australia Peter F. M. Choong

About the Editor

Peter F. M. Choong is the Sir Hugh Devine Chair of Surgery and Head of the Department of Surgery at the University of Melbourne. He is also a senior consultant in the Department of Orthopaedics at St. Vincent's Hospital Melbourne and Chair of the Bone and Soft Tissue Sarcoma Service at the Peter MacCallum Cancer Centre. He is the immediate Past Director and Professor of Orthopaedics at St. Vincent's Hospital, and Past President of the Australian Orthopaedic Association. He leads the Advanced Limb Reconstruction Research Program, and his team is a part of a national industry–university consortium recently awarded a multimillion-dollar grant from the Innovative Manufacturing Cooperative Research Centre for studying and translating innovative manufacturing solutions for the development of bespoke prostheses, and robotic-assisted image-guided bone tumour surgery.

Professor F. M. Choong's primary areas of research focus on improving the outcomes of arthritis surgery, studying the treatment of bone tumours and advanced limb reconstruction. He has received numerous research and achievement awards for his contribution to the advancement of surgery or to fundamental scientific research in the field. These include the RACS John Mitchell Crouch Award, the Paul Harris Fellowship from Rotary International, the Ivins Visiting Professorship (2003) and the Coventry Visiting Professorship (2014) from the Mayo Clinic. He was also awarded the AOA Research Excellence Award, the St. Vincent's Health Australia Excellence Award and the Research Excellence Award from the National Health and Medical Research Council of Australia. He has widely published almost 450 peer-reviewed articles in these areas.

Contents

Centre-Based Care for Bone and Soft Tissue Sarcoma

1

Olivia Imkyeong Jo and Peter F. M. Choong

1.1 Introduction

Bone and soft tissue sarcomas are rare tumours that constitute less than 1% of all cancers in adults [1]. Misrecognition, misdiagnosis and, as a consequence, inexpert attempts at management occur frequently [2]. With rare cancers such as sarcomas, the prognosis is improved when patients are managed at specialist centres with a multidisciplinary team [3]. Such centres are associated with better compliance with clinical practice guidelines, a better quality of diagnosis and management as well as a lower recurrence rate with notably less frequent reoperations compared to non-specialist centres [4]. This review provides the current evidence to support the multidisciplinary team approach to sarcomas and explains the operational structure of the multidisciplinary care at our centre.

1.2 The Rationale for Multidisciplinary Sarcoma Care

Sarcomas are rare tumours that require complex pathological diagnosis [5] and imaging interpretation [6–9]. Careful biopsy technique to ensure tissue extraction without contaminating healthy tissue is essential for optimal management of sarcomas. Surgical treatments of bone and soft tissue sarcomas are sophisticated and frequently require coordinated care from multiple surgical disciplines such as

O. I. Jo
Department of Surgery, University of Melbourne, Melbourne, VIC, Australia

P. F. M. Choong (✉)
Department of Surgery, University of Melbourne, Melbourne, VIC, Australia

Department of Orthopaedics, St. Vincent's Hospital Melbourne, Melbourne, VIC, Australia

Bone and Soft Tissue Tumour Service, Peter MacCallum Cancer Centre, Melbourne, VIC, Australia
e-mail: pchoong@unimelb.edu.au

P. F. M. Choong (ed.), *Sarcoma*, https://doi.org/10.1007/978-981-15-9414-4_1

orthopaedic oncology, general surgical oncology, thoracic surgery, plastic surgery and other anatomically indicated surgical disciplines. Chemotherapy is routinely used for many high-grade bone and soft tissue sarcomas and often entails multiple agents with significant toxicity. Radiation therapy is given for select tumours as an adjunct to surgery or as a solitary management option. The doses used for sarcomas are far greater than those used for more routine indications such as bone metastasis [10]. Together, the management of sarcomas mandates close cooperation of experts within the multidisciplinary team.

1.3 Diagnosis

Patients suspected of bone and soft tissue tumours should undergo a diagnostic work-up. This consists of clinical evaluation, local and systemic imaging of tumour extent and histological examination of the tumour. Radiographs can be helpful in revealing areas of calcification, soft tissue shadowing and bony destruction [11, 12]. Magnetic resonance imaging (MRI) is the modality of choice to determine the size and location of soft tissue lesion as well as the proximity to adjacent anatomic structures. Functional imaging, such as positron emission tomography (PET) [13] and bone scan [14], is often performed to decide the needle trajectory to target the most metabolically active area [14] within the lesion, to improve the overall diagnostic accuracy [15] and to assess for local recurrence [12].

Systemic staging is critically important for the management of sarcomas. A computed tomography (CT) scan of the chest should be obtained on initial presentation because sarcomas are known to metastasise to the lungs, and the findings of metastatic disease may alter the goals of treatment [12, 16]. In non-specialist centres, only 43% of patients with soft tissue sarcomas underwent radiological examination of the tumour, while 24% of patients were investigated for metastatic disease before treatment. This contrasts with specialist sarcoma centres where 100% of patients underwent local imaging of the tumours and 78% had systemic staging [17].

Biopsies allow for tissue diagnosis. In non-specialist centres, biopsies are often inadequately or inappropriately performed. Biopsies not performed by an expert may lead to delay in treatment from repeating a previously non-diagnostic biopsy, complications from improperly placed incision that confounds future surgeries and healthy tissue contamination [18]. Pre-referral biopsy can lead to increased local relapse and mortality as well as more radical surgery resulting in loss of function and long-term disability [19]. Incorrectly performed biopsy with poor techniques can lead to profound implications such as missing the chance of timely diagnosis of a potentially curable disease and adding morbidity to the definitive surgery.

Unlike many other cancers, in bone and soft tissue tumours, pathological interpretation requires understanding of the clinical presentation and radiological interpretation of aggressiveness due to their heterogeneous morphology [12]. Particularly, in low-grade cartilage bone tumours (Figs. 1.1, 1.2, 1.3, and 1.4), the specimen cannot be interpreted in isolation, but rather in the clinical and imaging context. The diagnosis made by the referring pathologist often exhibits significant discrepancies

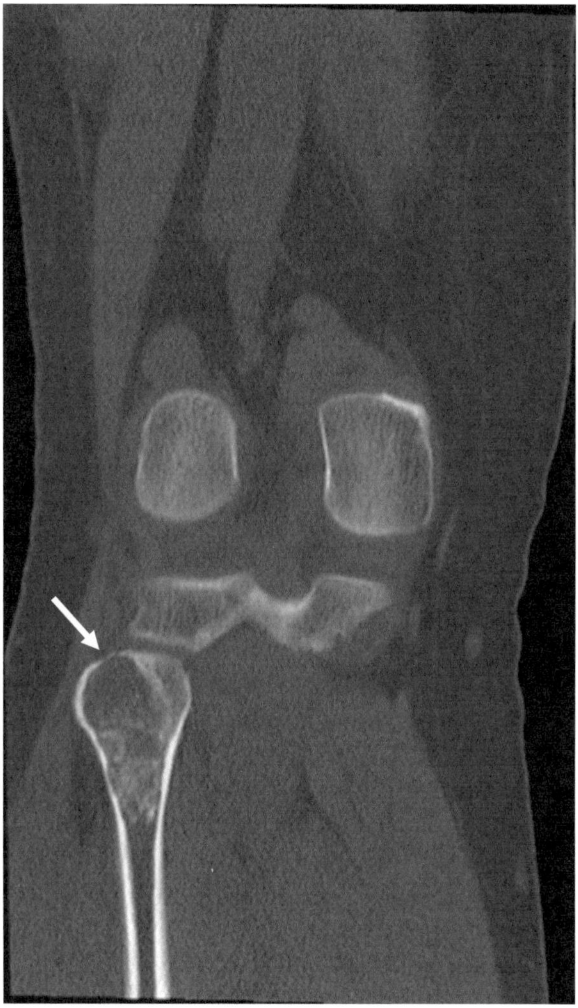

Fig. 1.1 Coronal computed tomography of proximal fibula of a 41-year-old female presenting with 2-week history of pain. Grade 1 chondrosarcoma. Image shows a chondroid lesion involving the proximal fibula. There is thinning of cortex without frank cortical breach (arrow)

from the final diagnosis by a musculoskeletal pathologist. Review of diagnosis by a specialist pathologist improves the accuracy of diagnosis in these rare and heterogeneous tumours [20] and is advised by current clinical practice guidelines [21–23]. The final diagnosis of sarcomas can be made collectively by experts following a discussion of all relevant clinical, imaging and histological findings.

1.4 Treatment of Bone Cancers

Primary bone cancers may be treated with resection, chemotherapy and radiation. Chemotherapy usually extends 10–12 weeks preoperatively, and significant toxicity is often associated. Specialist medical oncologic input is necessary to medically

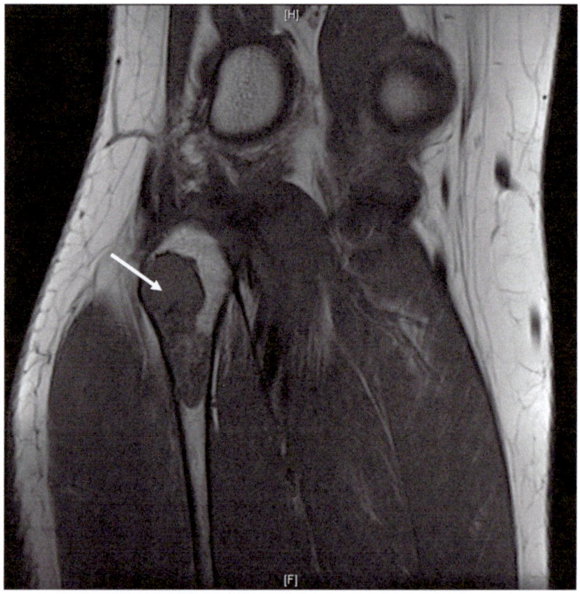

Fig. 1.2 T1 coronal sequence shows lobulated, expansile lesion of the right fibula head and neck (arrow), compatible with low-grade chondroid aetiology

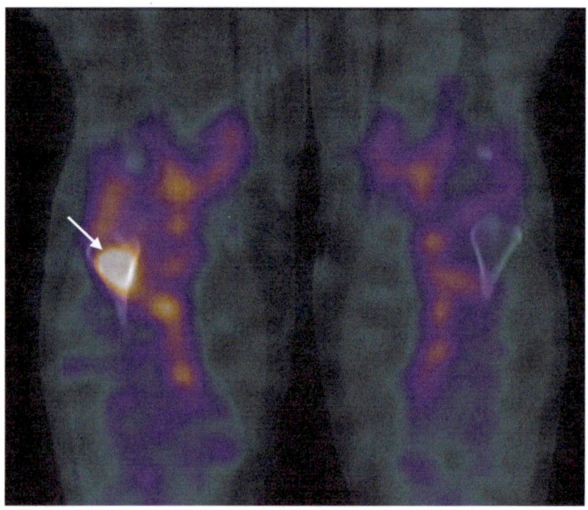

Fig. 1.3 Tc-99m DMSA (V) image demonstrates moderately intense tracer uptake uniformly within the chondroid abnormality of the proximal fibula (arrow). *Tc-99m DMSA (V)* technetium-99m dimercaptosuccinic acid

optimise patients for surgery and deal with any resultant toxicities. The surgical removal of the tumour is often complex and requires multiple surgical disciplines: orthopaedic oncology for resection of bone and skeletal reconstruction and plastic surgery for optimal tissue coverage. Effective communication and coordination between the disciplines prevent delay in providing the necessary care to patients. Pathological interpretation of the surgical specimen by the bone tumour pathologist regarding margins and degree of tissue necrosis is an important predictor of prognosis and guides subsequent management [10].

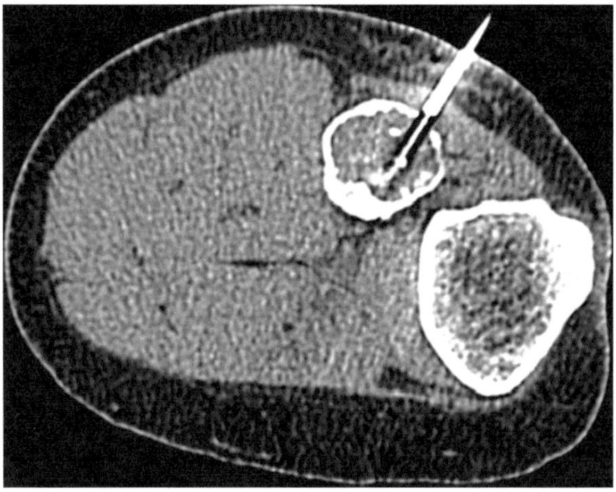

Fig. 1.4 Image-guided biopsy was carried out under computed tomography by a diagnostic radiologist through the shortest path to the tumour to minimise potential contamination. Optimal needle trajectory was determined upon discussion at the multidisciplinary meeting

1.5 Treatment of Soft Tissue Sarcoma

Currently, the mainstay treatment for soft tissue sarcoma is surgical removal of the entire tumour [10]. For localised sarcomas, a complete resection with a margin of several centimetres of healthy tissue to secure a free margin may achieve cure [24]. Unfortunately, unplanned soft tissue sarcoma excision occurs frequently without the utilisation of the multidisciplinary team, execution of necessary surgical margins or appropriate assessments of tumour diagnosis and local and systemic staging [1]. Unplanned surgery without a proper knowledge of the diagnosis is highly associated with residual disease or contamination of surrounding structures [25]. Positive excision margins have been reported to be as prevalent as 67–93% in patients treated outside of specialist centres [26–29]. Local recurrence rates at non-specialist centres are two to four times higher than those achieved in specialist centres [30–33]. Despite the tendency of excising potentially more aggressive and larger tumours [34], specialist hospitals showed better local control than community hospitals [1].

Due to the risks associated with incomplete excision, reoperation occurs frequently for patients initially treated inappropriately at non-sarcoma centres. Reoperation is often more complex and extensive [4]. The rates of plastic reconstruction and amputation were much higher in the re-excision group compared to the rates for patients who had appropriate initial resection. The required size of resection is increased at reoperation, thereby making the nature of reconstruction of defects more complex and increasing the need for tissue coverage [35]. As a result, these patients may experience greater surgical morbidity, potentially worse long-term functional outcomes [34] and significantly worse final results in terms of quality of surgery [4]. Nonetheless, re-excision has not been associated with worse local recurrence, metastasis-free survival nor overall survival [36–38].

With advantages of radiotherapy, the need to resect important neurovascular structures, or musculoskeletal structures, may be reduced, allowing for limb-sparing surgeries [39]. Radiation therapy pre- or post-limb-sparing surgery increases locoregional control in more than 90% of patients compared to conservative surgery without radiation therapy [4]. The role of chemotherapy in soft tissue sarcomas is controversial due to high toxicity and non-significant benefits to long-term survival and prognosis [12, 40]. Some evidence suggests chemotherapy can provide survival benefits in specific subtypes such as synovial sarcomas with metastasis [41, 42]. The decision to chemotherapy should be made on a case-by-case basis by medical oncologist with specific expertise.

1.6 Management of Metastatic Sarcoma

The decision of how to evaluate and treat suspicious nodules in the setting of a diagnosis of sarcoma (non-surgical, surgical or medical treatment with chemotherapy) must be carefully determined in the multidisciplinary setting with the treatment goals, prognosis and functional status of patient in consideration. The differentiation between metastatic nodules and other non-specific lung nodules or infection requires diagnostic radiologist comparing with previous scans. Definitive diagnosis may require biopsy to be taken by an interventional radiologist and interpreted by a pathologist. Patients with bone and soft tissue sarcomas with solitary metastasis to lungs or isolated lesion in the body are now treated more aggressively by thoracic surgeon, orthopaedic surgeon and other anatomically directed surgeons. This is due to the improved the prognosis for the patients [43].

1.7 Multidisciplinary Sarcoma Team and Clinic at St. Vincent's Hospital Melbourne and Peter MacCallum Cancer Centre

1.7.1 Sarcoma Clinic

Each patient referred to our sarcoma centre is triaged and receives scheduled appointments with orthopaedic or general surgical oncologists for initial investigation of bone and soft tissue mass. Concurrent appointments with medical oncologists and radiation oncologist can be organised on the same day and within the same building. This enables coordinated care, particularly for patients who travel a long distance. The services of another discipline are often able to be incorporated because the expectation for multidisciplinary needs for patients is embedded within the centre. Patients post definitive treatment of sarcomas must be followed up closely for early detection of potential recurrence of disease or metastasis. They are reviewed three to four monthly for the first 2 years with clinical examination and appropriate imaging (i.e. plain radiographs and MRI of the surgical site and CT of the chest) and six monthly for a further 2 years with a plan for yearly review for the following 4 years. Thus, a routine clinical follow-up spans at least 8 years.

1.7.2 Multidisciplinary Meeting

At St. Vincent's Hospital Melbourne, we have a weekly multidisciplinary meeting. Attendees include orthopaedic oncologists, medical oncologists, surgical oncologist, radiation oncologists, thoracic oncologist, plastic surgeon, musculoskeletal diagnostic radiologists, pathologists and administrative personnel (Fig. 1.5). Other disciplines may also bring relevant cases for discussion. Patients are presented with all relevant clinical, radiological and pathological findings. Specific questions are brought up and addressed with the unique input from different specialties. A consistent, comprehensive and institutional approach to manage sarcomas can prevent management instituted by a single provider within their own discipline. This also provides fantastic educational opportunities for specialists of one filed to learn about expertise and current advances that are outside of their field. Trainees are welcome to attend and observe a greater number of sarcoma cases than would otherwise encounter in a single non-sarcoma practice.

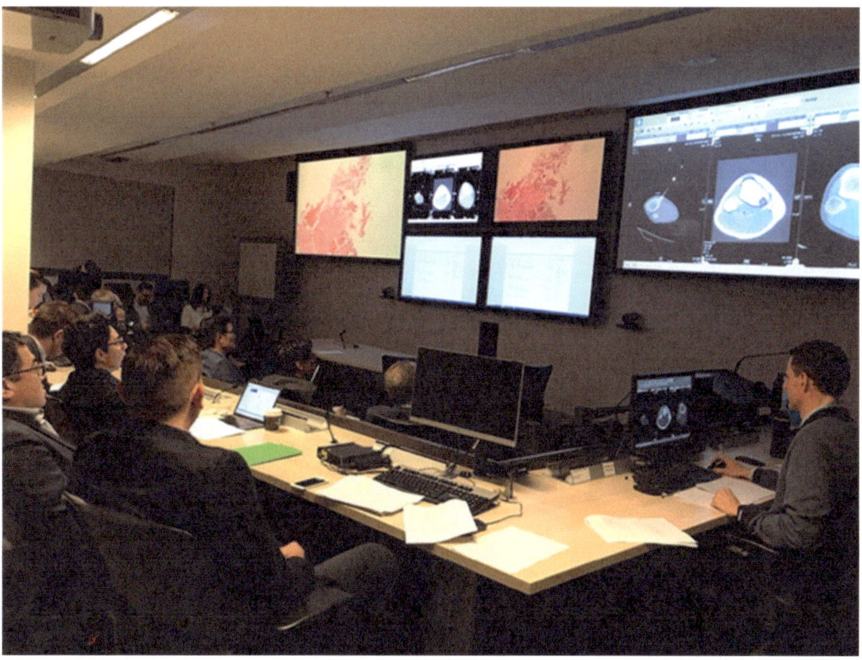

Fig. 1.5 St. Vincent's Hospital/Peter Mac Cancer Centre weekly multidisciplinary meeting. Orthopaedic oncologists, medical oncologists, radiation oncologists, thoracic surgeon, plastic surgeon, radiologists, pathologists, orthopaedic trainees and administrative staff are reviewing imaging

1.7.3 Clinical Trials

Clinical trials drive important advancements in the management of uncommon diseases like sarcomas. The multidisciplinary tumour team is often up to date with ongoing or new national and institutional trials and can provide an excellent platform for enrolling patients in appropriate clinical trials and maximising options [44].

1.8 Impact of Delayed Referral on Patient Outcomes

Delayed referral to a sarcoma centre occurs frequently and can be prolonged. Some causes for delayed referral include delayed presentation of patients to primary carer or non-compliance of referring hospitals with clinical practice guidelines [45]. Sixty-three percent of patients with delayed referral had been subjected to extensive imaging studies, and 34% received biopsy or surgery at local hospitals prior to referral [46]. Regardless of the cause of the delay, it has been shown to impact on patient management and prognosis [46, 47]. Only 28% of patients who were referred after undergoing inappropriate excision and developing local recurrences achieved disease-free survival as opposed to 73% of patients who were referred directly to a specialist centre [47]. Delayed referral was further associated with increased total number of operations and local recurrence rate [48]. However, there are conflicting evidence suggesting that the impact of delayed definitive treatment on overall survival or metastasis is not significant [49, 50].

1.9 Recommendation

The general recommendation is to refer patients with a tumour larger than 5 cm in size and lesions deep to or adherent to deep fascia directly to a sarcoma centre to be managed by a specialist sarcoma unit. Diagnostic investigations before referral are not required [51]. Patients treated at sarcoma centres with high patient load had greater survivorship even if they travelled further distances than those who stayed close to home and underwent treatment of sarcoma at a regional centre [4].

1.10 Conclusion

Due to the rarity of bone and soft tissue sarcomas, the likelihood of patients undergoing correct biopsy and imaging tests, initial curative management with wide margin and appropriate medical treatment is significantly higher at specialist centres with multidisciplinary team. Similarly, the rates of incomplete excision, reoperation and local recurrence are lower when patients receive treatments within a specialised sarcoma centre. Timely referral to a specialist centre equipped with a multidisciplinary team of experts before the commencement of any treatment would optimise management and reduce morbidity.

References

1. Kang S, et al. Unplanned excision of soft tissue sarcoma: the impact of the referring hospital. Surg Oncol. 2013;22(2):e17–22.
2. Blay J-Y, et al. Improved survival using specialized multidisciplinary board in sarcoma patients. Ann Oncol. 2017;28(11):2852–59.
3. Lazarides A, et al. Soft tissue sarcoma of the extremities: what is the value of treating at high-volume centers? Clin Orthop Relat Res. 2019;477(4):718–27.
4. Blay JY, et al. Improved sarcoma management in a national network of reference centers: analysis of the NetSarc network on 13,454 patients treated between 2010 and 2014. J Clin Oncol. 2016;34(Suppl 15)
5. Roitman PD, et al. Is needle biopsy clinically useful in preoperative grading of central chondrosarcoma of the pelvis and long bones? Clin Orthop Relat Res. 2017;475(3):808–14.
6. Crim J, et al. Can imaging criteria distinguish enchondroma from grade 1 chondrosarcoma? Eur J Radiol. 2015;84(11):2222–30.
7. Hicks RJ, Toner GC, Choong PF. Clinical applications of molecular imaging in sarcoma evaluation. Cancer Imaging. 2005;5:66–72.
8. Leddy LR, Holmes RE. Chondrosarcoma of bone. Cancer Treat Res. 2014;162:117–30.
9. Adigun IA, Rahman GA. A review of soft tissue sarcoma. Nigerian J Med. 2007;16(2):94–101.
10. Siegel GW, et al. The multidisciplinary management of bone and soft tissue sarcoma: an essential organizational framework. J Multidiscip Healthc. 2015;8:109–15.
11. Erwteman AS, Balach T. Clinical evaluation and management of benign soft tissue tumors of the extremities. Cancer Treat Res. 2014;162:171–202.
12. Nystrom LM, et al. Multidisciplinary management of soft tissue sarcoma. Sci World J. 2013;2013:852462.
13. Kay M, Simmonds P, Sundram F. The value of PET-CT in the management of sarcoma patients: 3 yr single centre experience in the South of England. Nucl Med Commun. 2012;33(10):1106–7.
14. Choong PF, et al. The role of thallium-201 and pentavalent dimercaptosuccinic acid for staging cartilaginous tumours. Int Semin Surg Oncol. 2004;1(1):10.
15. Andersen KF, et al. Volume-based F-18 FDG PET/CT imaging markers provide supplemental prognostic information to histologic grading in patients with high-grade bone or soft tissue sarcoma. Medicine (United States). 2015;94(51):e2319.
16. Clarkson P, Ferguson PC. Primary multidisciplinary management of extremity soft tissue sarcomas. Curr Treat Options Oncol. 2004;5(6):451–62.
17. Nijhuis PHA, et al. Soft tissue sarcoma—compliance with guidelines. Cancer. 2001;91(11):2186–95.
18. Avedian R. Principles of musculoskeletal biopsy. Cancer Treat Res. 2014;162:1–7.
19. Mankin HJ, Mankin CJ, Simon MA. The hazards of the biopsy, revisited. Members of the Musculoskeletal Tumor Society. J Bone Joint Surg Am. 1996;78(5):656–63.
20. Jalaludin ND, et al. Histopathological diagnoses in soft tissue tumours: an experience from a tertiary centre in Malaysia. Malays J Pathol. 2017;39(3):209–16.
21. Von Mehren M, et al. Soft tissue sarcoma, version 2.2016: clinical practice guidelines in oncology. JNCCN J Natl Compr Canc Netw. 2016;14(6):758–86.
22. Dangoor A, et al. UK guidelines for the management of soft tissue sarcomas. Clin Sarcoma Res. 2016;6:20.
23. Tan E, Iyer P, Soh SY. Non-rhabdomyosarcoma soft tissue sarcomas (NRSTS): a single-centre study in Singapore. Pediatr Blood Cancer. 2014;2:S384–5.
24. Luis AM. Multidisciplinary management of soft tissue sarcomas: it's time to make a team! Clin Transl Oncol. 2010;12(8):515–7.
25. Awad N, et al. Multidisciplinary approach to treatment of soft tissue sarcomas requiring complex oncologic resections. Ann Vasc Surg. 2018;53:212–6.
26. Bauer HCF, et al. Monitoring referral and treatment in soft tissue sarcoma: study based on 1,851 patients from the Scandinavian Sarcoma Group Register. Acta Orthop Scand. 2001;72(2):150–9.

27. Zacherl MMD, et al. Influence of prereferral surgery in soft tissue sarcoma: 10 years' experience in a single institution. Orthopedics (Online). 2012;35(8):e1214–20.
28. Randall RL, et al. Errors in diagnosis and margin determination of soft-tissue sarcomas initially treated at non-tertiary centers. Orthopedics. 2004;27(2):209–12.
29. Giuliano AE, Eilber FR. The rationale for planned reoperation after unplanned total excision of soft-tissue sarcomas. J Clin Oncol. 1985;3(10):1344–8.
30. Davis AM, et al. The impact of residual disease on local recurrence in patients treated by initial unplanned resection for soft tissue sarcoma of the extremity. J Surg Oncol. 1997;66(2):81–7.
31. Qureshi YA, et al. Unplanned excision of soft tissue sarcoma results in increased rates of local recurrence despite full further oncological treatment. Ann Surg Oncol. 2012;19(3):871–7.
32. Ueda T, et al. Influence of local recurrence on the prognosis of soft-tissue sarcomas. J Bone Joint Surg Br. 1997;79(4):553–7.
33. Bhangu AA, Beard JA, Grimer RJ. Should soft tissue sarcomas be treated at a specialist centre? Sarcoma. 2004;8(1):1–6.
34. Tan MTL, et al. Patterns of care of superficial soft tissue sarcomas: it is not always just a lump. Asia Pac J Clin Oncol. 2018;14(5):e472–8.
35. Traub F, et al. Influence of unplanned excisions on the outcomes of patients with stage III extremity soft-tissue sarcoma. Cancer. 2018;124(19):3868–75.
36. Fiore M, et al. Prognostic effect of re-excision in adult soft tissue sarcoma of the extremity. Ann Surg Oncol. 2006;13(1):110–7.
37. Manoso MW, et al. Outcomes of re-excision after unplanned excisions of soft-tissue sarcomas. J Surg Oncol. 2005;91(3):153–8.
38. Alamanda VK, et al. Primary excision compared with re-excision of extremity soft tissue sarcomas--is anything new? J Surg Oncol. 2012;105(7):662–7.
39. Clarkson PW, et al. Epineural dissection is a safe technique that facilitates limb salvage surgery. Clin Orthop Relat Res. 2005;438:92–6.
40. Frustaci S, et al. Ifosfamide in the adjuvant therapy of soft tissue sarcomas. Oncology. 2003;65(Suppl 2):80–4.
41. Ferrari A, et al. Synovial sarcoma: a retrospective analysis of 271 patients of all ages treated at a single institution. Cancer. 2004;101(3):627–34.
42. Lee SH, et al. High-dose ifosfamide as second- or third-line chemotherapy in refractory bone and soft tissue sarcoma patients. Oncology. 2011;80(3–4):257–61.
43. Nevala R, et al. Long-term results of surgical resection of lung metastases from soft tissue sarcoma: a single center experience. J Surg Oncol. 2019;120(2)
44. Grimer R, et al. UK guidelines for the management of bone sarcomas. Sarcoma. 2010;2010:317462.
45. Collin T, et al. Sarcomas in the groin and inguinal canal--often missed and difficult to manage. Ann R Coll Surg Engl. 2010;92(4):326–9.
46. Ashwood N, et al. Analysis of the referral pattern to a supraregional bone and soft tissue tumour service. Ann R Coll Surg Engl. 2003;85(4):272–6.
47. Abellan JF, et al. Nonreferral of possible soft tissue sarcomas in adults: a dangerous omission in policy. Sarcoma. 2009;2009:827912.
48. Gustafson P, Dreinhofer KE, Rydholm A. Soft tissue sarcoma should be treated at a tumor center. A comparison of quality of surgery in 375 patients. Acta Orthop Scand. 1994;65(1):47–50.
49. Han I, et al. Does delayed reexcision affect outcome after unplanned excision for soft tissue sarcoma? Clin Orthop Relat Res. 2011;469(3):877–83.
50. Goyal S, et al. Symptom interval in young people with bone cancer. Eur J Cancer. 2004;40(15):2280–6.
51. Billing V, et al. Simple guidelines for efficient referral of soft-tissue sarcomas: a population-based evaluation of adherence to guidelines and referral patterns. J Bone Joint Surg Ser A. 2012;94(14):1291–6.

The Epidemiology and Pathogenesis of Sarcoma

2

Wassif Kabir and Peter F. M. Choong

Sarcomas are a group of rare malignant neoplasms of mesenchymal origin which may occur in skeletal and extraskeletal tissue, including muscles, tendons, fat, synovium, fibrous tissue, blood vessels and the peripheral nervous system [1, 2]. Tumours of soft tissue and bone are characterised by a high degree of morphological, molecular and clinical heterogeneity. Sarcomas are classified by the World Health Organization (WHO) according to histological features into over 100 types, of which at least 70% are soft tissue sarcomas [2, 3]. The classification system for sarcomas is an evolving process, reflecting the advent of novel molecular, cytogenetic and immunohistochemical techniques which facilitate the identification of groups of sarcoma cells expressing tumour-specific markers [4]. These techniques play a pivotal role in the refinement of sarcoma diagnosis, which is currently based on tumour morphology, immunohistochemistry and clinic-pathological correlation [2].

2.1 Epidemiology of Sarcomas

Sarcomas represent fewer than 1 in 100 solid malignancies in adults but account for more than 1 in 5 solid malignant tumours in the paediatric population [5]. According to data from the Surveillance, Epidemiology and End Results (SEER) database [6], during the period between 1973 and 2008, soft tissue sarcomas occurred in higher

W. Kabir
Department of Surgery, University of Melbourne, Melbourne, VIC, Australia

P. F. M. Choong (✉)
Department of Surgery, University of Melbourne, Melbourne, VIC, Australia

Department of Orthopaedics, St. Vincent's Hospital Melbourne, Melbourne, VIC, Australia

Bone and Soft Tissue Tumour Service, Peter MacCallum Cancer Centre, Melbourne, VIC, Australia
e-mail: pchoong@unimelb.edu.au

P. F. M. Choong (ed.), *Sarcoma*, https://doi.org/10.1007/978-981-15-9414-4_2

frequencies than malignant bone cancers. In 1 year, 87% of sarcomas diagnosed were soft tissue sarcomas (STS), and the remaining 13% were malignant bone sarcomas. The most common malignant tumours of bone are osteosarcoma and chondrosarcoma, which cumulatively account for over 50% of bone cancer diagnoses [5]. Among STS, the category "other specified soft tissue sarcomas" was the most common, accounting for 51% of all STS. Kaposi sarcoma (9% of all sarcoma diagnoses) and fibrosarcomas (7% of all sarcoma diagnoses) were the two most frequent identifiable STS diagnosed in 2008, according to SEER data [5]. Overall, soft tissue sarcomas have an annual incidence of 6 per 100,000 persons [6]. In Europe, the estimated incidence of STS is 4 per 100,000 per year [7], while in England, the incidence of soft tissue sarcoma between 1979 and 2001 was 9.1 per million person-years at risk [8]. An increase in the overall incidence in STS has been recorded; however this may also reflect the advancement of diagnostic tools and greater research interest in the field of sarcomas.

The SEER database also shows the relationship between age and sarcoma incidence [6]. The mean ages at diagnosis for STS and malignant bone cancers were 58 and 40 years, respectively, in the 4-year period between 2004 and 2008 [9]. On the other hand, the average age of death in patients with STS and bone cancer were 65 and 58 years, respectively [9]. It is evident from results in the database that there is an increase in the rate of STS from infancy until 5 years of age. Although the incidence of STS is the lowest among young adults, this value rises gradually until age 50, after which the increase in incidence is more exaggerated. According to the SEER database, under 10 years of age, the incidence of STS was 0.9 per 100,000 children, and this increased to 18.2 per 100,000 adults over 70 years of age [1]. Malignant bone tumours have a relatively consistent incidence across all ages, with elderly individuals experiencing a slightly higher incidence. It is known, for example, that embryonal rhabdomyosarcoma is unique to young individuals, while undifferentiated pleomorphic sarcoma is primarily a tumour of older populations. Males are affected by STS more frequently than females, but the true variations in incidence according to gender and age groups are dependent on the histological type of sarcoma. The 5-year survival rate for STS has been reported as 50–60%; however there is significant variation in survival and prognosis for the various STS subtypes [10].

An investigation into the importance of race as a risk factor for sarcoma occurrence has revealed that Caucasians are much more commonly affected by Ewing's sarcoma than Asians, Africans and African Americans [11]. It is believed that this discrepancy in prevalence of Ewing's sarcoma between the different race groups reflects a genetic basis for the condition. Overall, Ewing's sarcoma has an incidence of 2.1 per million in the United States and is the second most common cancer of bone in children and adolescents [12]. Interestingly, people of Black ethnicity have the highest incidence of STS malignancies at 5.1 cases per 100,000 people, while Whites have a rate of 4.5 cases per 100,000 people, and American Indians/Asian Pacific Islanders have a lower incidence rate of 2.8 per 100,000.

Geographic variations in sarcoma incidence have also become evident. For instance, chondrosarcomas occur in greater rates in America compared to Asian countries [13]. A more detailed study of sarcoma incidence across various geographical regions, titled *Cancer Incidence in Five Continents, Volume XI,* shows that age-standardised incidence rates of osteosarcoma for both males and females do not in fact differ greatly between Asian countries and the United States, which was contrary to reports elsewhere [13]. Nevertheless, some interesting observations were made in this study, including the discovery that Japanese migrants living in "westernised" countries had a higher risk of osteosarcoma incidence relative to the overall population. For Japanese males, the incidence rate of osteosarcoma was 1.3 per 100,000 in California and 1.1 per 100,000 in Hawaii, in comparison to an incidence rate of 0.2–0.6 cases per 100,000 males in the general population across various continents [5]. Among females in Sondrio, Italy, a high incidence of osteosarcoma cases at 1.4 per 100,000 has also been discovered [5]. This finding is in contrast with the low incidence of 0.1–0.4 per 100,000 osteosarcoma cases among females in other regions of Italy [5]. Further epidemiological studies are required to uncover the significance of this finding which is presently unclear (Figs. 2.1 and 2.2 and Table 2.1).

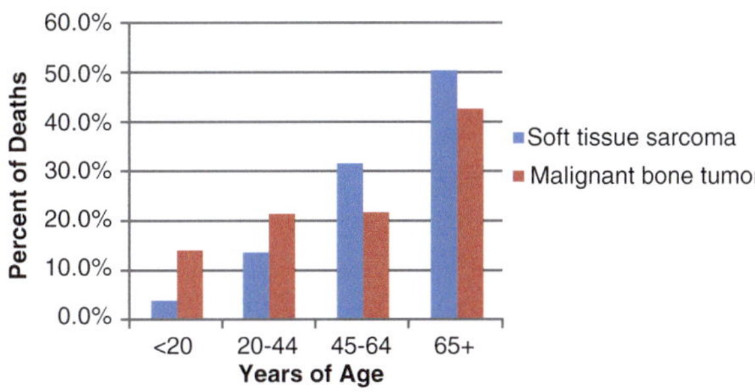

Fig. 2.1 Percentage of deaths according to age in patients suffering from sarcomas. The illustration was reproduced from Burningham et al. [5] with permission from the publisher Biomed Central

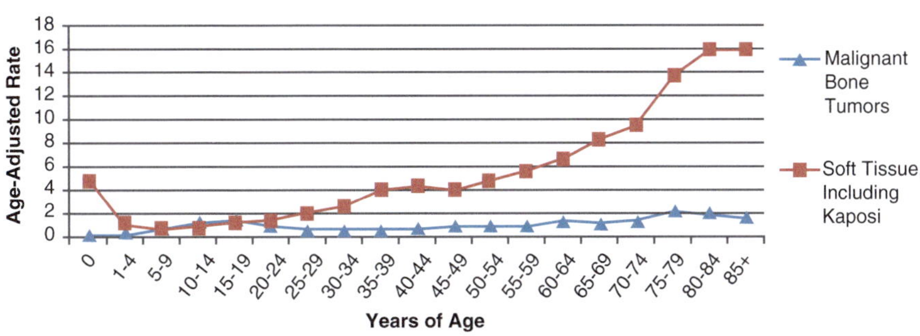

Fig. 2.2 Age-adjusted incidence rate of soft tissue sarcomas and malignant bone tumours. The illustration was reproduced from Burningham et al. [5] with permission from the publisher Biomed Central

Table 2.1 Occurrence of sarcomas identified by histological classification in 2008, according to data from the Surveillance, Epidemiology and End Results (SEER) database [5, 6]

Sarcoma types	Subtypes	Percentage (%)	
Malignant bone sarcomas	Osteosarcomas	4.0	12.7
	Chondrosarcomas	4.0	
	Ewing's sarcoma and other related sarcomas	2.0	
	Other specified malignant bone sarcomas	1.9	
	Unspecified malignant bone sarcomas	0.8	
Soft tissue sarcomas	Kaposi sarcoma	8.9	87.3
	Rhabdomyosarcomas	3.3	
	Fibrosarcomas, peripheral nerve sheath tumours, and other fibrous sarcomas	7.1	
	Other specified soft tissue sarcomas	51.2	
	Unspecified soft tissue sarcomas	16.8	

2.2 Pathogenesis of Sarcomas

2.2.1 Understanding the Origin of Sarcomas

It is postulated that sarcomas are derived from multipotent precursor cells of mesodermal tissues which have undergone malignant transformation [6]. There have been suggestions that subtypes of sarcomas arise from lineage-specific genetic mutations in mesenchymal stem cells (MSCs) that have not yet committed to a specific line of differentiation [14]. For example, the knock-out of p53 and RB genes in multipotent MSCs has been shown to induce osteosarcoma formation [15]. However, gene expression investigations have demonstrated that the cellular profiles of various soft tissue sarcoma groups are more similar to differentiated MSCs than undifferentiated MSCs [16]. Although the various histological grades and molecular phenotypes of sarcoma cells may be reflective of the stages of MSC differentiation during which oncogenic transformation occurs [14, 17, 18], histopathological findings suggest that sarcoma development is a more complicated process that could be better delineated through investigation of micro-RNA signatures [17]. Some findings suggest that perhaps sarcomas do not arise from differentiated MSCs nor directly from their expected precursors [17]. For instance, the diagnosis of rhabdomyosarcoma relies on the histological detection of rhabdomyoblasts and expression of muscle-related biomarkers. Despite showing features of skeletal muscle differentiation, rhabdomyosarcomas can develop in sites where skeletal muscle is absent. An explanation for this phenomenon can be derived from a study which showed that the activation of sonic-hedgehog signalling in adipocytes could generate embryonic rhabdomyosarcoma [19]. Hence, the transdifferentiation of mesenchymal progenitor cells is a probable mechanism through which sarcomas can develop from a variety of cell origins unrelated to their histologically observed differentiation status. Soft tissue sarcomas of uncertain differentiation commonly contain translocations resulting in fusion genes, though the association of these genes with particular cell types is unknown [18]. Owing to the histomorphological basis for the naming of sarcomas and the need to avoid confusion during interdisciplinary communication, the names of certain sarcomas are not indicative of their origin and pathobiology. Synovial sarcoma, for instance, is not associated with synovial joints and has been shown to resemble malignant peripheral nerve sheath tumours [20]. With regard to sarcomagenesis, there is a stronger emphasis on studying the histology, molecular signature and phenotype of the tissue rather than on the concept of histogenesis.

The most common sites of soft tissue sarcoma are deep tissues of the extremities such as deep fascia and skeletal muscle [4]. However, the head, neck, abdomen, trunk and retroperitoneum are also frequently affected. In the latest edition of the WHO Classification, soft tissue sarcomas are divided into 50 subtypes, including tumours of adipocytic, fibroblastic/myofibroblastic, skeletal muscle, pericytic (perivascular), smooth muscle, so-called fibriohistiocytic, vascular, chondroosseous and unknown differentiation [6]. These types are further divided into groups according to cell of origin and whether the tumour falls into benign, intermediate (locally aggressive), intermediate (rarely metastasising) or malignant categories of biological potential. Malignant sarcomas rarely originate from benign soft tissue tumours, except in the case of neurofibromas which may lead to malignant peripheral nerve sheath tumours in patients with type 1 neurofibromatosis. Moreover, the metastatic potential of malignant sarcomas is variable, such as dermatofibrosarcoma protuberans which has a very low frequency of metastasis. Soft tissue sarcomas of intermediate malignancy rarely metastasise but are known to have a high degree of recurrence.

The pathogenesis of soft tissue sarcomas is poorly understood, and their aetiology often remains unclear throughout the course of the disease [21]. There is, however, abundant evidence for the association between various genetic, molecular, immunological, infectious and environmental risk factors and the development of sarcomas. Identification of an exact cause of sarcoma is often complicated by extended periods of latency between time of exposure to risk factors and the development of the disease.

2.3 Genetic Predisposition Syndromes

Several inherited genetic syndromes have been linked with the development of bone and soft tissue sarcomas, primarily in children [22–26] (e.g. Li-Fraumeni syndrome, osteosarcoma, rhabdomyosarcoma and malignant peripheral nerve sheath tumours). However, many cases of sarcoma do not appear to be associated with cancer syndromes. An international genetic study found that 638 of 1162 sarcoma probands had pathogenic germline variants across 72 cancer-related genes including TP53, ATR, ATM, BRCA2 and ERCC2, and 217 subjects had 227 known or expected variants [27]. It was also found that the cumulative burden of multiple pathogenic variants in these genes were significantly associated with earlier age of cancer diagnosis. This study also found that among 911 families, recognisable genetic cancer syndromes were seen in only 17% [27]. This shows that a large number of both known and novel oncogenes or tumour suppressor genes are associated with sarcoma risk.

2.3.1 Li-Fraumeni Syndrome

Increased susceptibility for osteosarcoma, Ewing's sarcoma and rhabdomyosarcoma has been discovered in patients with Li-Fraumeni syndrome (LFS), an autosomal dominant condition with pathogenic mutations in the TP53 tumour suppressor gene. Between 25 and 33% of tumours in LFS patients are sarcomas [28, 29], which tend to arise at a younger age in LFS-affected patients than in patients unaffected by LFS. Data from the International Agency for Research on Cancer (IARC) database shows that 96% of sarcomas in LFS patients occur before 50 years of age, compared with 38% which occur before age 50 in the overall population [30]. Furthermore, almost 7% of paediatric soft tissue sarcoma patients are postulated to have LFS. A study of oncological patterns in families of children with soft tissue sarcomas found that about 33% of 151 families studied had a genetic predisposition syndrome and over 10% of the families had features consistent with LFS [22].

2.3.2 Retinoblastoma

Mutations in the retinoblastoma (RB) gene are known to predispose to soft tissue and bony cancers. Inheritance of a mutant copy of the RB gene and retinoblastoma of the bilateral type are linked to the development of late-onset osteosarcoma in patients suffering from retinoblastoma [31, 32]. In a longitudinal study of 1601 patients with RB, of which 963 had the inherited form, the cumulative frequency of a second cancer was 6 times higher for those with the inherited form versus the non-inherited form of RB. Sarcomas accounted for 60% of the second cancers [32].

In particular, retinoblastoma patients who receive chemotherapy or radiotherapy treatment could be at an increased risk of sarcoma development [33]. It has been reported that in patients with hereditary retinoblastoma who undergo radiotherapy, leiomyosarcomas are more likely to develop outside the field of radiation, whereas rhabdomyosarcoma, fibrosarcoma and pleomorphic sarcoma tend to arise within the radiation field [33–35]. A study which followed up 1601 retinoblastoma survivors demonstrated a statistically significant increase in the risk of soft tissue sarcomas in retinoblastoma patients compared to the general population, primarily for leiomyosarcoma which showed a 400-fold increase in risk [35]. Moreover, 78% of the leiomyosarcoma diagnoses were made over 30 years after the retinoblastoma diagnosis, which highlights a significant long-term risk of an additional malignancy in this cohort of patients [35].

2.3.3 Neurofibromatosis

Type 1 neurofibromatosis (NF1) is caused by mutations in the gene NF1 which undergoes a "double hit" inactivation phenomenon in which one allele is inactivated in the germline and the second allele is later knocked out by a somatic mutation, leading to development of the disease [36]. A large proportion of benign neurofibromas in NF1 may experience oncogenic transformation into malignant peripheral nerve sheath tumours (MPNSTs), which includes neurofibrosarcomas and malignant schwannomas [37, 38]. Up to 13% of NF1 patients will develop MPNSTs in their lifetimes [15]. In one study, the risk of this malignant transformation in NF1 patients was calculated to be 4.6% compared to 0.001% in the general population [39].

2.3.4 Other Sarcoma-Associated Genetic Syndromes

Patients with familial adenomatous polyposis (FAP), also known as Gardner syndrome, have a higher frequency of intra-abdominal desmoid tumours than the general population [40]. An increased risk of osteosarcoma has been discovered in patients with poikiloderma congenitale or Rothmund-Thomson syndrome—an autosomal recessive condition characterised by skeletal anomalies, short stature and unique skin changes, such as atrophy, telangiectasias and pigmentation. Other rare syndromes, such as Gorlin's syndrome, characterised by mutations in the PTCH1 gene [41, 42], and Costello syndrome which arises due to mutations in the HRAS gene [43], have been linked with the development of rhabdomyosarcomas.

2.4 Molecular Alterations in Sarcoma

During the past 25 years, karyotype analysis has been the basis for the molecular characterisation of sarcoma pathogenesis. In the domain of cytogenetics, the conceptual dichotomy between sarcomas with a simple karyotype and sarcomas with a complex karyotype has aided our understanding of different molecular aberrations that occur with respect to the genomic phenotype of the tumours. Sarcomas with simple genomes commonly exhibit transcriptional dysregulation and abnormal kinase signalling or epigenetic programming. It is possible to identify sarcomas in this group with tumour-specific molecular markers due to the presence of recurrent and predictable genomic rearrangements and activating point mutations. On the other hand, genomically complex sarcomas have non-recurrent and diverse rearrangements and gene amplifications. Therefore, the pathogenetic mechanisms of sarcoma are better characterised for those with simpler genomes. Transcriptional deregulation and deregulated signalling represent the two categories of pathobiology attributed to sarcomas with simple genomes. Conversely, sarcomas with complex genomes show highly heterogeneous, non-specific molecular alterations which promote oncogenesis through variable disruptions in cell biology, such as abnormal cell cycle regulation or genomic instability [44].

2.4.1 Sarcomas with Simple Karyotypes

Sarcomas with stable genomes generally have diploid karyotypes with a low frequency of mutations. When mutations or copy number variations occur, they do so in recognisable patterns, leading to tumour progression in a predictable manner. Mutations and balanced chromosomal rearrangements in known oncogenes and tumour suppressor genes are characteristic of genomically simple sarcomas. This group can be divided into five sub-categories according to the observed pattern of molecular genetic changes. These are (a) tumours with chimeric transcription factors, (b) tumours with deregulated kinase signalling, (c) tumours driven by oncometabolites and (d) tumours driven by primary epigenetic deregulation [2].

Fusion oncoproteins are often produced via the transcription of fusion genes which arise from chromosomal translocations in mesenchymal tumours. These oncoproteins can function as transcription factors that deregulate the expression of other genes normally involved in cell cycle processes [45]. In Ewing's sarcoma, for example, the gene fusions ESWR1-FLI1 (85% of translocations) and ESWR1-ERG (10% of translocations) are the best-known reciprocal translocations. ESWR1-ETS is another Ewing's sarcoma-related hybrid oncoprotein which has been shown to abnormally upregulate genes associated with cell proliferation, including PDGF-C, CCDN1 and c-MYC, downregulate cyclin-dependent kinase inhibitors, upregulate hTERT to allow cells to avoid senescence, repress apoptotic genes such as IGFBP-3, induce angiogenesis via VEGF overexpression and activate matrix metalloproteases which increases tumour metastatic potential [44]. Similarly, transcriptome sequencing of epithelioid haemangioma has shown that aberrant fusion of the FOS gene to various other genes such as ZFP36, resulting in loss of its trans-activation domain [46]. Epithelioid haemangioma presents as multifocal lesions, similar to epithelioid haemangioendothelioma, which is a low-grade angiosarcoma in which the WWTR1-CAMTA1 fusion gene drives tumorigenesis. In general, angiosarcomas rarely contain translocations. Rather, amplifications of oncogenes such as MYC, FLT4, PLCG1 and PTPRB are more common in primary and radiation-induced angiosarcomas [47]. Moreover, 10% of angiosarcomas of the breast contain mutations in KDR. Most of these genes are associated with increased angiogenesis.

Deregulated kinase signalling may be the main oncogenic driver in many sarcomas. Abnormal activation of receptor tyrosine kinases, such as KIT in gastrointestinal stromal tumours (GIST), and PDGFR in dermatofibrosarcoma protuberans are well-characterised examples of deregulated kinase signalling in sarcomas [48]. This knowledge has led to the clinically therapeutic pharmacological inhibition of KIT/PDGFRA in GIST patients. In up to 80% of GIST cases, KIT exhibits gain-of-function mutations which drive cell proliferation and survival [48]. Three major pathways are involved in KIT and PDGFRA-mediated tumorigenesis in GIST, namely, the PI3K/AKT/mTOR pathway, the RAS/RAF/MAPK pathway and the

JAK/STAT pathway [2]. The first two pathways are critical to GIST tumour proliferation and are further deregulated in advanced stages of this cancer. Although some KIT/PDGFRA mutations are associated with poor prognosis, the mutations in GIST provide more useful information regarding response to drug inhibitors than prognosis.

Epigenetic regulation and gene expression are two cellular functions that are commonly altered by mutations in metabolic enzymes leading to abnormal metabolic activity which can lead to oncogenic transformation in sarcomas. Approximately 50% of chondrosarcomas and up to 81% of patients with enchondromas show somatic mutations in isocitrate dehydrogenase [49]. These mutations allow abnormal enzymatic activity, such as the production of D-2-hydroxyglutarate (D2HG) from alpha ketoglutarate. D2HG, an oncometabolite, deactivates other oxygenase enzymes like TET2 to lead to DNA hypermethylation, particularly in chondral tumours [49]. D2HG also increases histone methylation through alternative pathways and consequently leads to an unstable epigenetic environment that has been shown to drive transdifferentiation of cells in bone towards a cartilage phenotype. Detection of IDH1 and IDH2 mutations can thus help to differentiate chondrosarcoma from chondroma and chondroblastic osteosarcoma. Mutations in IDH leading to oncometabolite generation have been reported in 86% of secondary central chondrosarcoma, up to 70% of primary central chondrosarcoma, 15% of periosteal chondrosarcoma, 54% of de-differentiated chondrosarcoma and up to 87% of Ollier-associated enchondromas [49]. In high-grade chondrosarcomas, however, IDH does not appear to be a requirement for ongoing tumour survival and growth [50, 51].

Some GIST tumours which do not show the characteristic KIT/PDGFRA mutations may contain mutations in one of the genes coding for succinate dehydrogenase (SDH) or mitochondrial complex II in the electron transport chain [52]. These mutations are associated with global DNA hypermethylation and are commonly seen in gastric GISTs affecting younger patients. Mutations in any SDH subunit is known to cause degradation of the B subunit specifically [52]. Therefore, immunohistochemical detection of SDH subunit B acts as a surrogate marker for the identification of mutations in SDH.

Primary epigenetic deregulation has been cited as one of the most important mechanistic factors in the development of various sarcomas. Mutations in genes which normally regulate chromatin structure, such as the SWI/SNF complex, the Polycomb group and PRC2 complex (involved in malignant peripheral nerve sheath tumours), are known to exacerbate pre-existing genomic instability in a range of tumour types [53]. However, epigenetic deregulation is now recognised as an increasingly common primary driver of oncogenesis in several tumours, for instance, SMARCA4 inactivation in thoracic sarcomas, SMARCB1 deletions in rhabdoid tumours [54], H3F3B gene mutations in 95% of chondroblastoma cases and H3F3A mutations in 92% of giant cell tumours of bone (GCTB) [47]. The latter two tumours are locally aggressive tumours which are more common in paediatric than adult populations. Importantly, the abnormalities in epigenetic programming that have been observed in some studies of sarcoma are thought to occur under the influence of chromosomal translocation-mediated hybrid oncoproteins, such as the SS18-SSX hybrid complex in synovial sarcoma, in which the oncoproteins disrupt the SWI/SNF chromatin remodelling complex [55]. In combination with immunohistochemical detection of mutant proteins, protein complexes and enzymes, next-generation sequencing for mutational variant analysis can also inform sarcoma diagnosis.

2.4.2 Sarcomas with Complex Karyotypes

The majority of sarcomas show diverse, non-specific genetic modifications on a background of highly complex genomes. These tumours are characterised by a high histological grade, cytological pleomorphism and variable differentiation signatures. With the exception of osteosarcomas and some radiation-induced sarcomas, which are more prevalent in children and adolescents than adults, most sarcomas with complex genomes occur more frequently in the older population [56]. High-grade myxofibrosarcoma, high-grade leiomyosarcoma, pleomorphic and undifferentiated liposarcoma, angiosarcoma and undifferentiated pleomorphic sarcoma are examples of tumours known to have complex genomes [2]. These sarcomas have a greater prevalence of gene copy number variations as opposed to single nucleotide polymorphisms [2]. Due to the high level of molecular heterogeneity in all sarcomas within this group, few tumour-specific markers are available for diagnostic use. Some of the postulated mechanisms of pathogenesis in genomically complex sarcomas include alterations in TP53 signalling, abnormal telomeric extension due to enzymatic modifications and inactivation of ATRX (a chromatin remodelling protein) and mutations in the Rb/E2F cell cycle regulatory pathway, which can engender unregulated cell proliferation and survival [2, 57].

Despite the difficulty in molecular characterisation of sarcomas containing complex unbalanced genotypes, a pattern in copy number alterations has been established in well-differentiated/de-differentiated liposarcoma (WD/DDLPS), which shows characteristic linear or ring-like neochromosomes formed from the accumulation of DNA from distinct parts of the genome [58]. Some of the genes contained within these neochromosomes include the CDK4 and MDM2 genes on chromosome 12, which are involved in progression of the cell cycle and repression of TP53, respectively [2]. Findings from research into the evolution of neochromosomes illustrate that the creation of these neochromosomes is a result of a series of intranuclear events involving the fragmentation, circularisation, amplification and linearisation of chromosome 12-derived genetic material [58]. Since the amplification of MDM2 and CDK4 is a recurrent feature of this disease, the abnormally excessive genetic and transcriptional products may be detected by fluorescence in situ hybridisation (FISH), immunohistochemistry or next-generation sequencing and therefore serve as diagnostic markers for WD/DDLPS.

Osteosarcoma is the most common primary high-grade tumour in humans, occurring predominantly in children and adolescents [59]. It is characterised by a high degree of genomic instability due to the presence of numerous chromosomal rearrangements, gene amplifications, mutations and deletions, the complexity of which contributes to the difficulty in the identification of genetic and molecular markers for this condition. However, molecular alterations in the RB and TP53 gene pathways (22% of osteosarcoma cases) are known to be common in high-grade bone cancers such as osteosarcoma [60]. At present, two cellular events are postulated to play a role in osteosarcoma pathogenesis. The first is chromothripsis, which describes the aberrant fragmentation and disordered assembly of chromosomes [61]. The second event is kataegis, which refers to a hypermutated area of the genome, and is observed in approximately half of all osteosarcoma cases [62]. These two phenomena may lead to the formation of osteosarcoma-associated onco-antigens, the detection of which could predict responses to cancer immunotherapy. Currently, high-grade sarcomas with complex genomes lack specific, recurrent molecular markers which can guide the management of these cancers (Table 2.2).

Table 2.2 Features of sarcomas containing simple karyotypes vs. complex karyotypes

Features	Sarcomas with simple karyotypes	Sarcomas with complex karyotypes
Karyotype	Simple, balanced	Complex, unbalanced High degree of genomic instability
Morphology	Relatively monomorphic	Pleomorphic, high-grade
Mutational rate	Low	High
Availability of molecular markers for diagnostic purposes	Clinically useful diagnostic markers (detectable using FISH, RT-PCR, NGS, immunohistochemistry)	Very limited
Common molecular/genetic alterations	Most molecular alterations are well characterised, e.g. chimeric transcription factors, deregulated kinase signalling, oncometabolite formation and epigenetic deregulation	Loss of tumour suppressor genes (especially TP53)
Clinical behaviour	Heterogeneous	Heterogeneous
Response to therapy	Clinically effective targeted therapies against deregulated kinases No effective therapy against hybrid transcription factors or aberrant epigenetic modifications	No targeted therapy Some respond to conventional chemotherapy and radiation therapy

FISH fluorescence in situ hybridisation, *RT-PCR* reverse transcriptase-polymerase chain reaction, *NGS* next-generation sequencing
Table was adapted from information summarised by Mariño-Enríquez et al. [2]

2.5 Infectious Risk Factors

Although the role of infectious agents in the development of sarcomas is not well understood, there is strong evidence for the association of certain viral infections with sarcoma pathogenesis [1]. In the context of a weakened immune system due to immunodeficiency syndromes, HIV infection or exposure to immunosuppressive pharmacotherapy following transplantation, human herpesvirus 8 and Epstein-Barr virus are known to cause Kaposi sarcoma [63] and a group of leiomyosarcomas, respectively [64]. There is insufficient evidence to support the role of oncogenic viruses in sarcomagenesis in the absence of immunosuppression.

2.6 Immunological Risk Factors

A weak immune system is unable to initiate and sustain strong innate or adaptive immune responses against tumour cell growth, malignant transformation, proliferation and invasion. As discussed previously, immunosuppressive medications as well as acquired and congenital immunodeficiency syndromes increase the risk of viral-mediated sarcoma pathogenesis, possibly by limiting the numbers of natural killer cells and T-cells involved in the destruction of nascent tumour cells. However, the underlying mechanism connecting immune deficiency to diverse cancer types remains to be fully uncovered. It has been suggested that acquired regional immunodeficiency in combination with chronic lymphedema, secondary to radical mastectomy (Stewart-Treves syndrome) or infectious conditions, may effect the development of rare angiosarcomas [65, 66].

2.7 Environmental Risk Factors

Several environmental risk factors are implicated in the development of sarcoma. These primarily include exposure to radiation, chemicals and a history of trauma.

2.7.1 Radiation Exposure

In the 1920s, published reports cited the increased prevalence of sarcomas in workers manufacturing radium watch dials. Over the last few decades, there has been increasing evidence for the increased risk of sarcoma in patients undergoing radiotherapy treatment for lymphoma, testicular cancer, ovarian cancer, breast cancer, lung cancer and other cancers. Although previous estimates suggested that approximately 0.5–5.5% of sarcomas are due to radiation [67], larger longitudinal population studies in patients who have undergone radiation therapy have demonstrated a lower frequency of sarcomas in this group, with an incidence of 0.8% at the most. A Swedish study of 122,991 breast cancer patients who received radiotherapy showed that breast cancer patients had at least a 0.13% risk of developing sarcoma at 10 years following radiation exposure [68].

In order to identify the cause of sarcoma as being due to radiation, several criteria must be met. These include documentation proving the development of sarcoma within the irradiated field, confirmation of sarcoma diagnosis by histology, a minimum 3-year period of latency between radiation exposure and sarcoma development and evidence that the region in which the sarcoma arose was unaffected prior to radiotherapy [69]. Post-radiation sarcomas typically arise in the margins of the field of radiation, however, which suggests that the mutagenic impact of radiation is highest at the periphery due to scatter radiation [70]. The vast majority of radiation-induced sarcomas develop in adult women, which is reflective of the high prevalence of female patients receiving radiotherapy for breast and gynaecological cancers. A clear dose-dependent correlation exists between the radiation dose and sarcoma incidence, with a high risk reported for individuals exposed to more than 5000 cGy and a negligible risk for those exposed to less than 10 Gy [71].

Radiation-induced sarcomas are known to be high grade and locally aggressive. A study of 160 post-radiation sarcomas at the Memorial Sloan-Kettering Cancer Center revealed that 87% of the tumours were high grade and the most common sarcoma subtype in this category was extraskeletal osteosarcoma with a prevalence of 21%, followed by malignant fibrous histiocytoma (16%) and angiosarcoma or lymphangiosarcoma (15%) [72]. Among the radiation-induced soft tissue sarcomas, 70% are undifferentiated pleomorphic sarcomas [1]. Since most post-radiation sarcomas are already very high grade at the time of detection, they are associated with a poor survival rate. The highest survival rate in this group is seen in patients who develop post-radiation sarcomas of the extremities (30% survival at 5 years), and the lowest rate is observed in patients with sarcomas in the vertebral column, pelvis and shoulder girdle (less than 5% survival at 5 years) [1, 73].

2.7.2 Chemical Exposure

Sarcomas have been associated with exposure to a range of different chemicals. Polyvinylchloride, use of thorotrast during carotid angiography (between 1930 and 1955) and inorganic arsenic and androgenic anabolic steroid medications have all been linked with the development of hepatic angiosarcoma (HAS) [74]. It is presumed that thorium dioxide, the main component of thorotrast solution, is sequestered by Kupffer cells of the liver, causing radiation injury to hepatic tissue, which leads to a range of hepatic malignancies. Moreover, chlorophenols, dioxin and phenoxyacetic herbicides have also been associated with sarcoma pathogenesis [75, 76]. German autopsy investigations from the 1940s and 1950s showed an increased incidence of liver disease, including HAS, due to the consumption of potassium arsenite and arsenic-contaminated water [74]. Despite a study by Leiss and Savitz which suggested a link between phenoxyacetic acid pesticides and soft tissue sarcomas in paediatric patients, additional investigations did not support this claim [77]. Nevertheless, studies in at least four countries including Sweden, Italy, the United

Kingdom and New Zealand provided strong evidence to conclude that the risk of soft tissue sarcomas in patients exposed to phenoxyacetic acid and chlorophenols in agricultural settings is about six times higher than the general population [78–80]. In certain animal models, benzene and o-nitrotoluene have also been shown to promote sarcomagenesis [81].

2.7.3 Trauma Exposure

Trauma has been cited as a rare causal factor in the development of soft tissue sarcomas in scar tissue secondary to surgery, fracture wounds, thermal and acid burns and implantation of metal or plastic prostheses following a long period of latency of at least several years [82]. Although soft tissue sarcomas are uncommonly detected during abdominal imaging following a history of abdominal trauma or pain, the vast majority of these tumours are asymptomatic. Furthermore, the connection between trauma and sarcoma appears to be more coincidental than aetiological in nature due to the liberal use of abdominal imaging in trauma patients.

References

1. Goldblum JR, Folpe AL, Weiss SW, Enzinger FM, Weiss SW. Enzinger and Weiss's soft tissue tumors. 6th ed. Philadelphia: Saunders/Elsevier; 2014. xiv, 1155 p.
2. Marino-Enriquez A, Bovee JV. Molecular pathogenesis and diagnostic, prognostic and predictive molecular markers in sarcoma. Surg Pathol Clin. 2016;9(3):457–73.
3. Fletcher CD. The evolving classification of soft tissue tumours—an update based on the new 2013 WHO classification. Histopathology. 2014;64(1):2–11.
4. Thway K. Pathology of soft tissue sarcomas. Clin Oncol (R Coll Radiol). 2009;21(9):695–705.
5. Burningham Z, Hashibe M, Spector L, Schiffman JD. The epidemiology of sarcoma. Clin Sarcoma Res. 2012;2(1):14.
6. Ferrari A, Sultan I, Huang TT, Rodriguez-Galindo C, Shehadeh A, Meazza C, et al. Soft tissue sarcoma across the age spectrum: a population-based study from the Surveillance Epidemiology and End Results database. Pediatr Blood Cancer. 2011;57(6):943–9.
7. Casali PG, Blay JY, ECECPo experts. Soft tissue sarcomas: ESMO Clinical Practice Guidelines for diagnosis, treatment and follow-up. Ann Oncol. 2010;21(Suppl 5):v198–203.
8. Alston RD, Rowan S, Eden TO, Moran A, Birch JM. Cancer incidence patterns by region and socioeconomic deprivation in teenagers and young adults in England. Br J Cancer. 2007;96(11):1760–6.
9. Howlader NNA, Krapcho M, Neyman N, Aminou R, Waldron W, Altekruse SF, Kosary CL, Ruhl J, Tatalovich Z, Cho H, Mariotto A, Eisner MP, Lewis DR, Chen HS, Feuer EJ, Cronin KA, Edwards BK. SEER cancer statistics review, 1975–2008. Bethesda: National Cancer Institute; 2011.
10. Jemal A, Siegel R, Ward E, Murray T, Xu J, Thun MJ. Cancer statistics, 2007. CA Cancer J Clin. 2007;57(1):43–66.
11. Worch J, Matthay KK, Neuhaus J, Goldsby R, DuBois SG. Ethnic and racial differences in patients with Ewing sarcoma. Cancer. 2010;116(4):983–8.
12. Grier HE. The Ewing family of tumors. Ewing's sarcoma and primitive neuroectodermal tumors. Pediatr Clin N Am. 1997;44(4):991–1004.
13. Guo W, Xu W, Huvos AG, Healey JH, Feng C. Comparative frequency of bone sarcomas among different racial groups. Chin Med J. 1999;112(12):1101–4.

14. Matushansky I, Hernando E, Socci ND, Mills JE, Matos TA, Edgar MA, et al. Derivation of sarcomas from mesenchymal stem cells via inactivation of the Wnt pathway. J Clin Invest. 2007;117(11):3248–57.
15. Lin PP, Pandey MK, Jin F, Raymond AK, Akiyama H, Lozano G. Targeted mutation of p53 and Rb in mesenchymal cells of the limb bud produces sarcomas in mice. Carcinogenesis. 2009;30(10):1789–95.
16. Genadry KC, Pietrobono S, Rota R, Linardic CM. Soft tissue sarcoma cancer stem cells: an overview. Front Oncol. 2018;8:475.
17. Danielson LS, Menendez S, Attolini CS, Guijarro MV, Bisogna M, Wei J, et al. A differentiation-based microRNA signature identifies leiomyosarcoma as a mesenchymal stem cell-related malignancy. Am J Pathol. 2010;177(2):908–17.
18. Nielsen TO, West RB, Linn SC, Alter O, Knowling MA, O'Connell JX, et al. Molecular characterisation of soft tissue tumours: a gene expression study. Lancet. 2002;359(9314):1301–7.
19. Hatley ME, Tang W, Garcia MR, Finkelstein D, Millay DP, Liu N, et al. A mouse model of rhabdomyosarcoma originating from the adipocyte lineage. Cancer Cell. 2012;22(4):536–46.
20. Ladanyi M, Antonescu CR, Leung DH, Woodruff JM, Kawai A, Healey JH, et al. Impact of SYT-SSX fusion type on the clinical behavior of synovial sarcoma: a multi-institutional retrospective study of 243 patients. Cancer Res. 2002;62(1):135–40.
21. Windham TC, Pisters PW. Retroperitoneal sarcomas. Cancer Control. 2005;12(1):36–43.
22. Hartley AL, Birch JM, Blair V, Kelsey AM, Harris M, Jones PH. Patterns of cancer in the families of children with soft tissue sarcoma. Cancer. 1993;72(3):923–30.
23. Li FP. Cancer families: human models of susceptibility to neoplasia--the Richard and Hinda Rosenthal Foundation Award lecture. Cancer Res. 1988;48(19):5381–6.
24. Li FP, Fraumeni JF Jr, Mulvihill JJ, Blattner WA, Dreyfus MG, Tucker MA, et al. A cancer family syndrome in twenty-four kindreds. Cancer Res. 1988;48(18):5358–62.
25. Zahm SH, Fraumeni JF Jr. The epidemiology of soft tissue sarcoma. Semin Oncol. 1997;24(5):504–14.
26. Zhang J, Walsh MF, Wu G, Edmonson MN, Gruber TA, Easton J, et al. Germline mutations in predisposition genes in pediatric cancer. N Engl J Med. 2015;373(24):2336–46.
27. Ballinger ML, Goode DL, Ray-Coquard I, James PA, Mitchell G, Niedermayr E, Puri A, Schiffman JD, Dite GS, Cipponi A, Maki RG. Monogenic and polygenic determinants of sarcoma risk: an international genetic study. Lancet Oncol. 2016;17(9):1261–71.
28. Evans SC, Lozano G. The Li-Fraumeni syndrome: an inherited susceptibility to cancer. Mol Med Today. 1997;3(9):390–5.
29. Varley JM, McGown G, Thorncroft M, Santibanez-Koref MF, Kelsey AM, Tricker KJ, et al. Germ-line mutations of TP53 in Li-Fraumeni families: an extended study of 39 families. Cancer Res. 1997;57(15):3245–52.
30. Ognjanovic S, Olivier M, Bergemann TL, Hainaut P. Sarcomas in TP53 germline mutation carriers: a review of the IARC TP53 database. Cancer. 2012;118(5):1387–96.
31. DerKinderen DJ, Koten JW, Nagelkerke NJ, Tan KE, Beemer FA, Den Otter W. Non-ocular cancer in patients with hereditary retinoblastoma and their relatives. Int J Cancer. 1988;41(4):499–504.
32. Yu CL, Tucker MA, Abramson DH, Furukawa K, Seddon JM, Stovall M, et al. Cause-specific mortality in long-term survivors of retinoblastoma. J Natl Cancer Inst. 2009;101(8):581–91.
33. Kleinerman RA, Stovall M, Tarone RE, Tucker MA. Radiotherapy and genetic susceptibility to cancer in a cohort of retinoblastoma patients. Ann Epidemiol. 2004;14(8):593.
34. Kleinerman RA, Schonfeld SJ, Tucker MA. Sarcomas in hereditary retinoblastoma. Clin Sarcoma Res. 2012;2(1):15.
35. Kleinerman RA, Tucker MA, Abramson DH, Seddon JM, Tarone RE, Fraumeni JF Jr. Risk of soft tissue sarcomas by individual subtype in survivors of hereditary retinoblastoma. J Natl Cancer Inst. 2007;99(1):24–31.
36. Colman SD, Williams CA, Wallace MR. Benign neurofibromas in type 1 neurofibromatosis (NF1) show somatic deletions of the NF1 gene. Nat Genet. 1995;11(1):90–2.

37. Brekke HR, Ribeiro FR, Kolberg M, Agesen TH, Lind GE, Eknaes M, et al. Genomic changes in chromosomes 10, 16, and X in malignant peripheral nerve sheath tumors identify a high-risk patient group. J Clin Oncol. 2010;28(9):1573–82.
38. Mertens F, Rydholm A, Bauer HF, Limon J, Nedoszytko B, Szadowska A, et al. Cytogenetic findings in malignant peripheral nerve sheath tumors. Int J Cancer. 1995;61(6):793–8.
39. Ducatman BS, Scheithauer BW, Piepgras DG, Reiman HM, Ilstrup DM. Malignant peripheral nerve sheath tumors. A clinicopathologic study of 120 cases. Cancer. 1986;57(10):2006–21.
40. Hizawa K, Iida M, Mibu R, Aoyagi K, Yao T, Fujishima M. Desmoid tumors in familial adenomatous polyposis/Gardner's syndrome. J Clin Gastroenterol. 1997;25(1):334–7.
41. Bale AE. Variable expressivity of patched mutations in flies and humans. Am J Hum Genet. 1997;60(1):10–2.
42. Hahn H, Wojnowski L, Zimmer AM, Hall J, Miller G, Zimmer A. Rhabdomyosarcomas and radiation hypersensitivity in a mouse model of Gorlin syndrome. Nat Med. 1998;4(5):619–22.
43. Gripp KW, Scott CI Jr, Nicholson L, McDonald-McGinn DM, Ozeran JD, Jones MC, et al. Five additional Costello syndrome patients with rhabdomyosarcoma: proposal for a tumor screening protocol. Am J Med Genet. 2002;108(1):80–7.
44. Bovee JV, Hogendoorn PC. Molecular pathology of sarcomas: concepts and clinical implications. Virchows Arch. 2010;456(2):193–9.
45. Hanahan D, Weinberg RA. Hallmarks of cancer: the next generation. Cell. 2011;144(5):646–74.
46. Antonescu CR, Chen HW, Zhang L, Sung YS, Panicek D, Agaram NP, et al. ZFP36-FOSB fusion defines a subset of epithelioid hemangioma with atypical features. Genes Chromosomes Cancer. 2014;53(11):951–9.
47. Behjati S, Tarpey PS, Sheldon H, Martincorena I, Van Loo P, Gundem G, et al. Recurrent PTPRB and PLCG1 mutations in angiosarcoma. Nat Genet. 2014;46(4):376–9.
48. Corless CL, Fletcher JA, Heinrich MC. Biology of gastrointestinal stromal tumors. J Clin Oncol. 2004;22(18):3813–25.
49. Amary MF, Bacsi K, Maggiani F, Damato S, Halai D, Berisha F, et al. IDH1 and IDH2 mutations are frequent events in central chondrosarcoma and central and periosteal chondromas but not in other mesenchymal tumours. J Pathol. 2011;224(3):334–43.
50. Suijker J, Baelde HJ, Roelofs H, Cleton-Jansen AM, Bovee JV. The oncometabolite D-2-hydroxyglutarate induced by mutant IDH1 or −2 blocks osteoblast differentiation in vitro and in vivo. Oncotarget. 2015;6(17):14832–42.
51. Suijker J, Oosting J, Koornneef A, Struys EA, Salomons GS, Schaap FG, et al. Inhibition of mutant IDH1 decreases D-2-HG levels without affecting tumorigenic properties of chondrosarcoma cell lines. Oncotarget. 2015;6(14):12505–19.
52. Killian JK, Kim SY, Miettinen M, Smith C, Merino M, Tsokos M, et al. Succinate dehydrogenase mutation underlies global epigenomic divergence in gastrointestinal stromal tumor. Cancer Discov. 2013;3(6):648–57.
53. Wilson BG, Wang X, Shen X, McKenna ES, Lemieux ME, Cho YJ, et al. Epigenetic antagonism between polycomb and SWI/SNF complexes during oncogenic transformation. Cancer Cell. 2010;18(4):316–28.
54. Lee RS, Stewart C, Carter SL, Ambrogio L, Cibulskis K, Sougnez C, et al. A remarkably simple genome underlies highly malignant pediatric rhabdoid cancers. J Clin Invest. 2012;122(8):2983–8.
55. Kadoch C, Crabtree GR. Reversible disruption of mSWI/SNF (BAF) complexes by the SS18-SSX oncogenic fusion in synovial sarcoma. Cell. 2013;153(1):71–85.
56. Guillou L, Aurias A. Soft tissue sarcomas with complex genomic profiles. Virchows Arch. 2010;456(2):201–17.
57. Liau JY, Lee JC, Tsai JH, Yang CY, Liu TL, Ke ZL, Hsu HH, Jeng YM. Comprehensive screening of alternative lengthening of telomeres phenotype and loss of ATRX expression in sarcomas. Mod Pathol. 2015;28(12):1545–54.
58. Garsed DW, Marshall OJ, Corbin VD, Hsu A, Di Stefano L, Schroder J, et al. The architecture and evolution of cancer neochromosomes. Cancer Cell. 2014;26(5):653–67.
59. Savage SA, Mirabello L. Using epidemiology and genomics to understand osteosarcoma etiology. Sarcoma. 2011;2011:548151.

60. Broadhead ML, Clark JC, Myers DE, Dass CR, Choong PF. The molecular pathogenesis of osteosarcoma: a review. Sarcoma. 2011;2011:959248.
61. Stephens PJ, Greenman CD, Fu B, Yang F, Bignell GR, Mudie LJ, et al. Massive genomic rearrangement acquired in a single catastrophic event during cancer development. Cell. 2011;144(1):27–40.
62. Chen X, Bahrami A, Pappo A, Easton J, Dalton J, Hedlund E, et al. Recurrent somatic structural variations contribute to tumorigenesis in pediatric osteosarcoma. Cell Rep. 2014;7(1):104–12.
63. Dourmishev LA, Dourmishev AL, Palmeri D, Schwartz RA, Lukac DM. Molecular genetics of Kaposi's sarcoma-associated herpesvirus (human herpesvirus-8) epidemiology and pathogenesis. Microbiol Mol Biol Rev. 2003;67(2):175–212, table of contents.
64. McClain KL, Leach CT, Jenson HB, Joshi VV, Pollock BH, Parmley RT, et al. Association of Epstein-Barr virus with leiomyosarcomas in young people with AIDS. N Engl J Med. 1995;332(1):12–8.
65. Dawlatly SL, Dramis A, Sumathi VP, Grimer RJ. Stewart-Treves syndrome and the use of positron emission tomographic scanning. Ann Vasc Surg. 2011;25(5):699 e1–3.
66. Shon W, Ida CM, Boland-Froemming JM, Rose PS, Folpe A. Cutaneous angiosarcoma arising in massive localized lymphedema of the morbidly obese: a report of five cases and review of the literature. J Cutan Pathol. 2011;38(7):560–4.
67. Davidson T, Westbury G, Harmer CL. Radiation-induced soft-tissue sarcoma. Br J Surg. 1986;73(4):308–9.
68. Karlsson P, Holmberg E, Samuelsson A, Johansson KA, Wallgren A. Soft tissue sarcoma after treatment for breast cancer—a Swedish population-based study. Eur J Cancer. 1998;34(13):2068–75.
69. Arlen M, Higinbotham NL, Huvos AG, Marcove RC, Miller T, Shah IC. Radiation-induced sarcoma of bone. Cancer. 1971;28(5):1087–99.
70. Pisters PW. Preoperative chemotherapy and split-course radiation therapy for patients with localized soft tissue sarcomas: home run, base hit, or strike out? J Clin Oncol. 2006;24(4):549–51.
71. Tucker MA, D'Angio GJ, Boice JD Jr, Strong LC, Li FP, Stovall M, et al. Bone sarcomas linked to radiotherapy and chemotherapy in children. N Engl J Med. 1987;317(10):588–93.
72. Brady MS, Gaynor JJ, Brennan MF. Radiation-associated sarcoma of bone and soft tissue. Arch Surg. 1992;127(12):1379–85.
73. Billings SD, McKenney JK, Folpe AL, Hardacre MC, Weiss SW. Cutaneous angiosarcoma following breast-conserving surgery and radiation: an analysis of 27 cases. Am J Surg Pathol. 2004;28(6):781–8.
74. Falk H, Herbert J, Crowley S, Ishak KG, Thomas LB, Popper H, et al. Epidemiology of hepatic angiosarcoma in the United States: 1964-1974. Environ Health Perspect. 1981;41:107–13.
75. Kogevinas M, Ferro G, Saracci R, Andersen A, Biocca M, Coggon D, et al. Cancer mortality in an international cohort of workers exposed to styrene. IARC Sci Publ. 1993;127:289–300.
76. Zambon P, Ricci P, Bovo E, Casula A, Gattolin M, Fiore AR, et al. Sarcoma risk and dioxin emissions from incinerators and industrial plants: a population-based case-control study (Italy). Environ Health. 2007;6:19.
77. Pahwa P, McDuffie HH, Dosman JA, McLaughlin JR, Spinelli JJ, Robson D, et al. Hodgkin lymphoma, multiple myeloma, soft tissue sarcomas, insect repellents, and phenoxyherbicides. J Occup Environ Med. 2006;48(3):264–74.
78. Balarajan R, Acheson ED. Soft tissue sarcomas in agriculture and forestry workers. J Epidemiol Community Health. 1984;38(2):113–6.
79. Eriksson M, Hardell L, Adami HO. Exposure to dioxins as a risk factor for soft tissue sarcoma: a population-based case-control study. J Natl Cancer Inst. 1990;82(6):486–90.
80. Hardell L, Lindstrom G, van Bavel B, Fredrikson M, Liljegren G. Some aspects of the etiology of non-Hodgkin's lymphoma. Environ Health Perspect. 1998;106(Suppl 2):679–81.
81. Rhodes MC, Bucher JR, Peckham JC, Kissling GE, Hejtmancik MR, Chhabra RS. Carcinogenesis studies of benzophenone in rats and mice. Food Chem Toxicol. 2007;45(5):843–51.
82. Piscitelli D, Ruggeri E, Fiore MG, Rossi R, Guerriero S. Undifferentiated high-grade pleomorphic sarcoma in a blind eye with a silicone prosthesis implant: a clinico-pathologic study. Orbit. 2011;30(4):192–4.

3 Anatomic Imaging of Bone and Soft Tissue Sarcoma

Marcus J. Pianta and Warren R. Perera

3.1 Plain Radiography

Radiographs are often one of the initial radiological investigations for tumour imaging. They are easily accessible and inexpensive and with minimal radiation exposure. They are well tolerated by patients and quick to perform so that motion artefact is minimised. Large soft tissue masses as well as smaller bone lesions are identifiable and whether there is any associated fat or mineralisation such as ossification or calcification. Complications including pathological fracture, bone destruction and new bone formation can also be observed.

Aggressive appearances include a hair-on-end or sunburst pattern, lamellation with a Codman's triangle and bone destruction, particularly over a short duration [1] although these can also be seen with non-tumour processes such as infection and trauma (Fig. 3.1a,b). More benign appearances include gradual and thick periosteal reaction and bone remodelling without destruction, as well as a clearly defined, narrow zone of transition [2]. Several views are desirable to better localise a lesion and help plan further cross-sectional imaging. Plain radiographs are also a mainstay of post-operative follow-up to assess bone union and graft integration as well as hardware positioning given they are minimally susceptible to metalware artefact.

3.2 Ultrasound

Ultrasound (US) is an easily accessible and non-invasive imaging modality that is frequently employed for initial investigations of palpable tumours. Its main uses are to confirm the presence of a mass and assess location, size and depth. It can demonstrate if a mass is cystic or solid and proximity to a joint. It has no established role

M. J. Pianta (✉) · W. R. Perera
Department of Medical Imaging, St. Vincent's Hospital Melbourne,
Melbourne, VIC, Australia
e-mail: warren.perera@svha.org.au

P. F. M. Choong (ed.), *Sarcoma*, https://doi.org/10.1007/978-981-15-9414-4_3

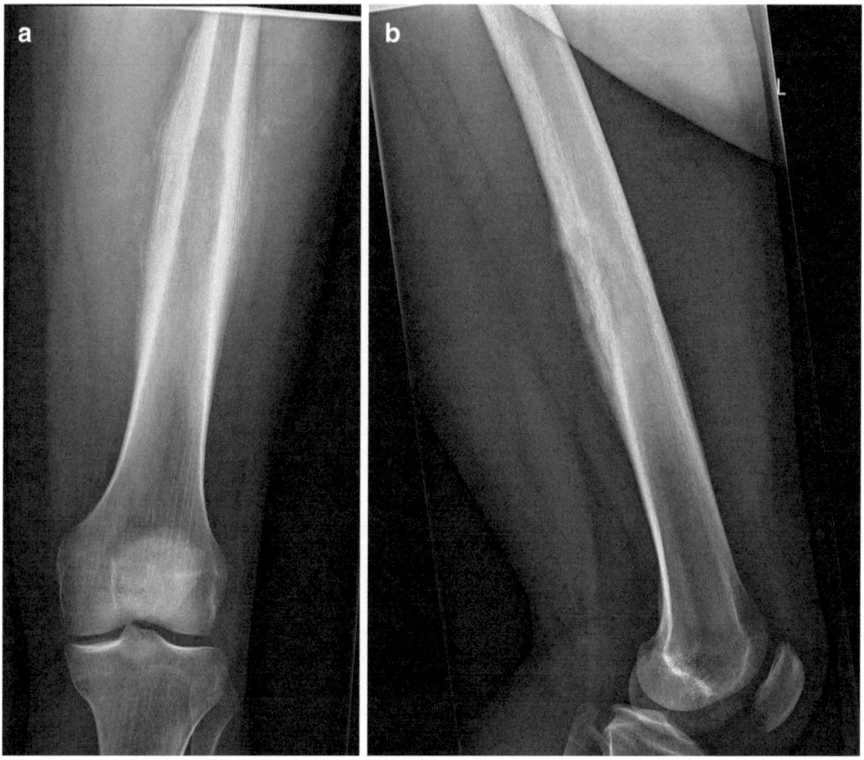

Fig. 3.1 (**a**) Anteroposterior and (**b**) lateral plain radiographs of the left femur in a 19-year-old male with a lamellated or onion-skin appearance of a distal left thigh Ewing's sarcoma. Note the large associated soft tissue mass with rim-mineralisation proximally and a Codman's triangle of aggressive periosteal reaction on the lateral view

in assessment of bone tumours [3]. It has a low specificity for characterising the nature of solid tumours [4, 5]. Sensitivity, specificity and accuracy can be improved in detection of soft tissue sarcoma and distinguishing between aggressive and benign lesions on ultrasound based on pattern of echotexture and vascularity [6].

Large tumours with internal heterogeneity that induce a mass effect and are located deep to the deep fascia raise suspicions of neoplasia on ultrasound examination. Vascularity of the lesion is reported as both useful and not useful in the literature and thus cannot be relied upon alone as a predictor of malignancy. Power and colour Doppler are used to determine the amount and pattern of vascularity of the mass. High-grade malignancies are often associated with increased peripheral flow due to angio-neo-genesis and also manifest central avascular areas due to necrosis [4]. In some cases, colour Doppler can also be employed to characterise the change in neovascularisation following adjuvant or neoadjuvant therapies although this tends to be the domain of functional imaging in most sarcoma centres.

Ultrasound can be used for image-guided fine needle or core biopsy of soft tissue masses, especially for superficial, small or precariously located masses where

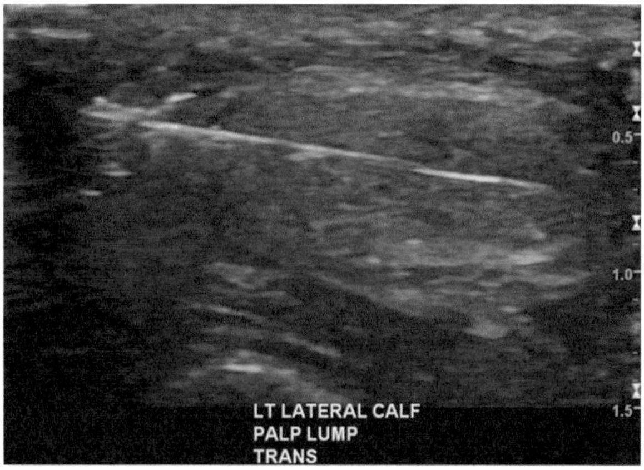

Fig. 3.2 Clear demonstration in a single ultrasound image of biopsy needle traversing the direct centre of a lesion in the calf. This is confirmed in real time by turning the probe 90° and confirming the position again in a transverse orientation

real-time imaging can be beneficial. Sampling that is clear of necrotic or haemorrhagic areas of the mass is preferred for histologic and other microscopic examinations. US can provide a high yield of tissue, representative of the mass (Fig. 3.2). Ultrasound also has a troubleshooting role in local tumour recurrence detection, especially when MRI is not suitable or degraded by artefact from metallic surgical hardware in prior reconstructive interventions.

Three-dimensional (3D) ultrasonography is a more sophisticated mode of ultrasonography which can enhance scanning planes providing spatially oriented and standardised views, previously not possible with ultrasound. This modality enables finer anatomical detail through multiplayer views, thus reducing operator dependence and allowing more consistent and reliable surveillance scans. This enhanced capability is likely to see greater adoption in soft tissue sarcoma work-up and management [4].

In current practice, if a soft tissue mass is a suspected malignancy, cross-sectional imaging by MRI, or at least CT if MRI is unavailable or contraindicated, should be performed prior to biopsy to allow local assessment and staging. This permits more accurate assessment using images not altered by intervention. It should be noted that soft tissue compartmental anatomy is better assessed on cross-sectional imaging, thereby permitting biopsy planning so other compartments are not unintentionally breached and contaminated.

3.3 Computed Tomography

Computed tomography (CT) is the most effective and accurate modality for evaluating osseous architecture. It also enables visualisation of anatomic structures in multiple planes. CT permits assessment of features such as cortical breakthrough and remodelling, periosteal reaction, bone lesion matrix, endosteal scalloping and pathological fracture. Subtle areas of mineralisation, extraosseous soft tissue extension or soft tissue gas can also be identified, features that are sometimes not as apparent on MRI. Artefacts can also be minimised in patients with metallic hardware from prior reconstructive surgery. Some soft tissue lesions can also be diagnosed depending on their tissue composition, i.e. fatty or cystic lesions. With the advent of multi-detector CT, CT angiography can readily and accurately demonstrate the vascular anatomy [4]. However, it is limited in the differentiation of subtle soft tissue differences.

CT is sensitive to calcification, both in bone and soft tissue lesions. If calcification is faintly evident on the initial plain film, CT may be more useful than MR in the characterisation of this and permit a more specific differential diagnosis. For example, the pattern of ossification in myositis ossificans is very different to the dystrophic calcification seen in some synovial sarcomas which is different to the osteoid matrix in osteosarcoma and the chondroid calcification that occurs in cartilage tumours.

Whilst MRI remains the mainstay for local staging of bone and soft tissue lesions, CT can be used for local staging if MRI is unavailable or contraindicated. CT is also currently the preferred modality for staging the chest to exclude pulmonary metastatic disease.

The rapid acquisition of images and its accuracy as a targeting mechanism makes CT an important enabler of techniques such as percutaneous aspiration and biopsy. Modern CT algorithms are now also being utilised to facilitate robot-assisted needle insertion where accuracy and safety are paramount [4].

3.4 Magnetic Resonance Imaging

MRI is an imaging technique which uses a magnetic field gradient to assess water and fat content of tissues and does not involve radiation. No single MRI sequence is adequate to assess a potential tumour, and scan protocols can vary in the time required to obtain depending on field of view, anatomy to be covered, clinical question and patient comfort. Most tumour scan protocols require a 30–40-min study, but some can be over an hour, particularly in cases of extensive tumour growth and intricate anatomy involvement. General principles of tumour assessment include imaging that is T1-weighted to best depict anatomy and compartments and T2-weighted with fat saturation to highlight pathology such as most tumours (Fig. 3.3), and post-contrast imaging is usually T1-weighted and performed also with fat saturation. In the setting of extensive metalware which distorts the magnetic field, fat saturation may not be applied in order to minimise the degrading effects of susceptibility artefact. In such cases, T1 pre- and post-contrast images need to be carefully compared to assess for contrast enhancement that may otherwise be obscured by adjacent bright T1 signal from fat or marrow.

Excellent contrast between soft tissues and bone can be achieved in order to assess anatomic compartments involved by a tumour, vessels and organs effaced or infiltrated, as well as surrounding abnormal signal which can suggest tumour spread, a biopsy tract or post-treatment changes. Additional ‘skip’ lesions within the bone, intra-/extraosseous extension and metastatic lymph nodes can also be evaluated.

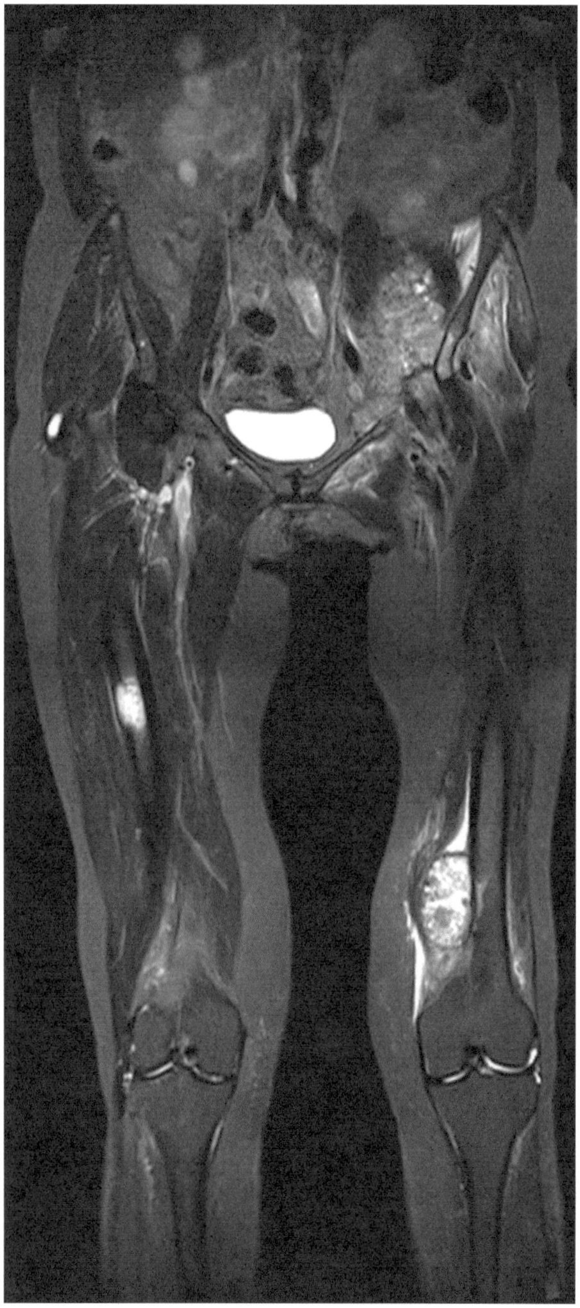

Fig. 3.3 Pelvis to below-knee MRI STIR (short-tau inversion recovery) image was performed for work-up of a left distal femur lesion in a 59-year-old female. Metastatic lesions are demonstrated of the mid-right femur and left ilium with large soft tissue component. Right trochanteric bursitis

The administration of a gadolinium contrast agent can improve lesion conspicuity, better demonstrate a 'tail' and tumour extension as well as evaluate post-treatment response such as necrosis, haemorrhage, recurrence or granulation [7]. More newly developed sequences can also provide further lesion information including diffusion-weighted imaging (DWI) [8] which demonstrates 'restriction' (high signal on DWI, low on apparent diffusion coefficient or ADC) in highly cellular lesions such as high-grade sarcoma and lymphoma, perfusion for blood flow [9, 10] in cases of tumour vs. oedema or granulation, use of chemical shift artefact [8] in fat-containing lesions where signal 'drop' occurs in out-of-phase images when compared to the T1-weighted in-phase images and less commonly MR spectroscopy [4] (MRS) to evaluate the presence of metabolites, particularly a choline peak in malignant tumours, although relatively non-specific.

3.5 Image Fusion

Image fusion is the process where a single image dataset is obtained from matching two or more image datasets. Image fusion is of use in sarcoma management as CT allows more detailed assessment of bone tumours, whilst MRI is the modality of choice for soft tissue assessment. Image fusion of both of these modalities permits the best of both of these modalities. Briefly, the process involves source images from two or more modalities which are segmented. An algorithm for fusion is performed, and the output images are obtained and taken as input for segmentation again to isolate the tumour alone from input images. This process occurs under the influence of various algorithms until the fused output image of both datasets (or modalities) is produced. There is already widespread use of image fusion via ^{18}F 2-fluoro-2-deoxy-D-glucose (^{18}F-FDG) positron emission tomography-computed tomography (PET-CT) with newer applications combining ^{18}F-FDG PET with MRI [11].

3.6 The Role of Pre-biopsy Imaging

Imaging before any intervention, including open or percutaneous biopsy, is essential for planning and prognostication, as well as to help inform the patient regarding possible diagnoses and treatment pathways. An assessment of intact soft tissue planes and structures can allow the procedure to be performed with minimal 'footprint', involving as few anatomical compartments as possible and be recorded (e.g. on a picture archiving and communication system (PACS)) for consideration in future treatment planning, including surgical resection [12]. Other than common initial investigations such as plain radiography and ultrasound, cross-sectional imaging techniques such as computed tomography (CT) and MRI better delineate anatomic compartments, tissue planes, neurovascular structures and the bone/soft tissue interface. Viable and more accessible portions of a tumour can also be accurately targeted to assist improving the outcomes of pre-treatment biochemical and molecular studies.

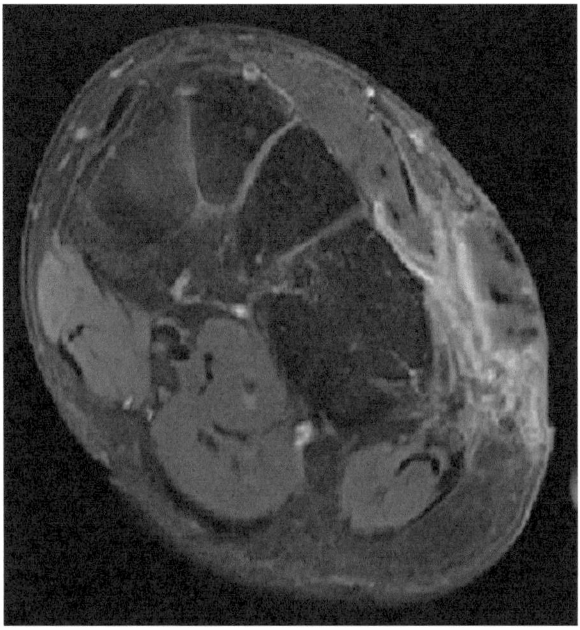

Fig. 3.4 Pre-biopsy MRI of the left foot in a 34-year-old male with inadequate excision (positive margins) of dermatofibrosarcoma protuberans (DFSP) at the lateral aspect. Coronal fat-saturated T1 post-contrast-enhanced images demonstrate haematoma overlying the lateral cuboid within the subcutaneous tissues, and there is an extensive contrast enhancement adjacent extending deep into the extensor musculature and along the superficial surface of the cuboid bone. It is unknown whether the original tumour was confined to the subcutaneous tissues and/or if the deep enhancement within muscle and on the bone is a result of inadvertent surgical exploration. This makes biopsy of a target lesion very difficult, and the subsequent management even more so

It is essential the pre-intervention anatomy and pathology are clearly identified, a task made more difficult in the setting of prior intervention, biopsy or surgery, which may be inadequate in cases of incomplete imaging evaluation [13] and can lead to compromise of future treatment due to inadvertent compartment contamination or alteration of anatomy (Fig. 3.4). Fascial disruptions, abnormal MRI signal in an anatomical compartment, seromas and surgical incision scars can all be observed on post-procedural imaging and must be taken into account when considering sites of likely residual or recurrent disease, as well as subsequent definitive treatment.

3.7 Image-Guided Biopsy: Technique

3.7.1 Approach: Broad Principles

Image-guided needle biopsy is now central to the staging and management plan of patients with solid tumours. The radiologist and the orthopaedic oncologic surgeon should take a team approach to percutaneous needle biopsy, especially when the lesion might be a primary sarcoma for which limb-sparing surgery would be considered. Image-guided needle biopsy has shown comparability with open biopsy for diagnosing musculoskeletal tumours, and the burden of complications and costs has also been shown to be lower [14].

The approach for needle biopsy is important because of the risk of local recurrence from tumour seeding along the biopsy track after core needle biopsy. In this regard, first principles require that the biopsy track be placed along the line of the planned incision to permit inclusion with the resection specimen [14].

Berger-Richardson et al. [16] note that there is a paucity of good-quality evidence regarding the incidence of needle track seeding of sarcoma. They estimated the incidence of needle track seeding at less than 1% for percutaneous biopsy of sarcoma located in the extremity, peritoneal cavity and retroperitoneum and most likely less in the modern era and use of coaxial biopsy needle kits. Nevertheless, they recommend needle biopsy trajectory should be carefully considered when planning percutaneous biopsy and the approach discussed with the treating surgical team.

3.8 Bone Biopsy

The lesion is viewed on all available imaging modalities often comprising of X-ray, CT, functional imaging and MRI. Based on this assessment, the most active part of the lesion (area of most functional tracer uptake or intravenous contrast enhancement) is selected for biopsy with the biopsy entry site and track trajectory aligning with the plane of the incision for potential surgery. Important adjacent structures such as neurovascular bundles are identified as well as compartmental boundaries to avoid unnecessary or accidental contamination. These are often best appreciated on MRI. CT is able to clearly delineate tumour invasion into the bone, thereby making it an excellent modality for demonstrating permeation, erosive changes and matrix calcification. Destructive bony lesions can be assessed for cortical thinning or destruction to allow ease of biopsy entry point; however the entry point for biopsy must still adhere to the surgical approach for limb-sparing surgical procedures [14].

Our bony lesion biopsies are performed under CT guidance given it is faster and more easily accessible than MRI and requires no specialised biopsy equipment. The patient's clinical data is optimised including coagulation profile and informed consent obtained. Risks discussed with the patient include but are not limited to infection, haemorrhage, neuropraxia and repeat biopsy [15]. Correct patient positioning for CT guidance is crucial for optimising the approach to the lesion, ensuring patient and interventionist comfort and confirming the trajectory point of the biopsy instrument [16]. Strict sterile technique, conscious sedation and local anaesthetic infiltration are employed to maximise comfort and care in relation to the procedure. Occasionally, general anaesthesia may be required, and this should be undertaken electively, for patients who have needle or claustrophobia, or who are intolerant or not responsive to narcotic or conscious sedation. Usual post-procedure precautions are observed, including observing the patient for at least 1 hour after the procedure.

We employ a coaxial technique for sampling multiple cores through a single puncture site in practically all bone lesion biopsies, which allows sampling with reduced exposure to radiation. In our institution, there are two biopsy needles that are used. For sampling osseous and chondroid lesions, we used the Bonopty Bone Biopsy System (AprioMed, Sweden) which employs a 14G penetration needle and 15G biopsy needle, whilst for dense osseous lesions, we use the Arrow OnControl Powered Bone Lesion Biopsy System (Teleflex, USA) which provides either a 10 or 11G access coaxial with 12 or 13G biopsy needle. To prevent slippage when drilling, an orthogonal approach to the plane of the cortex is planned. Once the coaxial needle is positioned against the lesion, the obturator is exchanged for the biopsy needle which is used to sample a core of the tumour (Fig. 3.5). Spring-loaded cutting needles are effective and efficient for sampling soft tissue components, and these may also be passed through the coaxial needle system manually (Fig. 3.6) [15].

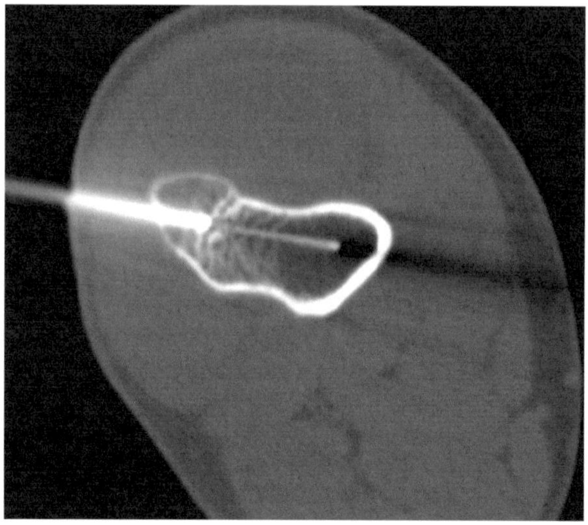

Fig. 3.5 Axial CT image with bone algorithm shows a bone biopsy, coaxial technique in the distal humerus. The smaller central needle can repeatedly access the bone for several samples, and a small gauge soft tissue biopsy needle can also be used when the lesion is particularly soft/fluid

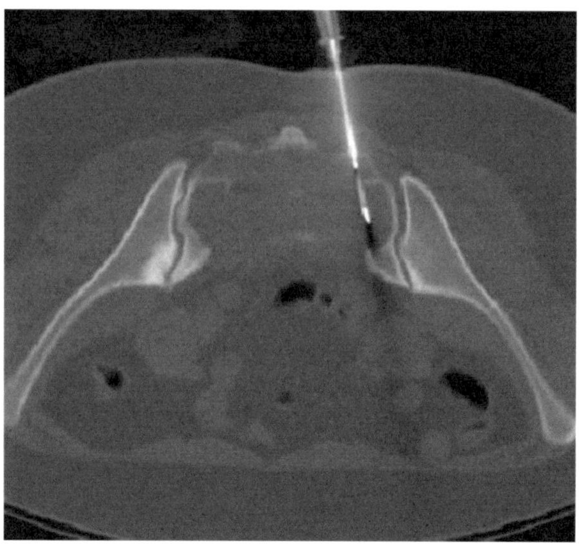

Fig. 3.6 Axial CT image in a case of sacral giant cell tumour of bone. Given the extensive bone replacement by soft tissue, a soft tissue needle was used to obtain an adequate sample

3.9 Soft Tissue Biopsy

The principles for image-guided biopsy of bone and soft tissue tumours are similar. In both cases the surgical approach aims to limit compartmental involvement. Thus, the biopsy track is positioned in a manner that allows its easy inclusion with the resected specimen. As always, the biopsy plane is discussed with the surgical team prior to the intervention to avoid inadvertent contamination of uninvolved compartments or vital structures [14].

We use of combination of CT and ultrasound as modalities of choice for soft tissue lesion biopsy. The technique under CT guidance is similar for bone lesions although the coaxial system employed is different as no bone penetration needle set is required.

Ultrasound offers real-time and multiplanar imaging, is cheap and readily available and is free from ionising radiation. Whilst operator dependent, the high spatial and contrast resolutions allow easier targeting of most but particularly small lesions that may be difficult to appreciate on non-contrast CT scans. The dynamic nature of this modality enables real-time visualisation and confirmation of the needle position to optimise safety and efficacy of the biopsy procedure [15]. Complications are the same as for CT-guided procedures, such as bleeding, infection and neuropraxia.

The procedure is done under local anaesthetic with sedation reserved for those lesions with clinical symptoms suggestive of nerve sheath tumours. Strict sterile conditions are again employed by the use of a sterile sheath overlying the probe and cord. Sterile gel may be placed within the sheath or on the biopsy site after sterile preparation. In our institution, we employ an 18-gauge needle core biopsy cutting needle with a coaxial system previously described (Fig. 3.7). For fatty or larger lesions, we use a 14-gauge needle to ensure an adequate specimen is obtained. Length and throw of the needle is selected based on the tumour location, size and depth. Typically, a 22-mm throw is employed; however sometimes a 15-mm throw is used when the lesion size is small and it's located adjacent to critical structures, i.e. neurovascular bundles.

The shortest biopsy path from the skin to the lesion is chosen when planning the biopsy trajectory. Local anaesthetic is infiltrated along the trajectory path under ultrasound guidance, and after a small skin incision, the coaxial needle is passed along the same longitudinal plane as the ultrasound transducer to allow visualisation of the coaxial needle. The biopsy needle is then inserted through the coaxial, and multiple core samples are taken under direct, real-time vision.

As with the CT-guided procedures, samples are sent to histopathology in 10% formalin or in normal saline for microscopy or flow cytometry depending on the differential diagnoses formulated pre biopsy. After the core biopsy has been performed, an ultrasound of the vicinity to rapidly identify any complications such as a hematoma is done. The patient is kept for observation, usually for 30 min and however up to an hour if conscious sedation is employed.

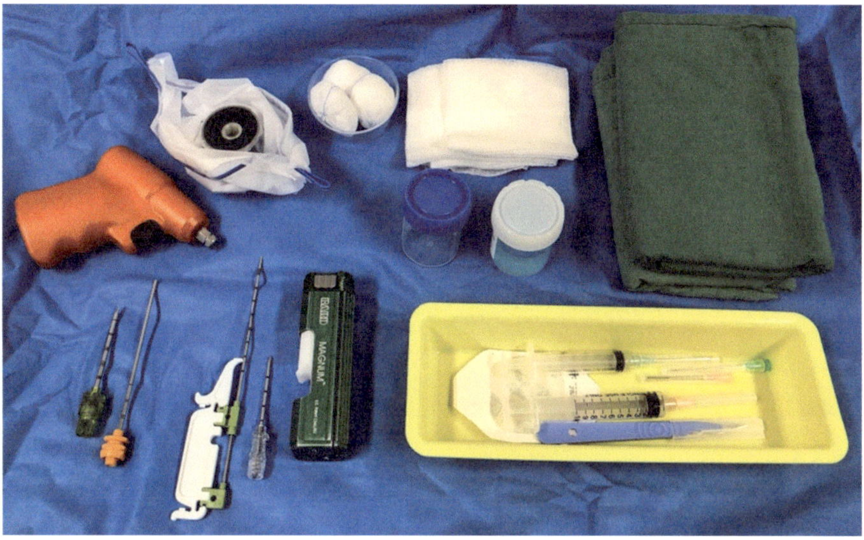

Fig. 3.7 Set up trolley with the range of equipment that can be used for biopsy, including battery-powered bone drill with sterile cover, coaxial and biopsy needles, spring-loaded soft tissue biopsy needle and coaxial, sterile and formalin specimen pots, kidney dish for sharps and drapes/gauze

3.10 Increasing Role of Interventional Radiology

Interventional radiology (IR) uses minimally invasive techniques to assist in preoperative lesion embolisation and diagnosis particularly of vascular lesions and malformations. Newer techniques are being employed for definitive lesion treatments whilst preserving organ function and in the management of pain, particularly in oligometastatic disease and to improve quality of life and prolong relapse intervals [17]. The IR team comprises a crucial and expanding role in multidisciplinary team discussions and tumour management.

Embolisation of soft tissue lesions such as vascular malformations, aneurysmal and simple bone cysts amongst other tumours can be performed definitively or as a preoperative measure [18]. Embolising agents are available with increasing efficacy and reduced side effects including sclerosants such as sodium tetradecyl sulphate foam, ethanol, polyvinyl alcohol particles, cyanoacrylate glue and intravascular coils, as well as chemotherapeutic agents. Cementoplasty can be performed to ablate a bone lesion such as metastasis to reduce pain [19] and restore an underlying supportive structure to avoid pathological fracture and without the resource requirements of an operating theatre (Fig. 3.8a, b). Ablation of lung metastases can also be performed repeatedly and with minimal morbidity.

Radiofrequency ablation can be efficaciously performed of osteoid osteomas, and alternate ablation techniques have also showed efficacy for other lesions including irreversible electroporation, microwave ablation and cryoablation [20].

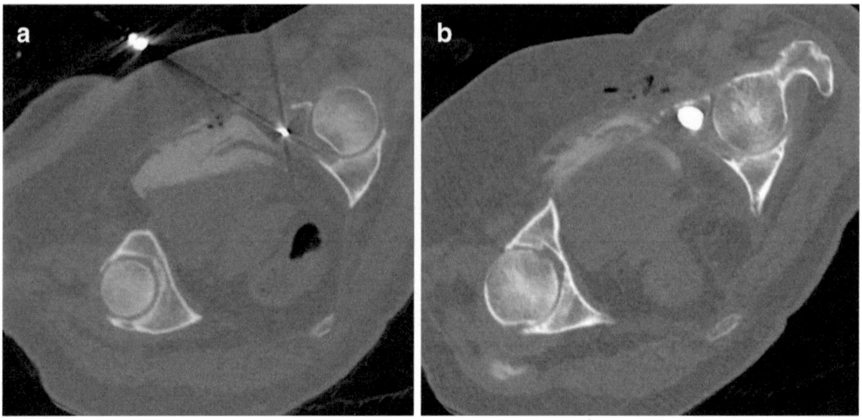

Fig. 3.8 Axial CT imaging demonstrates pre (**a**) and post (**b**) radiofrequency ablation and cementoplasty of a left acetabular renal cell carcinoma metastasis with pathological fracture and severe pain. Prior to the ablation, 5% dextrose solution with iodinated contrast was injected medial to the hip to displace the pelvic organs including bladder, and neurovascular structures, as well as into the hip joint for thermal insulation. Anterior approach has been used to access the lesion with a coaxial needle, through which an ablation probe was passed. Subsequently, bone cement (polymethyl methacrylate, PMMA) was injected for structural support

3.11 Artificial Intelligence

The requirement for continually increasing computing power in order to analyse imaging data and perform complex mathematical functions to generate images has led to early adoption of artificial intelligence (AI) and deep learning in radiology. Computer-aided diagnosis is becoming increasingly feasible, and complex algorithms are already being commonly used to improve imaging quality [20] by reducing artefacts and assisting in imaging analysis. Tumour volume analysis can aid in post-treatment response evaluation, whilst neurovascular mapping and organ segmentation can better clarify structures involved by tumour. Radiographic tumour appearances can also be matched to tumour biology, expected prognosis and treatment response [21]. Automation of and assistance with optimisation of workflows and flagging studies for the more immediate attention of radiologists and other clinicians can be achieved by incorporating factors such as increased tumour growth, presence of a skip lesion or metastatic disease and other unexpected findings.

References

1. Miller TT. Bone tumors and tumorlike conditions: analysis with conventional radiography. Radiology. 2008;246(3):662–74.
2. Helms C. Malignant bone and soft tissue tumors. In: Brant W, Helms C, editors. Fundamentals of diagnostic radiology. 3rd ed. Philadelphia: Lippincott, Williams & Wilkins; 2007. p. 1086–101.

3. Simon MA, Finn HA. Diagnostic strategy for bone and soft-tissue tumors. J Bone Joint Surg Am. 1993;75(4):622–31.
4. Aga P, Singh R, Parihar A, Parashari U. Imaging spectrum in soft tissue sarcomas. Indian J Surg Oncol. 2011;2(4):271–9.
5. Hung EH, Griffith JF, Ng AW, Lee RK, Lau DT, Leung JC. Ultrasound of musculoskeletal soft-tissue tumors superficial to the investing fascia. AJR Am J Roentgenol. 2014;202(6):W532–40.
6. Schulte M, von Baer A, Schultheiss M, Scheil-Bertram S. [Classification of solid soft tissue tumours by ultrasonography]. Ultraschall Med. 2010;31(2):182–90.
7. Nascimento D, Suchard G, Hatem M, de Abreu A. The role of magnetic resonance imaging in the evaluation of bone tumours and tumour-like lesions. Insights Imaging. 2014;5(4):419–40.
8. Davies A, Sundaram M, James S. Imaging of bone tumors and tumor-like lesions. Berlin: Springer; 2009.
9. Berquist TH. Magnetic resonance imaging of primary skeletal neoplasms. Radiol Clin N Am. 1993;31(2):411–24.
10. Gondim Teixeira PA, Renaud A, Aubert S, Ben Haj Amor M, Robin YM, Cotten A, et al. Perfusion MR imaging at 3-Tesla: can it predict tumor grade and histologic necrosis rate of musculoskeletal sarcoma? Diagn Interv Imaging. 2018;99(7–8):473–81.
11. Patel DB, Matcuk GR Jr. Imaging of soft tissue sarcomas. Chin Clin Oncol. 2018;7(4):35.
12. Barrientos-Ruiz I, Ortiz-Cruz EJ, Serrano-Montilla J, Bernabeu-Taboada D, Pozo-Kreilinger JJ. Are biopsy tracts a concern for seeding and local recurrence in sarcomas? Clin Orthop Relat Res. 2017;475(2):511–8.
13. Mesko NW, Wilson RJ, Lawrenz JM, Mathieu JL, Ghiam MK, Mathis SL, et al. Pre-operative evaluation prior to soft tissue sarcoma excision—why can't we get it right? Eur J Surg Oncol. 2018;44(2):243–50.
14. Liu PT, Valadez SD, Chivers FS, Roberts CC, Beauchamp CP. Anatomically based guidelines for core needle biopsy of bone tumors: implications for limb-sparing surgery. Radiographics. 2007;27(1):189–205; discussion 6.
15. Le HB, Lee ST, Munk PL. Image-guided musculoskeletal biopsies. Semin Intervent Radiol. 2010;27(2):191–8.
16. Berger-Richardson D, Swallow CJ. Needle tract seeding after percutaneous biopsy of sarcoma: risk/benefit considerations. Cancer. 2017;123(4):560–7.
17. Jiang C, Wang J, Wang Y, Zhao J, Zhu Y, Ma X, et al. Treatment outcome following transarterial chemoembolization in advanced bone and soft tissue sarcomas. Cardiovasc Intervent Radiol. 2016;39(10):1420–8.
18. Arrigoni F, Bruno F, Zugaro L, Splendiani A, Di Cesare E, Barile A, et al. Role of interventional radiology in the management of musculoskeletal soft-tissue lesions. Radiol Med. 2019;124(4):253–8.
19. de Baere T, Tselikas L, Gravel G, Hakime A, Deschamps F, Honore C, et al. Interventional radiology: role in the treatment of sarcomas. Eur J Cancer. 2018;94:148–55.
20. Yasaka K, Abe O. Deep learning and artificial intelligence in radiology: current applications and future directions. PLoS Med. 2018;15(11):e1002707.
21. Bi WL, Hosny A, Schabath MB, Giger ML, Birkbak NJ, Mehrtash A, et al. Artificial intelligence in cancer imaging: clinical challenges and applications. CA Cancer J Clin. 2019;69(2):127–57.

Nuclear Medicine and Molecular Imaging Techniques

4

Stephen M. Schlicht

Whilst anatomic techniques particularly CT and MRI form the mainstay in the evaluation, diagnosis and staging of musculoskeletal tumours, nuclear medicine/molecular imaging techniques provide unique metabolic and functional information complementary to structural imaging [1].

Bone and soft tissue tumours display a number of specific pathophysiological attributes including altered vascularity, osseous and cartilaginous matrix formation and altered metabolism allowing particular nuclear medicine techniques to uniquely highlight and characterise this altered tissue physiology.

4.1 Bone Scans

Bone scintigraphy using the most commonly used tracer technetium-99m (Tc-99m) methylene diphosphonate (MDP) is extremely sensitive in the detection of increased bone turnover and therefore is most useful in tumours characterised by increased osteoblastic activity. SPECT/CT hybrid techniques combine and co-register the metabolic imaging features with diagnostic CT allowing precise anatomic localisation and lesion characterisation whilst allowing whole-body assessment without increase in radiation dose.

Osteogenic sarcoma the most common primary malignant bone tumour typically demonstrates intense osteoblastic activity due to the formation of malignant osteoid and bone scintigraphy, for assessment of the primary lesion, presence of skip lesions and distant metastases, remains an important contributory staging modality (Fig. 4.1a, b). Osteosarcomatous distant metastases typically demonstrate increased bone tracer uptake and therefore maybe detected on whole-body views (Fig. 4.1b, c) [2].

S. M. Schlicht (✉)
Department of Medical Imaging, St. Vincent's Hospital Melbourne,
Melbourne, VIC, Australia
e-mail: stephen.schlicht@svha.org.au

P. F. M. Choong (ed.), *Sarcoma*, https://doi.org/10.1007/978-981-15-9414-4_4

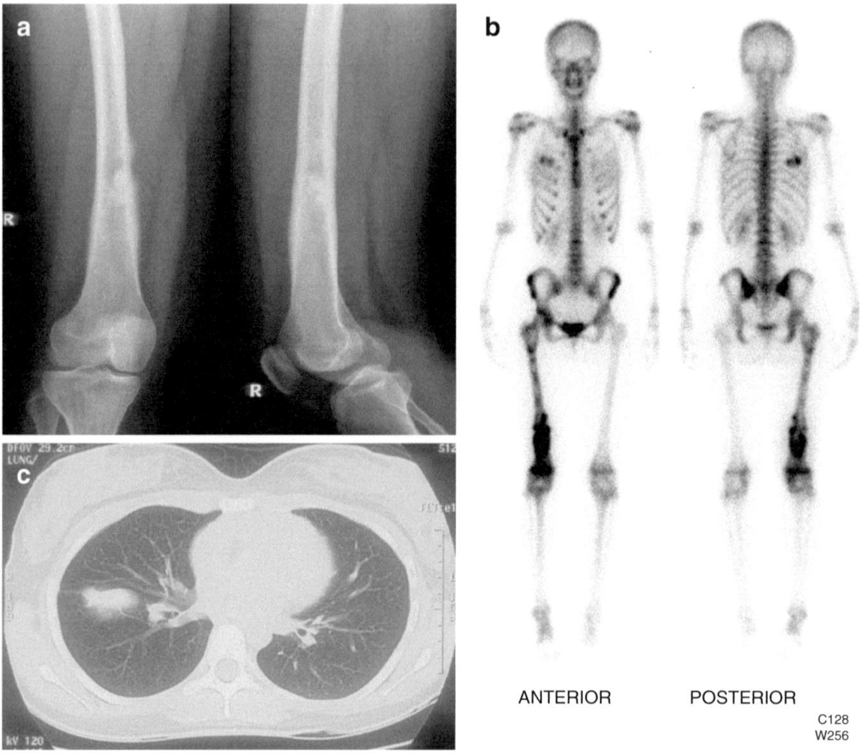

Fig. 4.1 (**a**) Plain X-ray demonstrating changes typical of osteogenic sarcoma of the right femur. (**b**) Delayed whole bone scan showing the tumour extending to involve the proximal right femur with uptake involving the right chest consistent with an osteogenic metastasis. (**c**) Axial CT slice of the chest confirming intra-parenchymal lung metastasis

Whilst highly sensitive, Tc-99m MDP suffers from very low specificity—less than 10% for the presence of malignant osteoid—and therefore will show increased accumulation in benign bone lesions and processes demonstrating increased bone turnover. These include osteoid osteoma, benign chondroid lesions and metabolic and degenerative conditions emphasising the need for correlation with structural imaging techniques including plain X-rays, CT and MRI.

Bone scintigraphy demonstrates reduced sensitivity in the detection of purely lytic lesions particularly in multiple myeloma though such destructive lesions may show increased marginal activity at the tumour/tissue interface (Fig. 4.2a–d).

4.2 Metabolic Imaging

4.2.1 Thallium-201 Scintigraphy

Tl-201 is a monovalent potassium analogue which is actively transported into tumour cells via the Na/K ATPase pump. Musculoskeletal tumours generally accumulate TL-201 according to their tumour grade and perfusion [3]. Thus the use of

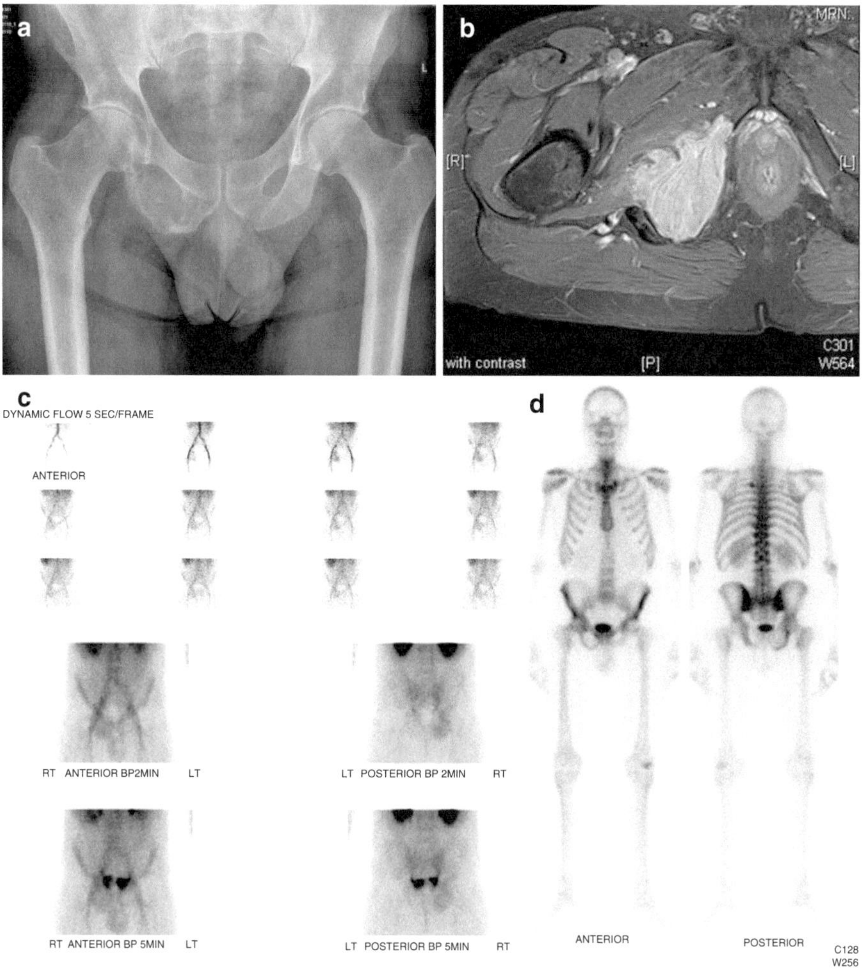

Fig. 4.2 (**a**) Middle aged patient with an expansile lytic lesion involving the right inferior pubic ramus and ischium. (**b**) Axial contrast-enhanced T1 MRI image showing marked enhanced and loss of the cortical margins in keeping with an aggressive lesion. (**c**) Immediate limited dynamic and blood pool images following injection of Tc-99m MDP showing increased vascularity and blood pool activity of the lesion. (**d**) Delayed whole-body views demonstrate only very subtle asymmetry of the right inferior pubic ramus and ischium typical of multiple myeloma. Focal uptake involving the posterior left fifth rib corresponds to a fracture

thallium scintigraphy in helping to differentiate benign from malignant lesions particularly where structural imaging maybe indeterminate can be very useful (Fig. 4.3a–e) [4].

Early and delayed planar images are obtained with delayed SPECT/CT images acquired of the tumour. The early images reflect tumour/lesion vascularity, and delayed images show tumour grade and viability depending on the amount of tracer retention and or washout of tracer (Fig. 4.4a–e). Caluser and colleagues in a study of 37 patients with sarcoma showed that when the lesion to normal tissue ratio of Tl

201 of the blood pool images exceeded lesion to normal tissue in the early blood pool images of a bone scan, this was 100% specific for sarcoma [5].

However it should be noted that TL-201 scans maybe positive in a number of histologically proven benign lesions particularly PVNS, fibromatosis and desmoid tumours, giant cell tumour of bone and granulomatous disease such as sarcoidosis and tuberculosis (Fig. 4.5a–c). Conversely false-negative scans maybe seen in predominately myxoid malignant lesions (Fig. 4.6a–e).

Other applications include identifying the most metabolically active part of the tumour prior to image-guided biopsy and assessing post-treatment responses. Sarcomas by their nature tend to demonstrate significant cellular heterogeneity with varied areas of viable tumour and necrosis. Delayed SPECT/CT images can precisely identify the most metabolically active parts of the tumour to give the correct histologic grade and show the areas of necrosis or cystic change which need to be avoided. The CT-guided biopsy images can be referenced directly to the SPECT/CT to ensure adequate and representative tissue samples to most accurately diagnose and grade the tumour [6].

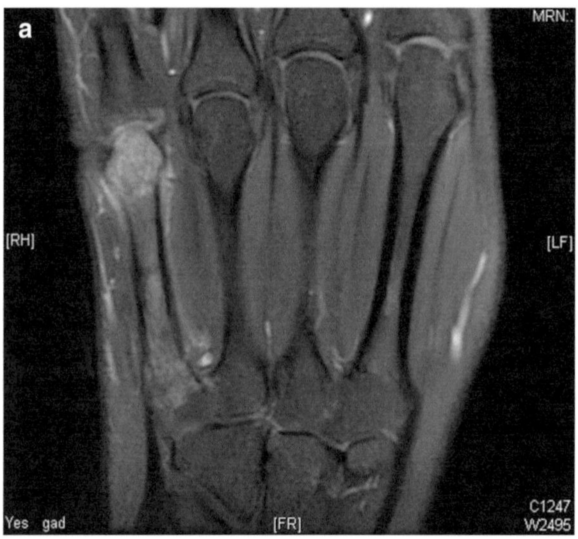

Fig. 4.3 (**a**) Post-contrast T1 coronal view of the left fifth metacarpal of an 18-year-old female showing enhancement of the bone and peri-lesional oedema thought to be most consistent with osteoblastoma on subsequent percutaneous biopsy. (**b**) Early planar Tl-201 images at 30 min showing intense uptake within the left fifth metacarpal. (**c**) Delayed planar Tl-201 images at 4 h show washout of tracer but with some persistent retention indicative of a vascular lesion. (**d**) Early planar Tl-201 images acquired 11 months later due to increasing clinical symptoms despite previous resection showing intense early uptake of tracer. (**e**) Delayed 4-h images demonstrating much more retention and activity compared to the scan 11 months previously in keeping with a high-grade histology. Repeat biopsy demonstrated osteogenic sarcoma

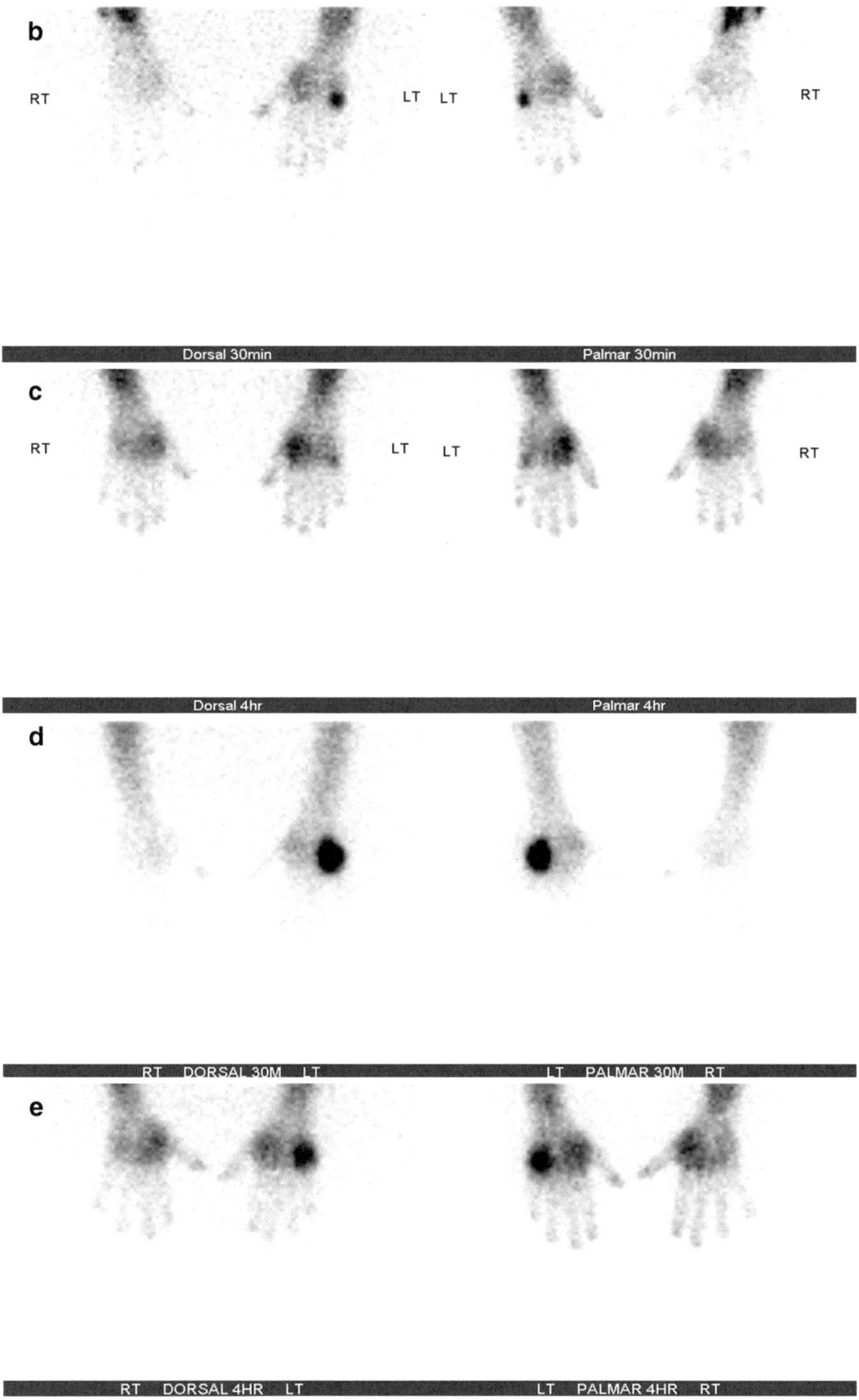

Fig. 4.3 (continued)

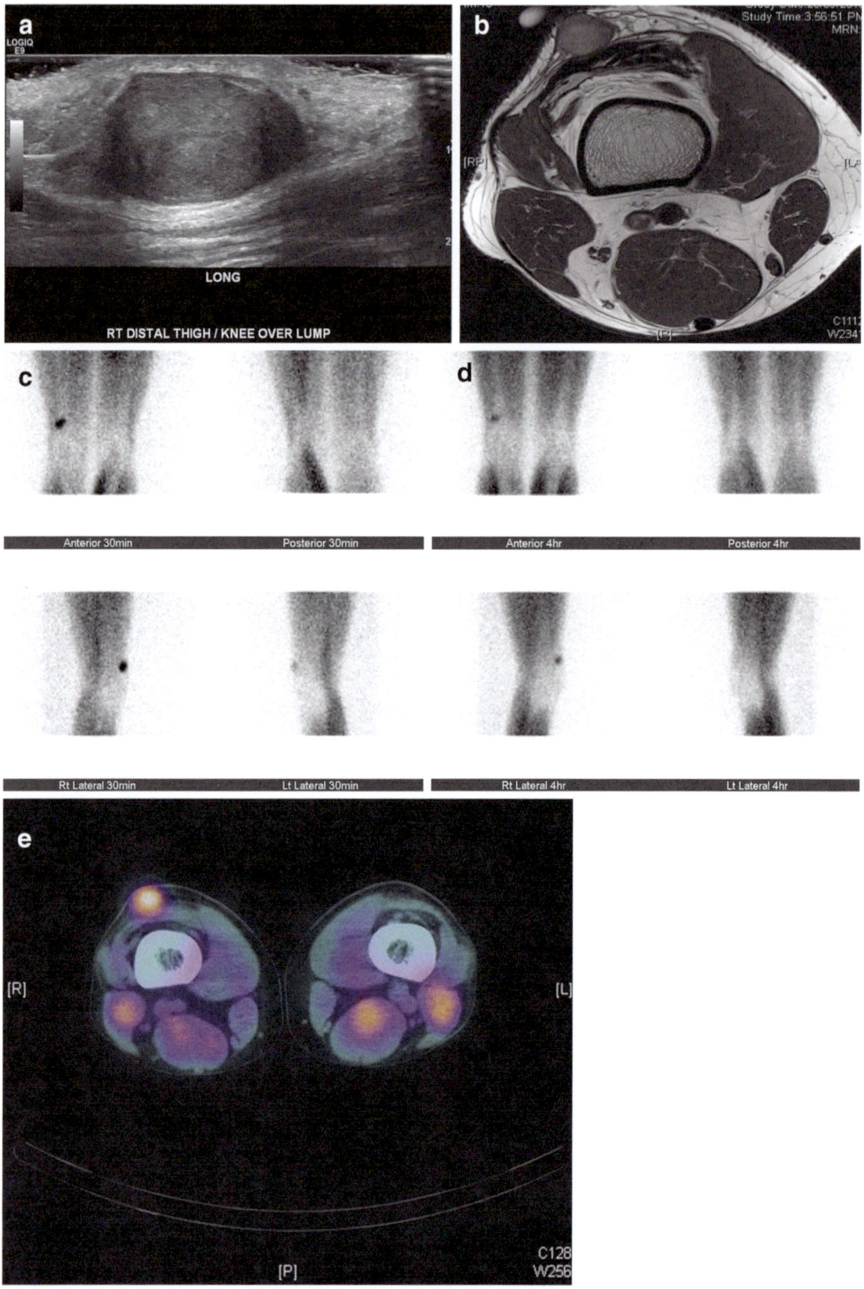

Fig. 4.4 (**a**) A 31-year-old male with a subcutaneous mass involving the right distal thigh thought on ultrasound to represent a lipoma. (**b**) T1-weighted axial MRI image confirms a solid subcutaneous mass but not following fat signal. (**c**) Early planar Tl-201 images showing intense early uptake (30 min). (**d**) Delayed planar Tl-201 images (4 h) demonstrate overall retention of activity consistent with a high-grade histology. (**e**) Delayed SPECT/CT Tl-201 image confirming uniform retention of tracer within the lesion confirmed to be high-grade pleomorphic sarcoma on percutaneous biopsy

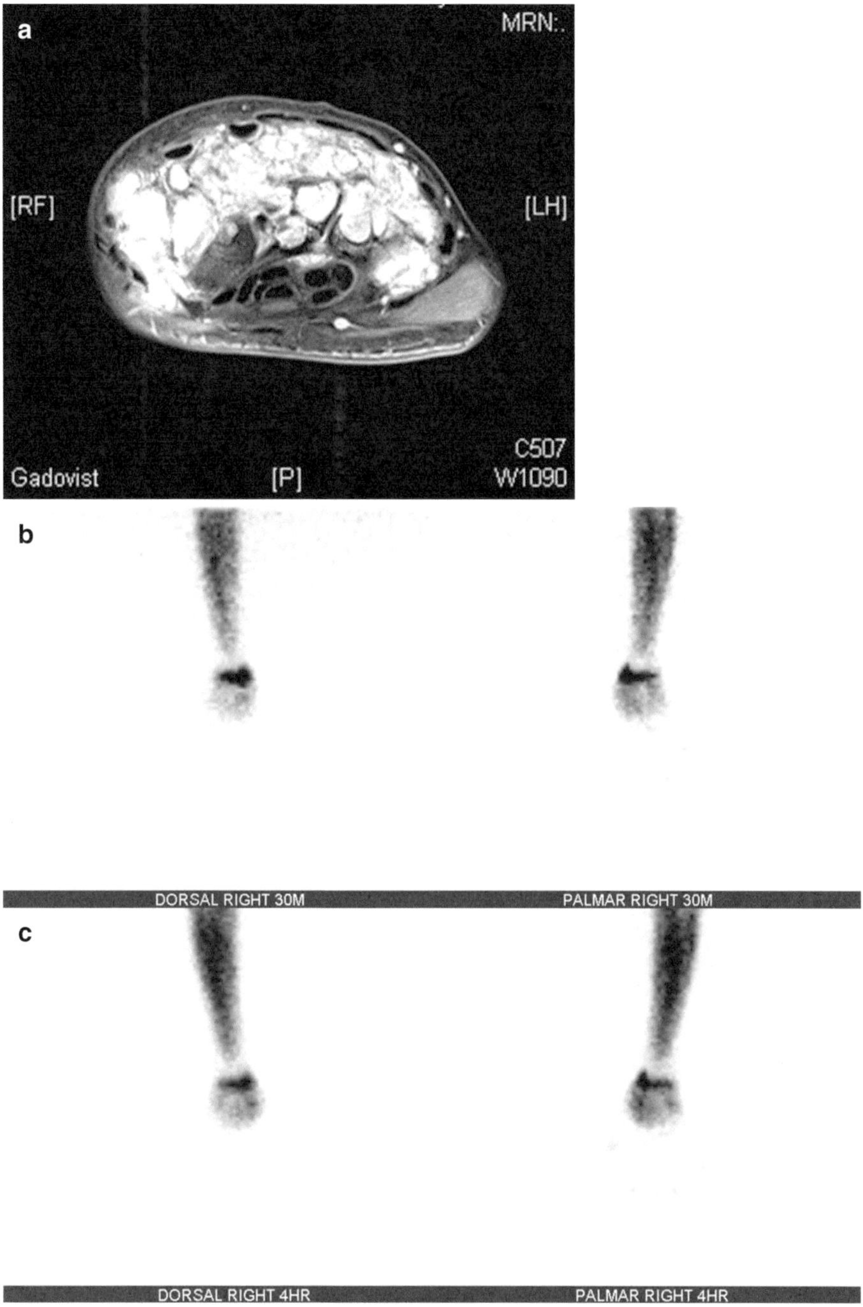

Fig. 4.5 (**a**) A 26-year-old female presenting with a diffuse soft tissue mass in the dorsal aspect of the right wrist, post-contrast T1-weighted axial image of the wrist demonstrates a diffusely enhancing mass with erosion of the underlying carpal bones. (**b**) Early planar Tl-201 images (30 min) show intense tracer uptake corresponding to the MRI mass. (**c**) Delayed Tl-201 images (4 h) demonstrate overall retention of tracer. Biopsy showed Pigmented villonodular synovitis—PVNS

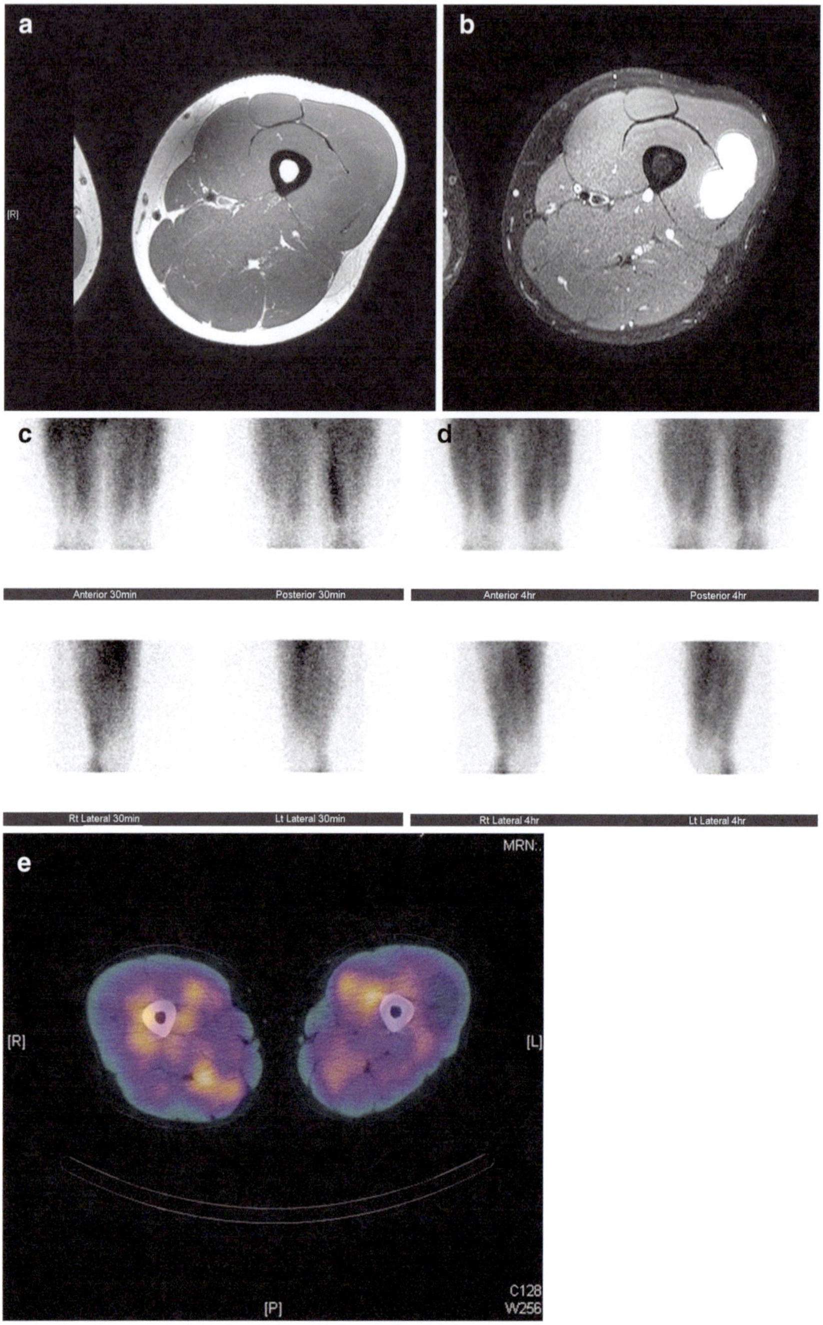

Fig. 4.6 (**a**) A 26-year-old male presents with a painless mass involving the lateral aspect of the left thigh. MRI T1 axial image demonstrates an isointense mass in the left vastus lateralis. (**b**) T2-weighted image shows high signal within the mass consistent with a myxoid lesion. (**c**) Early (30 min) and (**d**) delayed (4 h) planar Tl-201 images showing no appreciable uptake within the mass. (**e**) Delayed SPECT/CT Tl-201 axial image confirming the lesion appears photopaenic with no appreciable retention of tracer. Percutaneous biopsy demonstrated myxoid liposarcoma

4.2.2 Tc-99m Pentavalent Dimercaptosuccinic Acid (DMSA(V))

DMSA(V) mimics phosphate and accumulates in a range of neoplastic cells via hydrolysis [7]. It has been shown to concentrate in a variety of malignancies including thyroid and breast as well as bone tumours [8].

Chondrosarcoma is the second most common primary bone malignancy after osteosarcoma and constitutes approximately 25% of all primary bone tumours [9, 10]. Whilst high-grade lesions are usually apparent on structural imaging characterised by extensive bone destruction and extraosseous soft tissue, the distinction between lower-grade 1 and 2 chondrosarcoma and enchondroma can be difficult and problematic. Furthermore making the distinction even on histology may not be possible due to the relative paucity of malignant cells relative to the larger chondroid matrix in the lower-grade lesions [1].

Our experience has demonstrated a combination of Tc-99m DMSA(V) and Tl-201 to be the most useful functional imaging paradigm in assessing cartilage lesions. High-grade lesions typically demonstrate both Tl-201 and DMSA(V) uptake; low to intermediate lesions increased uptake of DMSA(V) only [1, 11]. Absence of DMSA(V) activity has been shown to have a negative predictive value of 100% such that a negative test effectively rules out chondrosarcoma (Fig. 4.7a–d) [6, 8].

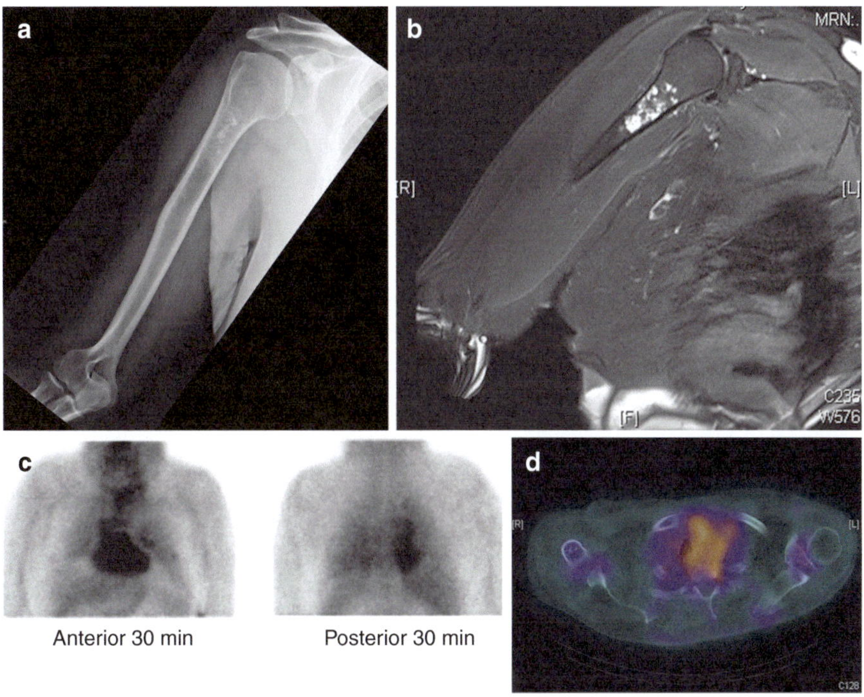

Fig. 4.7 (**a**) A 71-year-old male with right shoulder pain, plain X-ray demonstrating typical chondroid-type calcification involving the proximal right humerus. (**b**) T2 coronal MRI showing high signal consistent with cartilage. (**c**) Planar DMSA(V) images show no tracer uptake in the right humeral lesion. (**d**) SPECT/CT DMSA(V) image confirms no tracer activity within the lesion consistent with a benign enchondroma

4.2.3 18FDG PET/CT

18FDG acts as a glucose analogue with the degree of uptake increasing according to tumour grade relative to normal tissues. Thus the glycolytic activity of higher-grade tumours is greater than benign or low-grade lesions which can be quantified by the application of standardized uptake values (SUVs). Generally there is strong correlation between the SUVs and the pathological grade of the tumour reflecting cell mitotic activity and p53 overexpression [12]. This has led to the application of PET/CT in the application for use in initial diagnosis and biopsy planning, grading, staging and assessment of treatment response (Fig. 4.8a–d).

With the increasing emphasis on more tailored and targeted tumour-specific therapies, the unique metabolic information that molecular techniques such as PET/CT provide are becoming more important.

4.2.3.1 Initial Diagnosis

Whilst the sensitivity of PET/CT for detecting malignant lesions is high, PET/CT's principal utility in initial diagnosis is in the assessment of structurally indeterminate masses as most malignant tumour histology will demonstrate FDG uptake and accumulation [13]. Ioannidis and Lau showed using a SUV cut-off of 2, the sensitivity and specificity for the diagnosis of malignant soft tissue using 18FDG were 87% and 79% sensitivity and specificity, respectively [13]. The fact however that a number of benign lesions in particular PVNS, fibrous lesions and primary bone tumours such as giant cell tumour of the bone and fibrous dysplasia are FDG avid reduces its specificity and clinical utility even when the SUV is high (Fig. 4.9a–d) [14]. Similarly infective conditions particularly granulomatous may show high tracer uptake requiring careful correlation with structural imaging and multidisciplinary discussion to reach the correct diagnosis (Fig. 4.10a–d).

Like Tl-201 SPECT/CT, PET/CT is very useful in biopsy guidance allowing the most metabolically active portions of often large and structurally heterogeneous lesions to be appropriately targeted and sampled. The highly heterogeneous histologic grades seen particularly in the soft tissue sarcomas are directly reflected in the 18FDG spatial uptake distribution making it an ideal road map for biopsy planning and approach. The acquisition of whole-body views potentially provides the added evidence of coexistent metastatic disease determining prognosis and management decisions [14].

4.2.3.2 Staging and Restaging

PET/CT is complimentary to the conventional structural modalities of whole-body CT and MRI. It has been shown to be more accurate in the detection of distant bone metastases than bone scintigraphy in Ewing's sarcoma but less somewhat surprisingly in cases of metastatic osteosarcoma [15]. PET/CT has been shown to be more accurate in the detection of PET-avid distant soft tissue metastases than the conventional techniques of CT and MRI—in a study of 46 patients with diagnoses of Ewing's sarcoma, osteosarcoma and rhabdomyosarcoma, PET/CT was superior for

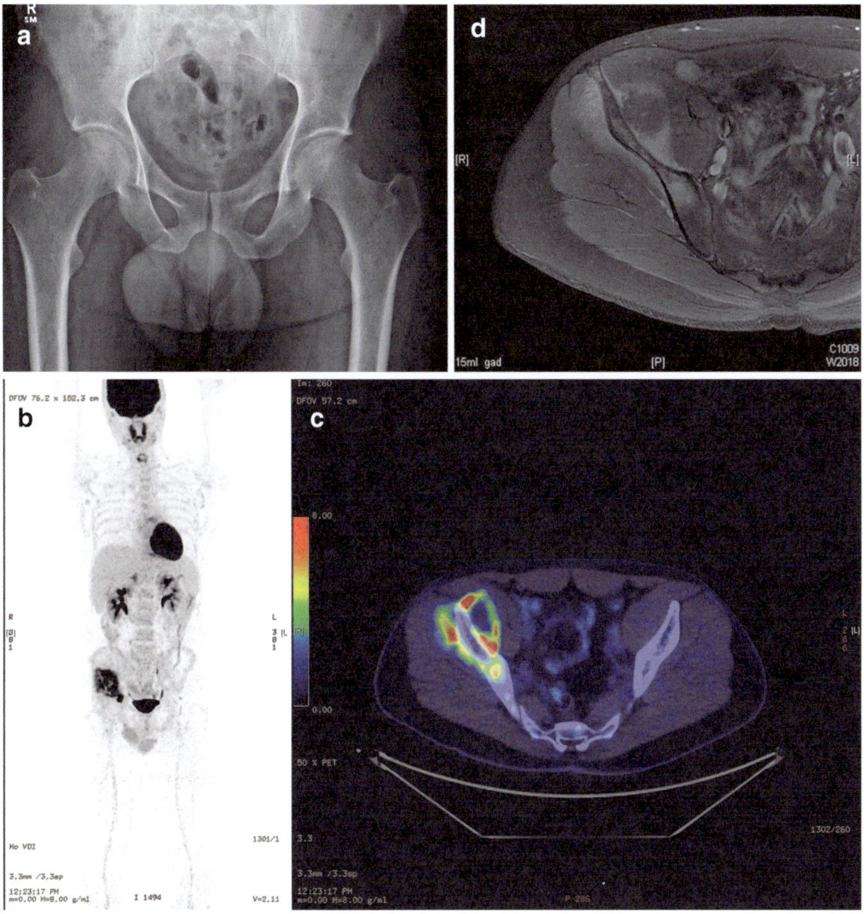

Fig. 4.8 (**a**) A 29-year-old male presents with right-sided pelvic and hip pain. X-ray initially reported as normal but demonstrates on review very subtle sclerosis involving the right iliac wing. (**b**) F18-FDG PET/CT whole-body MIP image demonstrates irregularly increased uptake involving the right hemi-pelvis and acetabulum. (**c**) F18-FDG axial fused images showing marginal activity within a soft tissue mass medial to the bony ileum consistent with viable active tumour and central photopaenia indicating tissue necrosis. Further viable tumour lies adjacent and lateral to the ileum. CT-guided biopsy targeting the areas of tracer uptake showed grade 3 chondrosarcoma. (**d**) Contrast-enhanced T1 MRI demonstrates areas of enhancement directly correspond to the areas of F18-FDG activity

detection of nodal disease, 95% versus 25% sensitivity and 90% versus 57% sensitivity for distant metastatic disease (Fig. 4.11a–c) [16].

PET/CT however is less sensitive for the detection of lung metastatic disease than conventional CT chest particularly for lesions less than 10 mm. However it may aid in helping to determine the nature of larger incidental lung nodules which do not demonstrate tracer uptake in the context of PET-avid disease elsewhere.

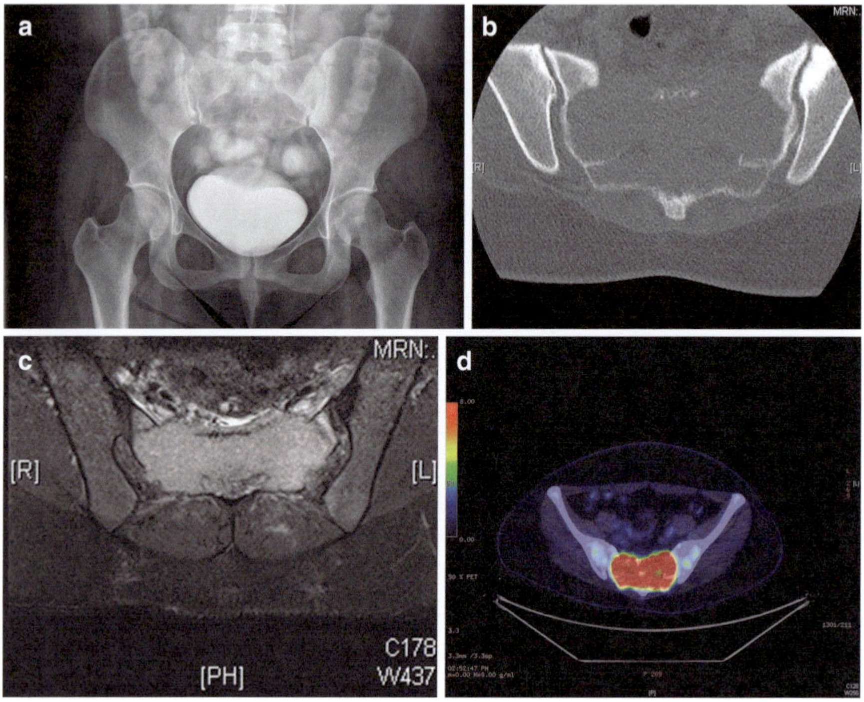

Fig. 4.9 (**a**) A 31-year-old female presents with lower back pain and paraesthesia with plain X-ray showing loss of cortical definition of the left sacral foramina and lucency. (**b**) Axial bone targeted CT image shows large soft tissue mass involving the sacrum with bony destruction consistent with an aggressive process. (**c**) T2 fat-saturated MRI axial image confirming the soft tissue mass without crossing the sacroiliac joints. (**d**) Corresponding F18-FDG fused axial image showing marked tracer uptake. Subsequent percutaneous CT-guided biopsy demonstrated giant cell tumour of the bone

A number of patients will develop local or distant recurrence following definitive initial treatment and management, and PET/CT plays an important role in the follow-up of these patients. Structural changes including fibrosis following radiotherapy and surgery and the presence of metal prostheses make interpretation of conventional imaging techniques difficult and frequently delay the diagnosis of recurrent disease. Multiple studies, including Johnson et al. who showed PET/CT detected all recurrences in 25 patients compared to CT and MRI alone, have demonstrated the high accuracy of PET/CT in detecting recurrent disease [17].

4.2.3.3 Response to Treatment/Prognosis

Studies have shown that PET/CT has a potential role in assessing tumour response to neoadjuvant chemotherapy regimens. Schulte et al. showed a direct correlation between glucose metabolism uptake and tumour regression on histology

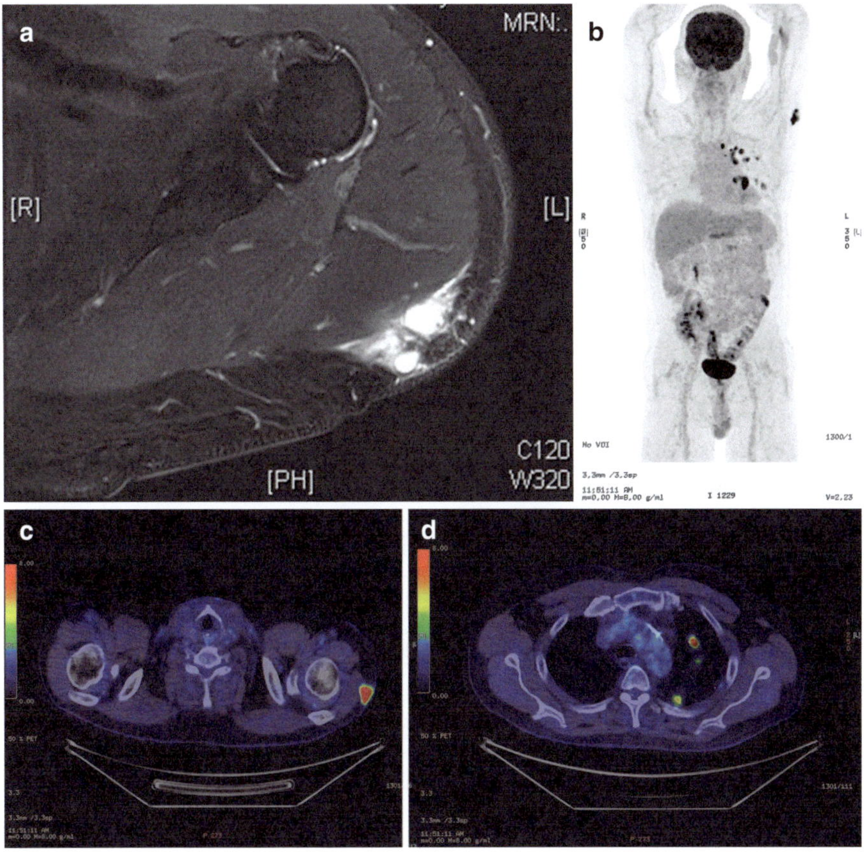

Fig. 4.10 (**a**) A 62-year-old Vietnamese male presented with a firm subcutaneous lump over the posterior aspect of the left shoulder. T2-weighted fat-saturated image shows an ill-defined solid subcutaneous mass ? soft tissue sarcoma. (**b**) F18-FDG MIP image demonstrates that the left shoulder mass is tracer avid with a number of PET-avid masses within the left lung raising the possibility of associated metastatic disease. (**c**) Fused axial PET/CT images confirming the index mass is metabolically active. (**d**) PET-positive lung parenchymal masses. Percutaneous biopsy of the left shoulder mass demonstrated *Cryptococcus neoformans* with the cavitating lung lesions consistent with associated lung parenchymal involvement

following therapy in patient with osteosarcoma [18]. Similarly, initial SUV max of the tumour in synovial sarcoma has been correlated with prognosis [19]. Eary et al. [20] have demonstrated that spatial heterogeneity as demonstrated by 18FDG uptake is independently predictive of patient outcome. Furthermore multiple groups have used tumour SUV to monitor treatment response with a 35% reduction in FDG uptake in the post-treatment scan compared to baseline predictive of histologic response [21–23].

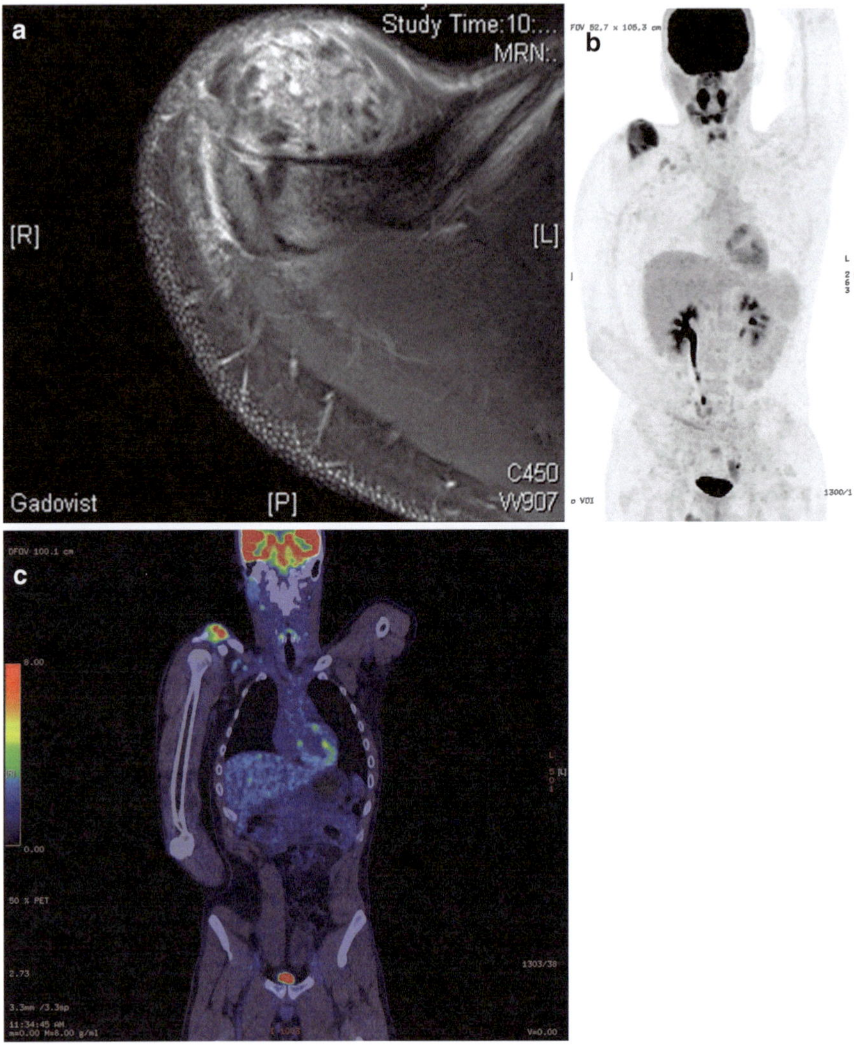

Fig. 4.11 (**a**) A 21-year-old male presents with a painless right shoulder mass. Axial contrast-enhanced T1-weighted MRI image shows a heterogeneously enhancing soft tissue mass. (**b**) F18-FDG MIP image shows irregular but marked tracer uptake within the mass with further focal fainter uptake within the right axilla. (**c**) Coronal fused PET/CT image confirming uptake in the right shoulder lesion with further activity seen in multiple axillary lymph nodes. Percutaneous biopsy of the right shoulder and lymph nodes demonstrated malignant epithelioid tumour with lymph node metastases

4.3 Conclusion

Functional imaging techniques provide unique metabolic information regarding bone and soft tissue tumours. Co-registering the information from conventional nuclear medicine and metabolic techniques with high-quality structural images further significantly contributes to the information and insights provided by the modalities individually. Such techniques can be utilised in the initial diagnosis, staging and monitoring of treatment response in this diverse and challenging group of tumours.

References

1. Hicks RJ. Functional imaging techniques for evaluation of sarcomas. Cancer Imaging. 2005;5:58–65.
2. Pevarski DJ, Drane WE, Scarborough MT. The usefulness of bone scintigraphy with SPECT images for detection of pulmonary metastases from osteosarcoma. AJR Am J Roentgenol. 1998;170:319–22.
3. Hicks RJ. Nuclear medicine techniques provide unique physiologic characterization of suspected and known soft tissue and bone sarcomas. Acta Orthop Scand Suppl. 1997;273:25–36.
4. Sugawara Y, Kikuchi T, Kajihara M, Semba T, Ochi T, Fujii T, Mochizuki T, Sakayama K, Nakata S. Thallium-201 scintigraphy in bone and soft-tissue tumors: a comparison of dynamic, early and delayed scans. Ann Nucl Med. 2005;19:461–8.
5. Caluser CI, Abdel-Dayem HM, Macapinlac HA, Scott A, Healey JH, Huvos A, Kalaigian H, Yeh SD, Larson SM. The value of thallium and three-phase bone scans in the evaluation of bone and soft tissue sarcomas. Eur J Nucl Med. 1994;21:1198–205.
6. Choong PF, Kunisada T, Slavin J, Schlicht S, Hicks R. The role of thallium-201 and pentavalent dimercaptosuccinic acid for staging cartilaginous tumours. Int Semin Surg Oncol. 2004;1:10.
7. Yokoyama A, Hata N, Horiuchi K, Masuda H, Saji H, Ohta H, Yamamoto K, Endo K, Torizuka K. The design of a pentavalent 99mTc-dimercaptosuccinate complex as a tumor imaging agent. Int J Nucl Med Biol. 1985;12:273–9.
8. Shinya T, Sato S, Kunisada T, Inai R, Yanai H, Ozaki T, Kanazawa S. Both a visual and a semiquantitative analysis for differentiating benign from malignant chondrogenic bone tumors using Tc-99m (V) DMSA scintigraphy: a prospective study. Nucl Med Commun. 2015;36:802–7.
9. Leddy LR, Holmes RE. Chondrosarcoma of bone. Cancer Treat Res. 2014;162:117–30.
10. Murphey MD, Walker EA, Wilson AJ, Kransdorf MJ, Temple HT, Gannon FH. From the archives of the AFIP: imaging of primary chondrosarcoma: radiologic-pathologic correlation. Radiographics. 2003;23:1245–78.
11. Kobayashi H, Kotoura Y, Hosono M, Sakahara H, Hosono M, Yao ZS, Tsuboyama T, Yamamuro T, Endo K, Konishi J. Diagnostic value of Tc-99m (V) DMSA for chondrogenic tumors with positive Tc-99m HMDP uptake on bone scintigraphy. Clin Nucl Med. 1995;20:361–4.
12. Folpe AL, Lyles RH, Sprouse JT, Conrad EU 3rd, Eary JF. (F-18) fluorodeoxyglucose positron emission tomography as a predictor of pathologic grade and other prognostic variables in bone and soft tissue sarcoma. Clin Cancer Res. 2000;6:1279–87.
13. Ioannidis JP, Lau J. 18F-FDG PET for the diagnosis and grading of soft-tissue sarcoma: a meta-analysis. J Nucl Med. 2003;44:717–24.
14. Toner GC, Hicks RJ. PET for sarcomas other than gastrointestinal stromal tumors. Oncologist. 2008;13(Suppl 2):22–6.
15. Franzius C, Sciuk J, Daldrup-Link HE, Jurgens H, Schober O. FDG-PET for detection of osseous metastases from malignant primary bone tumours: comparison with bone scintigraphy. Eur J Nucl Med. 2000;27:1305–11.
16. Volker T, Denecke T, Steffen I, Misch D, Schonberger S, Plotkin M, Ruf J, Furth C, Stover B, Hautzel H, Henze G, Amthauer H. Positron emission tomography for staging of pediatric sarcoma patients: results of a prospective multicenter trial. J Clin Oncol. 2007;25:5435–41.
17. Johnson GR, Zhuang H, Khan J, Chiang SB, Alavi A. Roles of positron emission tomography with fluorine-18-deoxyglucose in the detection of local recurrent and distant metastatic sarcoma. Clin Nucl Med. 2003;28:815–20.

18. Schulte M, Brecht-Krauss D, Werner M, Hartwig E, Sarkar MR, Keppler P, Kotzerke J, Guhlmann A, Delling G, Reske SN. Evaluation of neoadjuvant therapy response of osteogenic sarcoma using FDG PET. J Nucl Med. 1999;40:1637–43.
19. Lisle JW, Eary JF, O'Sullivan J, Conrad EU. Risk assessment based on FDG-PET imaging in patients with synovial sarcoma. Clin Orthop Relat Res. 2009;467:1605–11.
20. Eary JF, O'Sullivan F, O'Sullivan J, Conrad EU. Spatial heterogeneity in sarcoma 18F-FDG uptake as a predictor of patient outcome. J Nucl Med. 2008;49:1973–9.
21. Benz MR, Czernin J, Allen-Auerbach MS, Tap WD, Dry SM, Elashoff D, Chow K, Evilevitch V, Eckardt JJ, Phelps ME, Weber WA, Eilber FC. FDG-PET/CT imaging predicts histopathologic treatment responses after the initial cycle of neoadjuvant chemotherapy in high-grade soft-tissue sarcomas. Clin Cancer Res. 2009;15:2856–63.
22. Evilevitch V, Weber WA, Tap WD, Allen-Auerbach M, Chow K, Nelson SD, Eilber FR, Eckardt JJ, Elashoff RM, Phelps ME, Czernin J, Eilber FC. Reduction of glucose metabolic activity is more accurate than change in size at predicting histopathologic response to neoadjuvant therapy in high-grade soft-tissue sarcomas. Clin Cancer Res. 2008;14:715–20.
23. Schuetze SM, Baker LH, Benjamin RS, Canetta R. Selection of response criteria for clinical trials of sarcoma treatment. Oncologist. 2008;13(Suppl 2):32–40.

Biopsy

5

Peter F. M. Choong

5.1 Background

In his treatise on bone sarcomas [1], Ewing stated that "Abundant clinical material, wide clinical experience, and knowledge of the embryology, physiology and pathology of bone, are the more essential qualifications for successful investigation in this field". His comments highlighted the core principle today that for a rare tumour such as sarcoma, the best efforts come from where clinical material, knowledge and experience are the greatest, namely, tumour centres. Moreover, he believed strongly that surgeon, radiologist and pathologist (and later radiation oncologist) needed to work strongly together for success in this endeavour. Ewing went on to propose a novel concept for its day that a tumour could be defined not only by its microscopic appearance but also its responsiveness to treatment [2]. In all, Ewing was a man ahead of his time who highlighted the importance of the diagnosis in good treatment of sarcoma.

Diagnosing a sarcoma is critical for its effective and successful treatment. Inadvertent excision following poor knowledge of the sarcoma behaviour, erroneous assumptions based on clinical findings alone, the absence of good anatomic imaging or lack of appreciation for a poor correlation between anatomic and histologic findings often leads to sub-optimal patient outcomes such as more complex re-excisional surgery including amputation, a higher local recurrence rate, the potential for greater metastatic events and a higher risk of death from disease [3].

Safe, representative and appropriate biopsy is required for the diagnosis of sarcoma. Safety is a key issue because inappropriate biopsy may lead to post-biopsy

P. F. M. Choong (✉)
Department of Surgery, University of Melbourne, Melbourne, VIC, Australia

Department of Orthopaedics, St. Vincent's Hospital Melbourne, Melbourne, VIC, Australia

Bone and Soft Tissue Tumour Service, Peter MacCallum Cancer Centre, Melbourne, VIC, Australia
e-mail: pchoong@unimelb.edu.au

P. F. M. Choong (ed.), *Sarcoma*, https://doi.org/10.1007/978-981-15-9414-4_5

bleeding with the carriage of sarcoma cells by haematoma beyond the original confines of the tumour. Inexpert surgery may lead to the opening of tissue planes permitting further contamination of otherwise virgin tissue whose inclusion within the subsequent definitive operative field may result in extensive surgery. This latter event creates an even greater dilemma if contaminated haematoma involves vital anatomic structures such as nerves, vessels and joints for which sacrifice may result in significant functional consequences such as altered limb function or even amputation [4].

Representative tissue is critical for an accurate diagnosis [5, 6]. Ensuring that the target for biopsy (bone and soft tissue) will have the highest chance of delivering representative tissue is a major requirement of the treating team. To achieve this, adequate and meaningful imaging is required prior to biopsy. Such imaging including anatomic (X-rays, computed tomography, magnetic resonance imaging) and functional (nuclear bone scans, thallium scans and positron emission tomography) scans allow for the most metabolically active tissue to be identified and the most highly necrotic areas to be avoided (Fig. 5.1). Targeting of specific areas for

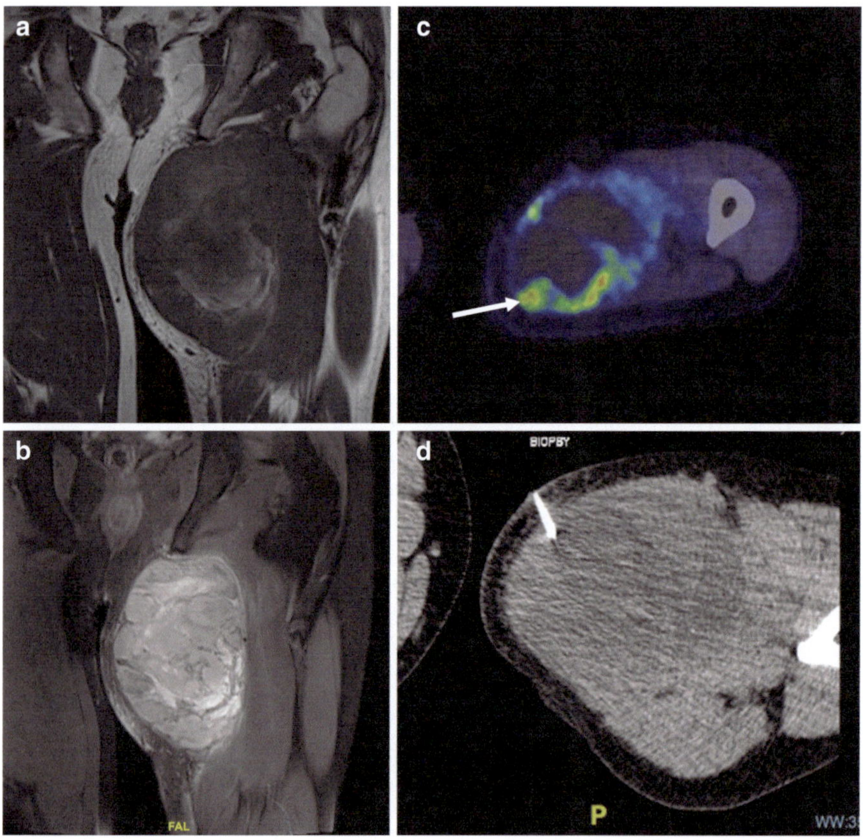

Fig. 5.1 (**a**) T1 coronal view of large adductor sarcoma. (**b**) Fat saturation proton density coronal image of large adductor sarcoma. (**c**) PET image of adductor sarcoma demonstrating central necrosis with focal activity along the periphery of the tumour. Metabolically active tumour targeted for biopsy (white arrow). (**d**) CT-guided biopsy of targeted tumour with high metabolic activity and avoiding area of central necrosis

needle biopsy is best achieved with CT guidance [7, 8], and a snapshot of the needle in situ not only assists the surgeon in locating the biopsy site and planning the surgical approach but also for allowing discussion regarding representativeness of the biopsy should a discrepancy between histological and anatomic findings emerge.

Appropriate biopsy refers to the optimal location of the biopsy entry site [9]. There is genuine concern about the nature of seeding along the biopsy tract which has opened up the debate of open versus percutaneous biopsy [10]. This is of importance when planning the surgical approach, as well as when attempting to avoid contaminating important neurovascular and articular structures. Biopsy tracts are conventionally placed along incisions lines taken to approach the tumour such that the biopsy tract may be included in the resection margin (Fig. 5.2). In one study of 180 patients comparing open versus percutaneous biopsy, 32% of open and 0.8% of percutaneous biopsies were associated with biopsy track seeding [11]. Although open biopsy may allow access to larger tissue samples, the tissue that is only accessible is directly below the incision to avoid unnecessary dissection of the tumour. In this regard, the tissue directly below the incision has to contain representative tissue if it is to be a meaningful biopsy. Guided core needle biopsy, however, allows tissue to be accessed at a distance from the puncture site in multiple directions from a single puncture point (Fig. 5.3). This applies for both bone and soft tissue tumours [5, 6, 12, 13]. It is thought that the co-axial nature of needle biopsy may also help to minimise the degree of track seeding.

5.2 Who Should Have a Biopsy?

Anyone with a radiographic abnormality of bone, with persistent pain that is not responsive to simple analgesics and which is worse at night, should be suspected of having a possible malignant bone tumour. Anyone with a lump engaging the deep

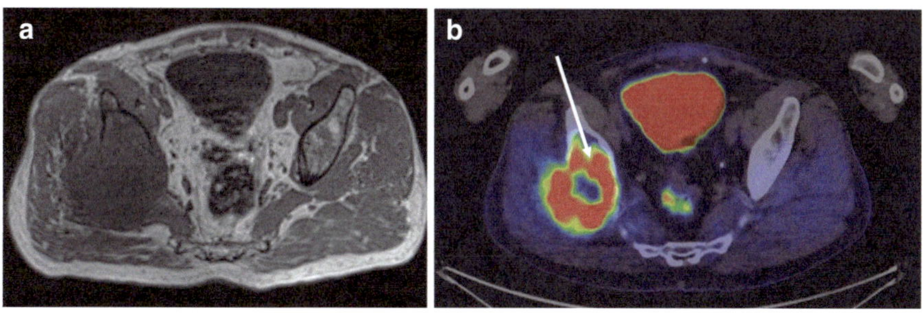

Fig. 5.2 (**a**) MR image demonstrating large periacetabular osteosarcoma. Biopsy through the buttock will potentially endanger the gluteal flap. (**b**) PET scan demonstrating hypermetabolic lesion with central necrosis. Arrow indicates that a CT-guided transosseous biopsy through the anterior inferior iliac spine will be able to target metabolically active tissue; avoid the area of central necrosis and remain in line with a standard ilio-femoral incision

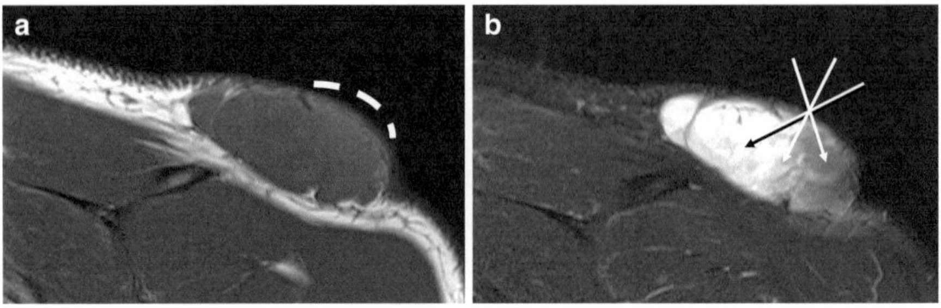

Fig. 5.3 (**a**) T1 MRI demonstrating large subcutaneous sarcoma. In order to minimise dissection, open biopsy can only sample tissue directly beneath the skin incision (dashed line). (**b**) T2 fat-saturated MRI demonstrating heterogeneous signal within subcutaneous sarcoma. Through a single entry point on the surface, multiple core needle biopsies may be obtained to sample different regions of the sarcoma

fascia or deep to the deep fascia and greater than 5 cm in diameter should be suspected of having a soft tissue sarcoma until proven otherwise [14]. Except in rare circumstances, imaging modalities alone are not reliable when determining the histology of a bone or soft tissue abnormality. It is critical that patients presenting with the above symptoms and signs should be considered for biopsy. Decisions to recommend a biopsy should follow discussions with clinicians from a centre specialising in sarcoma care.

5.3 Where Should the Biopsy Be Undertaken?

Ideally, all biopsies should be undertaken at a centre specialising in sarcoma management. At these centres, there will be the resources to ensure that the tissue is handled appropriately and expeditiously between the time of biopsy and histological examination. Because of the multidisciplinary nature of sarcoma care, there will be a designated team of pathologists who are experts in analysing and interpreting the histological findings and who will be in close contact with the other members of the multidisciplinary team regarding the case. In certain circumstances, it may be practical that subcutaneous tumours or large sarcomas be subjected to biopsy outside of a tumour centre. In these circumstances, it is advisable that biopsy occur after discussion with experts from a centre specialising in sarcoma management.

5.4 What Investigations Should Be Undertaken Before Biopsy?

Biopsy will induce a tissue artefact through inflammation, bleeding, haematoma and oedema. Depending on the extent of the biopsy artefact, imaging studies may not be able to differentiate what is attributable to the tumour or biopsy. Such confounding may lead to over- or under-diagnosis of sarcoma. It is therefore preferable that all imaging studies (anatomic and functional) should be completed prior to biopsy. This is particularly important where MRI is concerned, as the sensitivity of MRI to detect inflammation or trauma leaves it vulnerable to post-traumatic artefact, making it difficult to interpret MRI findings after biopsy.

5.5 Who Should Perform the Biopsy?

Conventionally, open biopsies are best performed by surgeons who will be leading the definitive surgical management of the tumour. This is because decisions as to the site of the biopsy incision need to be made in the context of the potential approach to resecting the entire tumour with wide margins. Ideally, the biopsy track will be excised en bloc with the operative specimen. Sarcoma surgeons are best placed to decide the safest approach to tumour resection and hence the position of the biopsy incision.

Percutaneous core needle biopsies are usually performed by radiologists who are expert in this technique. Those with the greatest experience are usually associated with a tumour centre and are familiar with the requirements to mitigate inadvertent complications such as misplaced biopsy sites and sampling poorly representative areas. Radiologists who work in conjunction with a multidisciplinary sarcoma team will be familiar with the requirements and use of various pieces of equipment required for sampling of bone and soft tissue tumours.

5.6 Placement of the Biopsy Entry Site (Figs. 5.4, 5.5, and 5.6)

Key considerations

1. Avoid locations that may contaminate neurovascular structures. Sampling near a major neurovascular structure may accidentally lead to contamination of important nerves and vessels requiring subsequent resection. This may lead to loss of muscle function or viability of parts distal to the biopsy site. For example, biopsies through the flexor fossae; posterior and lateral aspects of the deltoid where the axillary nerve enters and courses through the muscle, respectively; the centre of the buttock muscle where the gluteal vessels enter; and the anterior abdominal wall should be avoided or, at least, require careful discussion and contemplation.
2. Avoid transgressing joint cavities. For example, sampling tumours around the anterior distal femur and thigh may inadvertently involve the suprapatellar pouch. Contamination of a joint cavity may require sacrifice of that joint as well as more complex extra-articular resections if the bone is the primary site. Biopsies in the forearm may involve the flexor bursae which span from the palm to the upper forearm, and haematoma within these bursae may cross-contaminate the hand and the forearm.

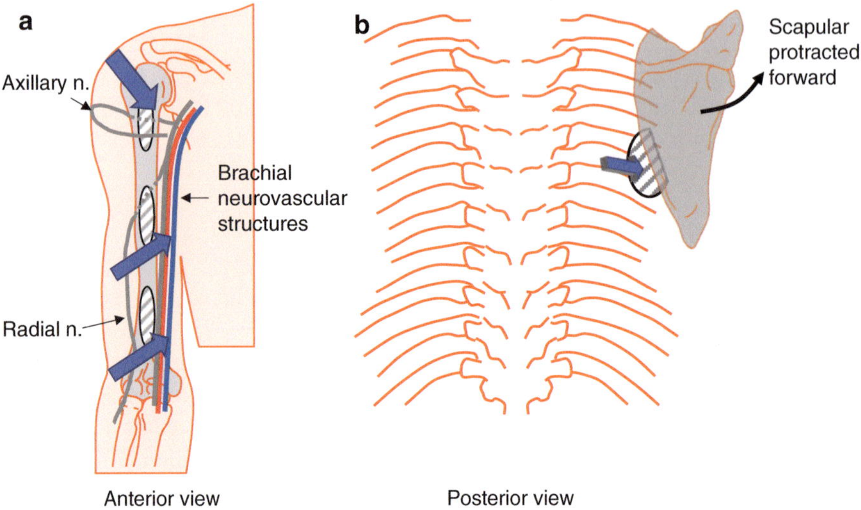

Fig. 5.4 Biopsy of tumours of the upper limb and shoulder girdle. (**a**) Tumours of the humerus should be approached from the front to avoid important neurovascular structures. As the axillary nerve enters the deltoid muscle from behind, it is safer to position proximal humeral biopsies from the front. Mid-shaft humeral biopsies may be approached from the front to avoid the radial nerve as it courses in the spiral groove. Anterior midline biopsy of distal humeral tumours can avoid the posterior interosseous nerve and the medial brachial neurovascular structures. (**b**) Protracting the scapular forwards will allow access to subscapular lesions

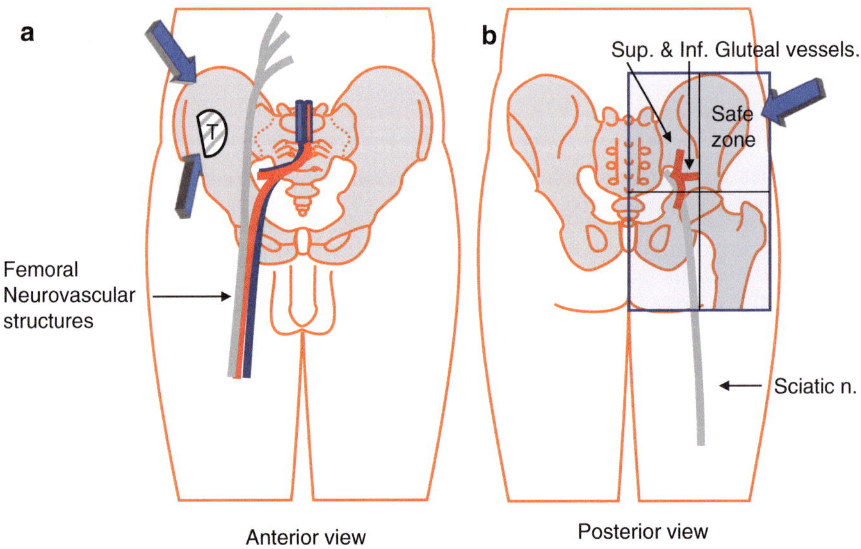

Fig. 5.5 (**a**) Tumours of the boney pelvis should be approached along the line of the iliac crest which conforms to the standard ilio-inguinal or ilio-femoral incision normally used in surgical approaches to pelvic tumours. (**b**) The buttock can be divided into quadrants. The upper inner quadrant contains the vessels to the gluteal flap, the lower inner quadrant contains the sciatic nerve, and the lower outer quadrant contains the hip joint. The upper outer quadrant is the safe zone. Positioning the biopsy is critical for avoiding these important structures

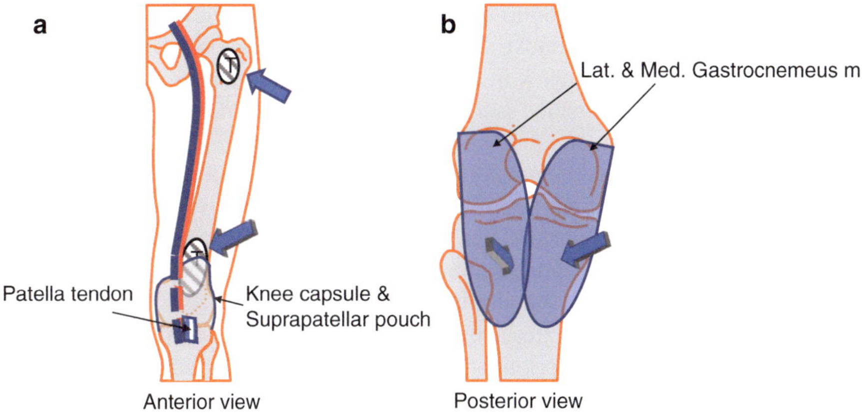

Fig. 5.6 (**a**) Biopsy of femoral lesions should be from a lateral approach to avoid the hip capsule and femoral neurovascular structures proximally and the knee joint and suprapatellar pouch distally. The patella tendon is vulnerable from anterior approaches, and the femoral vessels are vulnerable as they pass through the adductor hiatus medially. (**b**) Biopsy of proximal tibial tumours may occur through the gastrocnemii to avoid tumour spillage

3. Avoid areas which may inadvertently compromise muscle function. For example, laterally placed tumours of the deltoid will need biopsy from a more anterior direction to avoid involvement of the axillary nerve as it tracks forwards on the deep surface of the muscle.
4. Use single entry versus multiple biopsy sites.
5. Bone tumours are more challenging than soft tissue tumours to biopsy.
6. Some sites can be very difficult if not impossible to biopsy without great morbidity, e.g. inner wall of acetabulum, and diagnosis may be based on anatomic and radiologic characteristics as well as the behaviour of the tumour rather than on biopsy tissue.
7. Biopsy of very superficial tumours may result in ulceration and secondary infection.

5.7 Biopsy Technique

5.7.1 Open Biopsy

Open biopsy of a suspected sarcoma should be undertaken in centres expert in the management of sarcoma. In exceptional circumstances, biopsy may be undertaken after appropriate advice from experts at a tumour centre.

1. Tourniquet—If possible, a tourniquet should be used to minimise haematoma formation and to maintain a dry field for adequate visualisation of the biopsy site.
2. Selection of biopsy site—After thorough review of the anatomic and functional imaging, the biopsy site most likely to yield representative tissue is selected.
3. Special attention is paid to areas of necrosis, cyst formation or haemorrhage as these sites are unlikely to yield tumour tissue or the findings may be spurious.

4. Plan site of biopsy incision to coincide where possible with surgical incision that will be used for definitive resection. If biopsy incision cannot align with surgical incision, then have it in a position that can be included with the operative specimen without undue sacrifice of normal or important structures.
5. Direct incision down onto tumour. Ensure haemostasis on the way in. Achieve adequate exposure, but be careful not to damage or dissect side wall or create planes of dissection around the tumour. This is to minimise the operative footprint. Careful use of blunt self-retaining retractors will aid with exposure.
6. Sample tissue directly under the incision line. Do not dissect away from the incision line to minimise the surgical footprint.
7. Send tissue to pathology fresh for examination. Ideally, frozen section of the tissue should be obtained prior to closure to ensure that representative tissue has been obtained.
8. While awaiting the results of the frozen section, it may be useful to place haemostatic material such as Surgicel® into wound under compression.
9. If the results of the frozen section are satisfactory, release the tourniquet, and confirm haemostasis.
10. Once haemostasis is confirmed close in layers with direct suture of the fascia overlying the tumour, followed by fat and skin. Dissolvable subcuticular sutures should suffice. Only employ a subcutaneous drain if it is clear that a haematoma will develop post-operatively.
11. Resist the temptation to infiltrate the area with local anaesthetic as this may serve to increase the size of the surgical footprint and may inadvertently spread tumour cells.
12. Apply a compressive bandage. Elevate and rest the limb if relevant. Avoid unnecessary strenuous activity over the following 48 h to minimise haematoma formation.

5.7.2 Percutaneous Biopsy

1. Ideally, this would be performed under CT guidance in a sterile field.
2. Careful pre-biopsy instillation of local anaesthetic is often needed in the absence of a general anaesthetic in the radiology suite. Avoid approaching the biopsy site with the anaesthetic, but instead inject local anaesthetic in an arc from a distance proximally that would numb the dermatome involved.
3. Once the tumour biopsy site has been confirmed by laser cross-hairs and marked, a stab incision is made for the introduction of a co-axial sheath (soft tissue) or co-axial drill instrument (bone) with an obturator in position.
4. This is directed down to and where appropriate through the tumour to the planned end-point. With soft tissue tumours, a firing mechanism is deployed which fires the biopsy needle through the co-axial device a set distance. For bone, the biopsy needle within the protective sheath is hand-drilled through the bone. The biopsy needle is then extracted and tissue harvested. Additional cores may be taken in a diverging array from the puncture site to ensure adequate sampling within the tumour.

5. On completion of the biopsy, the needle and protective sheath are removed and pressure applied to the area for several minutes.
6. Occasionally, a bone tumour may bleed through the protective sheath. In this case, haemostatic material, e.g. Gelfoam®, may be inserted down the protective sheath to tamponade the bleeding. An adhesive dressing can then be applied.

5.7.3 What Tests Should Be Ordered on the Biopsy Material?

All tissue should be sent fresh to pathology for examination. The pathologist (sarcoma) should be forewarned of the biopsy and any special instructions conveyed prior to the biopsy. Tests routinely requested include:

1. Histology and immunohistochemistry to confirm sarcomatous nature of tumour.
2. Culture and antibiotic sensitivities if infection is part of the differential diagnosis.
3. Flow cytometry if lymphoma is suspected.
4. Molecular pathology tests looking for signature abnormalities, e.g. evidence of translocation, gene amplification, gene expression.
5. Chromosomal analysis if this is available or pertinent to the case.

5.7.4 How Should the Results of the Biopsy Be Interpreted?

The biopsy result should be interpreted in the context of the radiologic findings and once all the pathological tests have been performed. The imaging and pathology findings should be concordant, and the extent of this should be the subject of a regular multidisciplinary tumour conference at which the opinions of sarcoma clinicians, radiologists and pathologists are used to inform the final diagnosis. If there is any discordance between clinical presentation, biopsy result and radiologic findings, then any discrepancy will need debate to arrive at a consensus opinion. Under such conditions, a re-biopsy may be in order, and this should part of the multidisciplinary team discussions.

References

1. Ewing J. Neoplastic disease; a treatise on tumours. 2nd ed. Philadelphia: W.B. Saunders Company; 1922. 1054 p.
2. Huvos AG. James Ewing: cancer man. Ann Diagn Pathol. 1998;2(2):146–8.
3. Charoenlap C, Imanishi J, Tanaka T, Slavin J, Ngan SY, Chander S, et al. Outcomes of unplanned sarcoma excision: impact of residual disease. Cancer Med. 2016;5(6):980–8.
4. Mankin HJ, Mankin CJ, Simon MA. The hazards of the biopsy, revisited. Members of the Musculoskeletal Tumor Society. J Bone Joint Surg Am. 1996;78(5):656–63.
5. Trieu J, Schlicht SM, Choong PF. Diagnosing musculoskeletal tumours: how accurate is CT-guided core needle biopsy? Eur J Surg Oncol. 2016;42(7):1049–56.
6. Trieu J, Sinnathamby M, Di Bella C, Pianta M, Perera W, Slavin JL, et al. Biopsy and the diagnostic evaluation of musculoskeletal tumours: critical but often missed in the 21st century. ANZ J Surg. 2016;86(3):133–8.

7. Chang IJ, Ilaslan H, Sundaram M, Schils J, Subhas N. CT-guided percutaneous biopsy of sclerotic bone lesions: diagnostic outcomes. Skelet Radiol. 2018;47(5):661–9.
8. Chang YY, Chen CK, Yeh YC, Wu MH. Diagnostic feasibility and safety of CT-guided core biopsy for lung nodules less than or equal to 8 mm: a single-institution experience. Eur Radiol. 2018;28(2):796–806.
9. Liu PT, Valadez SD, Chivers FS, Roberts CC, Beauchamp CP. Anatomically based guidelines for core needle biopsy of bone tumors: implications for limb-sparing surgery. Radiographics. 2007;27(1):189–205; discussion 6.
10. Oliveira MP, Lima PM, da Silva HJ, de Mello RJ. Neoplasm seeding in biopsy tract of the musculoskeletal system. A systematic review. Acta Ortop Bras. 2014;22(2):106–10.
11. Barrientos-Ruiz I, Ortiz-Cruz EJ, Serrano-Montilla J, Bernabeu-Taboada D, Pozo-Kreilinger JJ. Are biopsy tracts a concern for seeding and local recurrence in sarcomas? Clin Orthop Relat Res. 2017;475(2):511–8.
12. Wallace AN, McWilliams SR, Wallace A, Chang RO, Vaswani D, Stone RE, et al. Drill-assisted biopsy of the axial and appendicular skeleton: safety, technical success, and diagnostic efficacy. J Vasc Interv Radiol. 2016;27(10):1618–22.
13. Wallace AN, Pacheco RA, Vyhmeister R, Tomasian A, Chang RO, Jennings JW. Fluoroscopy-guided intervertebral disc biopsy with a coaxial drill system. Skelet Radiol. 2016;45(2):273–8.
14. Rydholm A, Berg NO. Size, site and clinical incidence of lipoma. Factors in the differential diagnosis of lipoma and sarcoma. Acta Orthop Scand. 1983;54(6):929–34.

Bone Tumour Pathology

6

Vanessa Tran and John Slavin

6.1 Introduction

Bone tumours encompass an extensive range of lesions, which present in the human skeletal structure. Despite their extreme rarity, bone sarcomas include a broad, heterogeneous list of tumour subtypes that have various, distinct clinical and pathological characteristics. In addition to primary mesenchymal lesions, the bone can also give rise to many other non-sarcomatous tumours, including tumours of haematopoietic origin and metastatic bone disease, and these therefore must also be included in the differential list. The diagnostic challenge for pathologists, therefore, is twofold: (1) these tumours are uncommon and infrequently encountered in clinical practice, which presents a challenge to inexperienced pathologists, and (2) the broad histological spectrum of bone tumours can cause diagnostic confusion. Accurate diagnosis is essential in prognostication of disease and ensuring appropriate treatment. For this reason, bone cancers are best managed in a multidisciplinary team at expert tertiary referral centres [1].

6.2 Epidemiology

Malignant neoplasms of the bone are very rare tumours that comprise only 0.2% of the tumour burden [2]. A primary tumour of the bone, however, including benign lesions, is relatively common. Its lack of clinical significance means that the precise incidence of such tumours is unknown [3]. It can be estimated that for every one case of bone cancer, there are at least 10,000 cases of benign bone tumours [4]. In

V. Tran (✉)
Department of Surgery, University of Melbourne, Melbourne, VIC, Australia

J. Slavin
Department of Anatomical Pathology, St. Vincent's Hospital Melbourne, Melbourne, VIC, Australia
e-mail: john.slavin@svha.org.au

P. F. M. Choong (ed.), *Sarcoma*, https://doi.org/10.1007/978-981-15-9414-4_6

2019, there were 255 new diagnoses of bone cancer in Australia and 101 deaths [5]. As a collective entity, these tumours demonstrate a bimodal age distribution with peaks in the second and seventh decades of life and a slight predilection for males [6].

6.3 Classification

The World Health Organization (WHO) classification of tumours of the bone categorises bone tumours according to their presumed line of differentiation [6]. Within each of these 12 subgroups, the tumours can be further sorted into benign, intermediate (locally aggressive) and malignant subtypes. Benign tumours generally respond well to local excision or curettage and have minimal risk of recurrence. Intermediate tumours are also known as locally aggressive or rarely metastasising lesions and described as tumours that may infiltrate and recur locally but lack metastatic potential. The malignant type denotes the most aggressive group of tumours, which demonstrate both local recurrence risk and distant metastasis.

6.4 Grading and Staging

Malignant bone tumours can be further stratified by their risk of metastasis. The grade of a tumour uses its histological features to predict the clinical behaviour of the sarcoma. There are various grading systems that categorise bone sarcomas into either two, three or four tiers; however, unlike the FNCLCC grading system in soft tissue tumours, consensus is lacking. Broadly speaking, the pathological diagnosis of a bone tumour will determine its grade [6]: low-grade lesions (<25% risk of metastasis) and high-grade lesions (>25% risk of metastasis) [7–9]. The stage of a bone tumour also provides prognostic information based on clinical and pathological information. The favoured system is the American Joint Committee on Cancer (AJCC) staging system [10]. This incorporates information regarding the size of the tumour, the involvement of regional lymph nodes, the presence of distant metastases and its histological grade.

6.5 Diagnostic Approach

Prompt evaluation and diagnosis are essential to the management of patients with bone tumours. However, due to their rarity within the general population and the presentation of non-specific symptoms, delays in diagnosis are common [11]. In the 2006 NICE guidelines, it was recommended that all patients with bone sarcomas be managed in a multidisciplinary team setting at a specialist referral centre [1]. Thus, prompt recognition and referral is paramount.

When a bony lesion is suspected on clinical assessment, imaging is an essential next step. Plain X-rays remain a valuable investigation for bone tumours and should be the first investigative choice. Radiological findings can be used to differentiate between osteosarcomas, Ewing sarcoma, giant cell tumours (GCTs) as well as non-sarcomatous lesions, such as osteomyelitis [12]. Computed tomography (CT) is often the next step in assessing the diagnosis. Magnetic resonance imaging (MRI) is extremely useful when further characterisation of a lesion and its surrounding soft tissue is required, as well as for the process of local staging and surgical planning [13]. If malignancy is suspected or diagnosed, computed tomography (CT) of the chest should be ordered to assess the presence of pulmonary metastases [12].

Achieving a definitive diagnosis requires a sample of the tissue to be examined by pathologists. A biopsy, therefore, is the next key stage in diagnosis of a suspicious lesion. Appropriate sampling of the tissue is crucial since inadequate tissue samples may prevent accurate pathological analysis.

The biopsy tract should be carefully considered as it will require excision along with the tumour, if confirmed as a malignant lesion [14]. Fine-needle aspiration (FNA) is the least invasive option and allows for cytologic evaluation of a lesion. Needle core biopsy provides a larger sample of intact tissue and provides higher diagnostic yield when compared with FNA [15–17]. Open biopsy provides the most sensitive results of all biopsy techniques; however, it is a more invasive procedure, with higher complication risks [18, 19].

6.6 Osteogenic Tumours

Osteogenic tumours, otherwise known as bone-forming tumours, encompass both benign and malignant tumours that histologically recapitulate osteoid or bone tissue. The WHO classification of tumours of the bone describes ten subtypes of osteogenic tumours, as listed in Table 6.1, which reflects the various natural history and pathological features of each tumour.

6.6.1 Benign Osteogenic Lesions

Osteoma is a benign tumour of the bone that is frequently asymptomatic and discovered only incidentally. They primarily arise in the skull bones, including the calvarium, facial bones and jaw bones, and rarely occur anywhere else [20]. While

Table 6.1 Summary of subtypes of bone-forming tumours [3]

Benign tumours	Malignant tumours
Osteoma	Central
Osteoid osteoma	Low-grade central osteosarcoma
Osteoblastoma	Conventional osteosarcoma
	Telangiectatic osteosarcoma
	Small cell osteosarcoma
	Surface
	Parosteal osteosarcoma
	Periosteal osteosarcoma
	High-grade surface osteosarcoma

typically slow-growing, large osteomas may obstruct the paranasal sinuses, causing symptoms of headache, nasal discharge or exophthalmos [21, 22]. If resected, these tumours reveal a well-circumscribed lesion that attach broadly to the underlying bone. The tissue is primarily composed of dense, compact bone with areas of trabecular bone that contain a fibrous stroma with few cells. These tumours, if asymptomatic, do not require any treatment.

Osteoid osteoma and osteoblastoma are both benign tumours, distinguished arbitrarily by their size, that are characterised by the production of osteoid or mature bone [23]. The more commonly encountered lesion is osteoid osteoma, which primarily occurs in children and adolescents, more commonly in males [24, 25]. Osteoid osteoma arises most commonly in the femur and tibia classically causing unrelenting pain that is worse at night and effectively relieved by non-steroidal anti-inflammatory drugs (NSAIDs) [26, 27]. Osteoblastomas, on the other hand, appear primarily in the posterior arch of the vertebral column and do not cause the same intensity of pain [24]. Both tumours appear macroscopically as round, red lesions with a gritty texture. By definition, osteoid osteomas do not exceed 20 mm in greatest diameter, and osteoblastomas are larger than 20 mm [6]. The histological characteristics are indistinguishable between both types of tumours [24, 28]. These tumours typically present as a solitary lucent nidus of osteoblastic activity surrounded by a hypervascular, sclerotic bone [26]. Some tumours may have more than one central nidus, and this is more common in osteoblastoma than osteoid osteoma [29, 30]. The prognosis is very favourable for both tumours with almost negligible risk of recurrence, although larger lesions may require surgical excision.

6.6.2 Osteosarcoma

Osteosarcoma or osteogenic sarcoma is the most common primary bone malignancy. It most commonly occurs in children between 10 and 20 years of age but also has a smaller peak in incidence after 60 years of age, with a slight predilection for males [31–33]. Certain genetic syndromes have been associated with the development of osteosarcoma, including inherited retinoblastoma [34], Li-Fraumeni syndrome [35] and Rothmund-Thomson syndrome [36]. Within the adult population, there are additional risk factors for secondary osteosarcoma, including Paget's disease [37] and previous exposure to ionising radiation [38]. These tumours often arise in the metaphyseal portion of long bones, with the most common sites being the femur (most commonly distal), tibia, humerus and pelvis, which collectively account for up to 80% of all cases [39, 40]. Lesions have also been described in almost all other bones in the body, including extraskeletal sites in extremely rare cases [41].

As shown in Table 6.2, osteosarcoma comprises seven subtypes, which each reflect a distinct pattern of clinical features and behaviours. Broadly speaking, these subtypes can be grouped into central and surface tumours. Low-grade, conventional, telangiectatic and small cell osteosarcomas are typically intramedullary lesions, while parosteal, periosteal and high-grade osteosarcomas occur on the bone surface [42]. Table 6.2 summarises the osteosarcoma subtypes by location and grade.

Table 6.2 Summary of osteosarcoma subtypes by location and grade [3]

	Central (intramedullary)	Surface
Low grade	Low-grade central osteosarcoma (fibrous dysplasia-like and desmoplastic fibroma-like)	Parosteal osteosarcoma
Intermediate grade		Periosteal osteosarcoma
High grade	Conventional osteosarcoma Telangiectatic osteosarcoma Small cell osteosarcoma	High-grade osteosarcoma

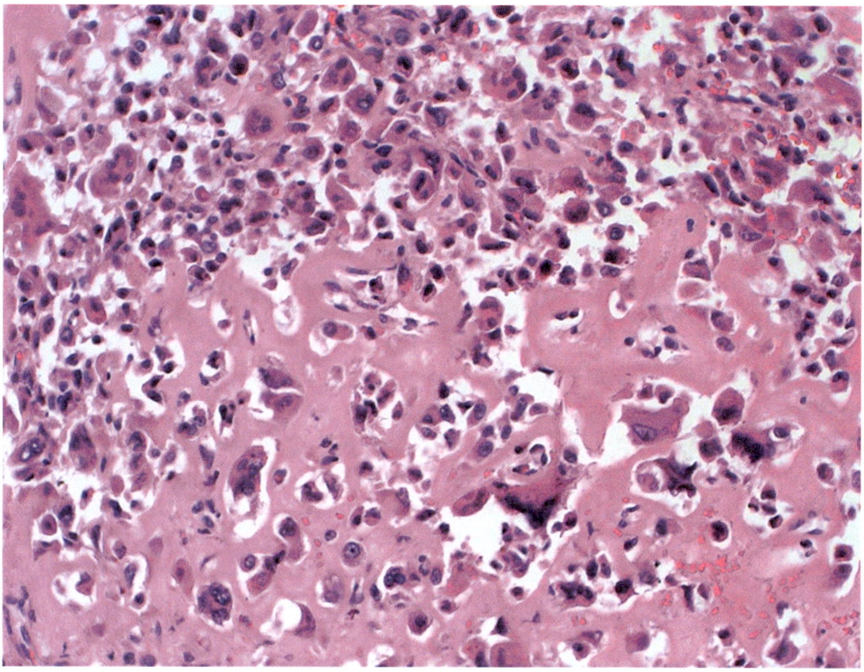

Fig. 6.1 Osteosarcoma containing osteoblasts set in an osteoid matrix

6.6.2.1 Central (Intramedullary) Osteosarcoma

Conventional osteosarcoma is the most common variant, accounting for 80–90% of all osteosarcomas. This is a high-grade, intramedullary tumour that primarily arises in the childhood population [39, 40]. Conventional osteosarcoma can be further classified into histological subtypes, primarily osteoblastic, chondroblastic and fibroblastic, although this does not seem to reflect any appreciable difference in prognosis or clinical behaviour [43, 44]. The tumour demonstrates highly atypical, pleomorphic spindle- or polyhedral-shaped cells, with occasional mitotic figs [42, 43, 45]. Osteoblastic subtypes (76–80% of cases) have a predominant bone or osteoid extracellular matrix (ECM) (Fig. 6.1); chondroblastic subtypes (10–13%) have a high-grade hyaline cartilaginous ECM; and fibroblastic subtypes (10%) show high-grade spindle cells in its ECM [43].

Telangiectatic osteosarcoma is a rare subtype of central osteosarcoma. Like conventional osteosarcoma, it primarily arises in the second decade of life and demonstrates a male preponderance [46]. In one-quarter of cases, patients will present with a pathological long bone fracture [47]. Macroscopic examination of this tumour reveals a characteristic multicystic lesion with haemorrhage into the cavities [48]. Radiological and histological examination can both resemble aneurysmal bone cysts (ABCs) due to the cystic nature of the tumour. However, identification of highly atypical, pleomorphic cells with focal osteoid formation point towards a diagnosis of telangiectatic osteosarcoma.

Small cell osteosarcoma is even rarer, accounting for only 1.5% of all osteosarcomas [49–51]. Although still predominantly a tumour of childhood, it is also encountered in the older population. Epidemiological studies suggest a slight female predilection [49–52]. It often forms lytic lesions within the metaphysis of long bones with an associated large soft tissue mass that may mimic Ewing sarcoma [14, 51, 53]. Microscopic examination reveals small, round, blue malignant cells with a background osteoid matrix and occasionally characteristic spindling of tumours cells [45, 51]. To compound its histological similarity with Ewing sarcoma, these tumours also demonstrate positivity to CD99, and thus, misdiagnosis may occur [54–56]. Immunohistochemical staining for FLI-1 is therefore important in these contexts, as it is frequently positive in Ewing sarcoma but negative in small cell osteosarcoma [57, 58]. The overall prognosis for small cell osteosarcoma is worse than conventional osteosarcoma [49, 51].

Low-grade central osteosarcoma demonstrates a more favourable prognosis compared with its high-grade counterparts described above. These tumours most commonly arise in the knee, either in the distal femur or proximal tibia [59–61], affecting patients in the third or fourth decade of life [6, 62]. They arise within the intramedullary cavity and often cause cortical destruction. The lesion itself is grey-white with a firm, gritty texture and poorly circumscribed margins. Disruption of the bony cortex may extend into the adjacent soft tissue [60, 63]. Microscopic examination demonstrates a paucicellular, fibroblastic proliferation of spindle cells arranged in interlacing fascicles. These cells demonstrate a uniform in appearance with only mild nuclear atypia and only occasional mitotic figures. The background is abundantly collagenous and there is variable osteoid formation. Karyotypic analyses of low-grade central osteosarcomas may demonstrate supernumerary ring chromosomes that contain amplified sequences of chromosome 12q13–15 [64–66]. Detection of MDM2 and CDK4 amplification, therefore, can be useful in distinguishing these tumours from benign fibrous and fibro-osseous lesions, including fibromatosis, fibrous dysplasia and myositis ossificans [67, 68].

6.6.2.2 Surface Osteosarcoma

Parosteal osteosarcoma is low-grade juxtacortical osteosarcoma and is the most common surface osteosarcoma. About 70% of cases arise in the posterior aspect of the distal femur, and as a result, these patients often present with a painless, slow-growing mass and restriction in knee flexion [69]. Arising from the cortex, these are firm, ossified masses with lobulated borders. A cartilage cap on the tumour surface is present in 25% of cases, which may mimic osteochondroma [70]. The presence of any softer areas is suspicious of dedifferentiation to high-grade osteosarcoma, which has been reported in 16–43% of cases [69, 71, 72]. Similar to low-grade central osteosarcoma, MDM2 and CDK4 amplification is often encountered, and their detection by immunohistochemistry may be of diagnostic utility [67, 68, 73]. In general, prognosis is favourable in parosteal osteosarcoma with overall 5-year survival at approximately 91% [69]. However, the presence of dedifferentiation confers a worse prognosis that is similar or only slightly better than conventional osteosarcoma [61, 69, 71, 72].

For every three parosteal osteosarcomas, there is only one case of periosteal osteosarcoma, making it an extremely rare tumour. This tumour has a preponderance to arise in the diaphysis or diaphyseal/metaphyseal junction of long bones, predominantly in the anteromedial aspect of the distal femur and proximal tibia [74–76]. The gross specimen reveals a broad-based, sessile lesion encased in a well-circumscribed pseudocapsule. The cartilage appears atypical, and there is often a myxoid background with some areas of calcification [77].

High-grade surface osteosarcoma is an even more infrequent variant than periosteal osteosarcoma, accounting for less than 1% of all osteosarcomas [78]. This tumour arises in an age group similar to that of conventional osteosarcoma and also appears histologically similar to conventional osteosarcoma [79]. Resected specimens demonstrate a well-circumscribed, lobulated lesion on the cortical surface of the bone with extension into the soft tissue and disruption of the underlying cortex. Histological examination reveals that of a high-grade spindle cell tumour with atypical features, similar to what is seen in conventional osteosarcoma [79].

6.7 Chondrogenic Tumours

Chondrogenic or cartilage-forming tumours, which encompass both benign and malignant lesions, are the most common primary bone neoplasm. Its prevalence is largely accounted for by the benign tumours, namely, osteochondroma and enchondroma. There are many subtypes of chondrogenic tumours, of which several selected types will be discussed below. Table 6.3 lists the cartilaginous tumours defined by the WHO classification.

Table 6.3 Summary of subtypes of cartilaginous tumours [3]

Benign	Malignant
Osteochondroma	Chondrosarcoma
Chondroma	Primary chondrosarcoma
Enchondroma	Secondary chondrosarcoma
Periosteal chondroma	Periosteal chondrosarcoma
Chondromyxoid fibroma	Dedifferentiated chondrosarcoma
Subungual exostosis and bizarre parosteal osteochondromatous proliferation	Mesenchymal chondrosarcoma
Synovial chondromatosis	Clear cell chondrosarcoma
Chondroblastoma	

6.7.1 Benign Cartilaginous Tumours

Chondromas encompass a group of benign tumours that are thought to arise from displaced embryonic growth plate cartilage [80]. They can be subdivided by the location in which they arise: enchondromas, which involve the medullary cavity, and periosteal chondromas, which arise on the surface of bone. Enchondromas typically involve the bones of the hand, while the much rarer periosteal chondroma favours the long bones [81]. These tumours rarely exceed 5 cm in greater diameter [82, 83]. As these tumours are treated by curettage rather than en bloc excision, they are often received in fragments, and a gross description is therefore unavailable. Microscopically, they appear as a hypocellular tumour of abundant blue hyaline cartilage, which lack any evidence of atypia. Some cases of periosteal chondroma demonstrate more cellularity and some nuclear pleomorphism. The main differential diagnosis for enchondromas is low-grade chondrosarcoma. Assessment of the radiological and histological features is important in these cases to rule out features of malignancy. Features suspicious of low-grade chondrosarcoma would include new lucencies, periosteal reactions or soft tissue masses on imaging or hypercellularity, atypia, mitoses and myxoid changes under the microscope [84].

Chondromyxoid fibroma is a very rare benign cartilaginous tumour [85]. While its prognosis is very favourable, even for recurrent tumours, it can be misdiagnosed as chondrosarcoma [80]. This tumour most commonly presents with the symptom of pain and affects patients of any age but most commonly the second and third decades of life [86–88]. The lesions are lobulated, semitranslucent and blue-grey in colour, with well-circumscribed borders and clear separation from adjacent bone. Histologically, the ill-defined lobules have a hypocellular centre of stellate or spindle-shaped tumour cells in a chondromyxoid background [85].

6.7.2 Malignant Cartilaginous Tumours

Chondrosarcoma encompasses a heterogeneous class of cartilaginous bone tumours that include conventional chondrosarcomas and rarer entities of dedifferentiated, mesenchymal and clear cell chondrosarcoma. Conventional chondrosarcoma, unlike conventional osteosarcoma, is a disease of adulthood and typically affects patients in their fifth to seventh decades of life, with a slight male preponderance [89]. These tumours can be further subdivided into primary conventional chondrosarcomas (arise de novo), secondary central chondrosarcoma (arise from enchondroma) or secondary peripheral chondrosarcoma (arise from osteochondroma). The most common site of occurrence is the pelvis, although this tumour can arise at any site that has undergone endochondral ossification [6]. Macroscopic examination of primary chondrosarcoma reveals a blue-white translucent mass with a lobular surface that resembles hyaline cartilage. The tumour may involve the intramedullary space or erupt through the cortex into adjacent soft tissues. At the microscopic level, lobules of blue hyaline cartilage can be seen, along with atypical chondrocytes of varying sizes and shapes, which contain enlarged, hyperchromatic nuclei (Fig. 6.2).

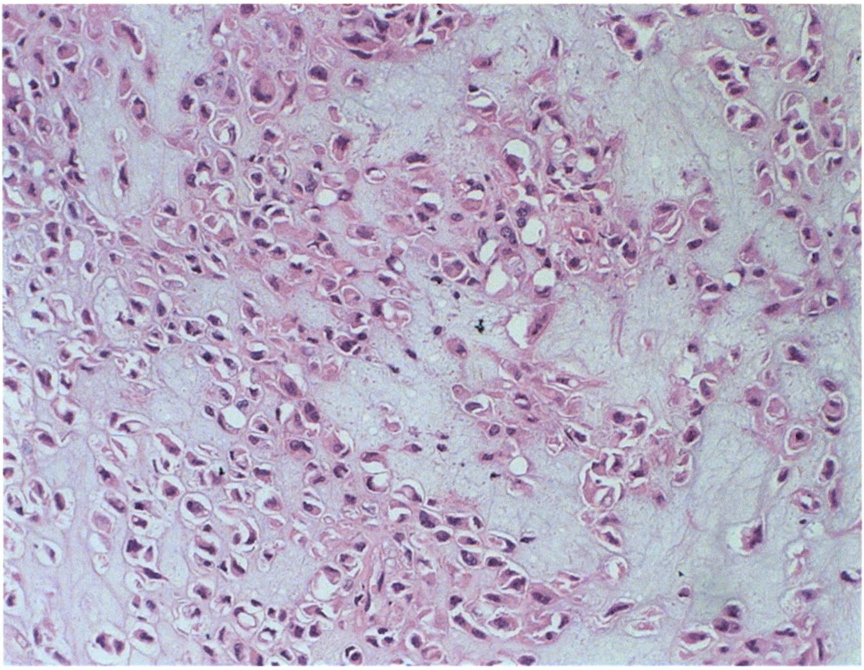

Fig. 6.2 Chondrosarcoma with malignant chondrocytes set in a chondroid matrix

Grading of primary chondrosarcomas [1 to 3] based on histological features can provide important prognostic information about local recurrence and metastasis [90, 91]. Grade 1 tumours demonstrate subtle atypia, with moderate cellularity and plump, uniform nuclei. These tumours can be difficult to differentiate from enchondromas [92, 93]. Grade 2 tumours demonstrate greater cellularity and more nuclear atypia, often with mitotic figures and areas of necrosis. Grade 3 tumours are pleomorphic with increased cellularity and frequent mitoses against a chondroid matrix background [94]. The most important differentials to exclude are enchondromas and chondroblastic osteosarcomas. Radiological information, particularly destruction of the cortex, is a useful clue, and more recently, detection of IDH mutations by immunohistochemistry has been used to confirm diagnosis [80, 95–97].

Rare variants of chondrosarcoma include dedifferentiated chondrosarcoma, mesenchymal chondrosarcoma and clear cell chondrosarcoma. These encompass distinct entities of tumours that display a chondrogenic line of differentiation but have varying clinical characteristics and behaviours. Dedifferentiated chondrosarcoma has a distinct biphasic morphology characterised by a low-grade chondrosarcoma juxtaposed to an area of dedifferentiated, high-grade sarcoma of non-cartilaginous histology [98, 99]. This subtype frequently metastasises to the lungs and confers median survival of less than 1 year, making it the worst prognosis of the three chondrosarcoma variants described here [100–102]. Mesenchymal chondrosarcoma is another biphasic tumour, comprising well-differentiated hyaline cartilage components amongst areas of poorly differentiated small round cells. This tumour may be misdiagnosed as other small round blue cell tumours, such as Ewing sarcoma. Immunohistochemistry may be useful in distinguishing mesenchymal chondrosarcoma from Ewing sarcoma, with the detection of SOX9 positivity with negative FLI-1 staining [58, 103]. Clear cell chondrosarcoma is another variant that shows the characteristic presence of tumour cells with clear cytoplasm and may be mistaken for chondroblastoma, GCT and even renal cell carcinoma. Immunohistochemistry is strongly positive for S100 and type II and X collagens [104].

6.8 Fibrogenic Tumours

Fibrosarcoma of the bone describes a malignant tumour of fibroblastic differentiation [6]. This tumour shares histological similarities with many other sarcomas, including liposarcoma, rhabdomyosarcoma, synovial sarcoma, malignant peripheral nerve sheath tumour and fibromatosis. Given this confusion, previous epidemiological studies are likely to have included non-fibrosarcomas and overestimated its incidence [6, 105]. Macroscopic examination of fibrosarcomas demonstrates a firm, collagenous mass with well-circumscribed borders. Histologically, the tumour demonstrates a predominance of uniform spindle cells without significant pleomorphism, arranged in a distinctive fibrosarcomatous 'herringbone' pattern, which may be present in other tumours. In order to make a diagnosis of fibrosarcoma, histological and cytogenetic features must be further evaluated to exclude possible differential diagnoses. The tissue should firstly be evaluated for malignant osteoid or cartilage, which would suggest a diagnosis of osteosarcoma or dedifferentiated chondrosarcoma [6]. These lesions are aggressive, with risk of local recurrence and lymph node and distant metastasis [106].

6.9 Giant Cell Tumour of the Bone

GCTs are named after the osteoclast-like giant cells that characterise its histology. These benign, locally aggressive tumours represent approximately 20% of benign bone tumours and 5% of all primary bone tumours, primarily presenting between 20 and 45 years of age [46, 107–110]. On gross examination, GCTs often lie in an eccentric location within the bone, resulting in thinning of the cortex. The lesions themselves are often well-defined and reddish-brown in colour due to the areas of haemorrhage. Histological examination reveals the presence of many giant cells, which resemble normal osteoclasts, with variable number of nuclei, prominent nucleoli and eosinophilic cytoplasm. These multinuclear giant cells are evenly spread amongst round-, oval- or spindle-shaped mononuclear cells. Mitotic activity variable in GCT, however, the presence of atypical mitotic figures, would suggest a differential diagnosis of another sarcoma or malignancy that is associated with giant cells [6].

The most common treatment for GCT is intralesional curettage; however, this has reported recurrence rates of up to 40% [107, 111–114]. The local recurrence rate declines with complete en bloc excision. One concern with local recurrence is the increased risk of the so-called 'benign' pulmonary metastases, which occur in approximately 2% of GCTs [115–117]. These pulmonary lesions respond well to surgical treatment, while some have even shown spontaneous regression and, however, still carry a risk of mortality if disease progression occurs [116, 118, 119].

It is known that the stromal tumour cells of GCT express high levels of receptor activator of nuclear factor-kappa B ligand (RANKL) [120–125]. In normal tissue, RANKL is produced by osteoblasts and binds to its receptor, RANK, which is found on the surface of mature and precursor osteoclasts. The interaction between RANK and RANKL plays a crucial role in the differentiation and activation of osteoclasts [126–128]. In this way, through the RANK-RANKL interaction, the neoplastic stromal cells in GCT are also able to induce the recruitment and formation of osteoclasts, a key component of its pathogenesis. Understanding this mechanism has prompted the investigation into the utility denosumab, a monoclonal antibody to RANKL, originally developed for the treatment of osteoporosis and metastatic bone disease, as a chemotherapeutic agent for GCT [108, 124].

6.10 Ewing Sarcoma

Ewing sarcoma is a unique entity and is classified under 'miscellaneous tumours' in the WHO classification of tumours of the bone [6]. This represents the second most common type of bone sarcoma in childhood, primarily affecting patients in the second decade of life [129]. Patients typically present with non-specific symptoms of pain, fever, weight loss and leucocytosis, which can mimic osteomyelitis [130]. Over half of patients present with a mass in the affected area and few (16%) with a pathological fracture [6]. Ewing sarcoma primarily affects the long bones of the upper and lower limbs, although the pelvis, ribs and spine are also commonly implicated [2, 131, 132]. Extraskeletal manifestations can also occur in Ewing sarcoma, with up to 30% arising in the soft tissue [133].

Macroscopically, Ewing sarcoma is often a grey-tan mass with areas of haemorrhage and necrosis. The borders are destructive with infiltrative margins [134]. The round cell morphology of Ewing sarcoma presents a diagnostic challenge as many differential diagnoses, including soft tissue tumours and other non-sarcomatous lesions, need to be considered. Ewing sarcoma can be subdivided into three groups based on its histology: classical Ewing sarcoma, primitive neuroectodermal tumour (PNET) and atypical Ewing sarcoma. Classical Ewing sarcoma, the most common subtype, displays dense sheets of uniform, small round blue cells with pale pink cytoplasm and indistinct cytoplasmic membranes (Fig. 6.3) [135]. Tumours with evidence of neural differentiation are diagnosed as PNET. This involves either detection of Homer-Wrist rosettes, which are clusters of cells arranged around a solid neurofibrillary process, or positive staining for CD99 [136, 137]. Atypical

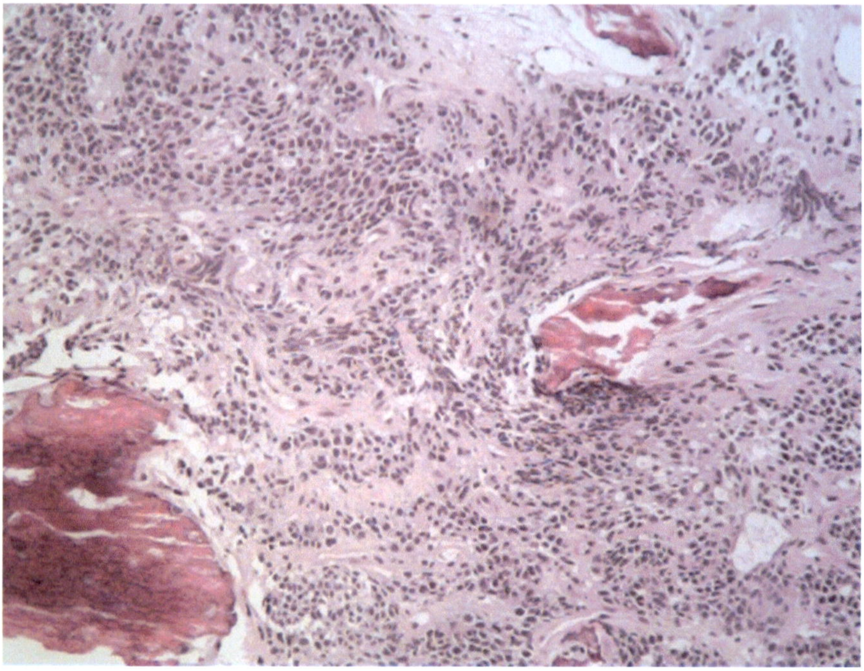

Fig. 6.3 Ewing's sarcoma with nests of small cells with scant cytoplasm replacing the bone

Ewing sarcoma is the term designated for any tumours that deviate from the description of classical Ewing sarcoma. Such deviations include nuclear pleomorphism, irregular nuclear membranes or prominent nucleoli [135, 138–140]. Immunohistochemistry can be extremely useful in the assessment of Ewing sarcoma. CD99 is a highly sensitive but non-specific marker in Ewing sarcoma, demonstrating a strong, diffuse membranous pattern of staining [135, 138]. Notably, however, other round cell tumours also demonstrate CD99 positivity, including lymphomas, mesenchymal chondrosarcoma, small cell osteosarcoma and desmoplastic round cell tumour, which presents a potential diagnostic pitfall [56, 141–143]. Other markers, including FLI-1 and ERG, are also non-specific markers that demonstrate frequent positivity in Ewing sarcoma but also in lymphoma and other sarcomas [57, 135, 144–146].

Cytogenetic analyses of Ewing sarcoma demonstrate a recurrent balanced translocation involving the EWSR1 gene on chromosome 22q12. The fusion partners are referred to as the ETS family of transcriptional regulators, with the most common being FLI-1, which accounts for 85–90% of all translocations [147–149]. Other members of the ETS family include ERG, ETV and FEV [150–152]. Fluorescence in situ hybridisation (FISH) or reverse transcriptase-polymerase chain reaction (RT-PCR) can be used to detect these translocations, which may be particularly useful in the differential diagnosis of small round blue cell tumours [153–156].

6.11 Tumours of Haematopoietic Origin

6.11.1 Plasma Cell Myeloma (Multiple Myeloma)

Plasma cell myeloma (PCM), also known as multiple myeloma, is a haematological malignancy that results from the clonal proliferation of plasma cells within the bone marrow. It is one of the most common haematological malignancies, accounting for approximately 15% of all cases [157]. This is primarily a disease of older age, with the median age of diagnosis being 66–70 years [158–160]. The common bones affected reflect the sites of normal haematopoietic cell production. This primarily encompasses the axial skeleton, namely, the vertebrae, ribs, skull, pelvis, femur, clavicle and scapula [161]. The infiltrative and lytic nature of PCM within the affected bones results in the symptom of bone pain or a pathological fracture, as well as hypercalcaemia and anaemia [162].

Diagnosis of PCM is currently based on the International Myeloma Working Group (IMWG) criteria [163]. In addition to clinical assessment and laboratory investigations, a bone marrow aspirate or biopsy is required to assess the plasma cells. The WHO describes various morphological patterns encountered in PCM, including interstitial, nodular, focal, obliterative and fibrous patterns [6]. In PCM, the clonal plasma cells are typically well-differentiated, with characteristic round nuclei that are located eccentrically in a cell with abundant basophilic cytoplasm (Fig. 6.4). Immunohistochemical analysis demonstrates strong, uniform positivity

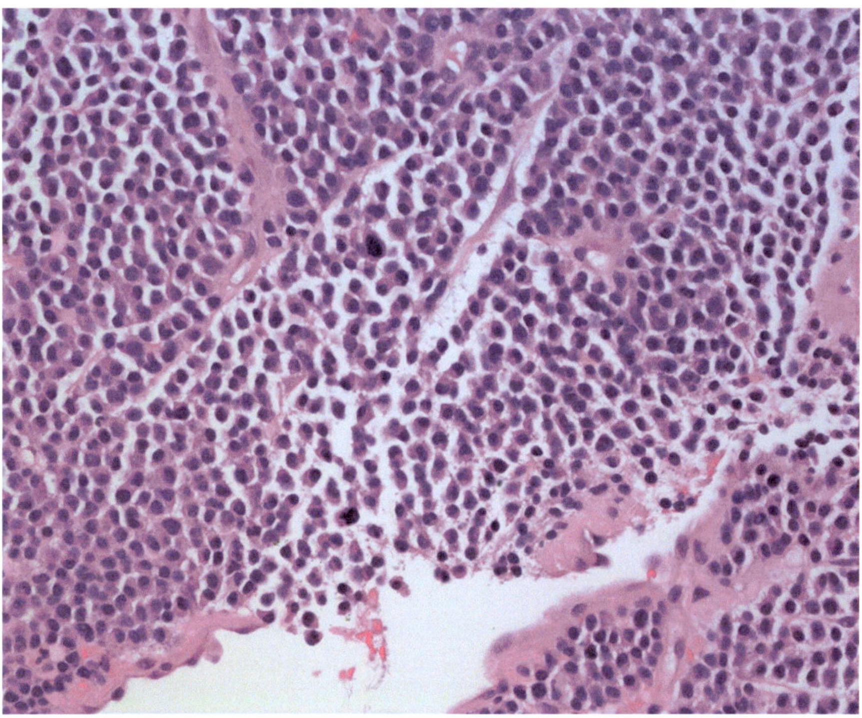

Fig. 6.4 Myeloma containing sheets of plasma cells

Table 6.4 Summary of stage and criteria of Revised International Staging System (R-ISS) for multiple myeloma [175]

Stage	Criteria
I	Serum β_2-microglobulin <3.5 mg/L Albumin >3.3 g/dL Standard-risk chromosomal abnormalities Normal LDH
II	Not stage I or III
III	Serum β_2-microglobulin $\leq$5.5 mg/L High-risk chromosomal abnormalities: del17p, t(4;14) or t(14;16) High LDH

to plasmacytic markers CD138 (syndecan-1) [164–166], CD38 [167, 168] and MUM1 [169]. Quantification of the clonal plasma cells can be performed in multiple ways. The traditional method involves the differential counting of May-Giemsa-stained smears. More recent methods involve using CD138 immunostaining [170–172] and flow cytometry [173]. Based on these investigations, the diagnosis of PCM can be concluded if clonal plasma cell population comprises 10% or more of the total cells in the bone marrow.

Staging of PCM is based on the International Staging System (ISS), which stratifies PCM into three prognostic groups. The initial ISS was based on the serum β_2-microglobulin and albumin levels [174], and it has since been revised to include additional biochemical and cytogenetic variables, as shown in Table 6.4 [175].

6.11.2 Solitary Plasmacytoma of the Bone

Solitary plasmacytoma of the bone (SPB) is also tumour of monoclonal plasma cells that, unlike PCM, occurs in the absence of systemic manifestations. SPB occurs in a slightly younger age group, with a median age of diagnosis of 55 years [176, 177]. Histologically, these lesions demonstrate a proliferation of plasma cells. Immunohistochemistry is useful in identifying SPB in histologically ambiguous cases [6]. The immunoprofile of SPB is similar to that of PCM, with strong positivity to CD138 and MUM1.

6.11.3 Primary Non-Hodgkin Lymphoma of the Bone

Primary lymphoma of the bone (PLB) is an uncommon bone tumour that accounts for 7% of all bone malignancies [46, 178, 179]. It is defined as a malignant proliferation of lymphoid cells, resulting in at least one mass within the bone, that occurs in the absence of any lymph node involvement or any other extranodal lesions [6, 180, 181]. Patients, often between 40 and 55 years of age, present with local bone pain, with or without an associated soft tissue mass or swelling [180]. The femur, spine and pelvic bones are the most commonly affected sites [182, 183]. Diffuse large B-cell lymphoma (DLBCL) represents the greater proportion of PLB; however, others, such as follicular lymphoma, small cell lymphoma and anaplastic large cell lymphoma, have also been described [182–185]. Gross descriptions of these tumours are not widely understood, since needle biopsy is performed to confirm diagnosis, followed by chemotherapy and radiotherapy as treatment. The histological appearance of the tumour will reflect the type of lymphoma present. DLBL demonstrates a characteristic destructive growth pattern centrally, which fills up the marrow spaces between the bony trabeculae. The cells are pleomorphic with large, irregular, multilobulated nucleoli. Immunohistochemistry demonstrates CD20 positivity in all primary lymphomas as it is a marker of B-cells. In DLBCL, PAX5 is also positive.

6.12 Langerhans Cell Histiocytosis

Langerhans cell histiocytosis (LCH) describes a group of benign bone tumours of 'undefined neoplastic nature' characterised by the clonal proliferation of Langerhans-type cells. LCH affects people of all ages, though most common in those under 30 years of age, and is twice as likely to affect males as females [186, 187]. It is known to arise in the bones of the skull, ribs, femur, pelvis and mandible, often causing pain and swelling to the affected area. The tumour demonstrates a proliferation of Langerhans cells, which are medium to large cells with abundant eosinophilic to clear cytoplasm and indistinct cytoplasmic borders. The nuclei are oval-shaped and have prominent, irregular folds and grooves. These cells exist on a background of inflammatory cells, including lymphocytes, eosinophils, neutrophils and plasma cells. The presence of atypical mitosis and marked pleomorphism is an unusual features and should raise suspicion for Langerhans cell sarcoma [188, 189]. Immunohistochemistry reveals positivity for dendritic markers CD1a, S100 and CD207 (langerin), which also reflects the immunoprofile of normal epidermal Langerhans cells [190, 191]. Consideration of the histological and immunohistochemical features can be extremely useful in separating LCH from its common mimics. Common differential diagnoses include Rosai-Dorfman disease, which does not express CD1a or CD207 [192, 193], and Erdheim-Chester disease, which contains foamy histiocytes and is negative for CD1a and S100 [194, 195].

References

1. National Institute for Health and Clinical Excellence. Improving outcomes for people with sarcoma: the manual. London: National Institute for Health and Clinical Excellence; 2006.
2. Howlader NJhscgc, based on November SEER data submission, posted to the SEER web site. SEER Cancer Statistics Review, 1975-2008. Bethesda, MD: National Cancer Institute; 2011.
3. Fletcher CD, Bridge JA, Hogendoorn PC, Mertens F. WHO classification of tumours of soft tissue and bone, vol. 2003. Lyon: IARC; 2013. p. 305–10.
4. Rosenberg AE. Bone sarcoma pathology: diagnostic approach for optimal therapy. Am Soc Clin Oncol Educ Book. 2017;37:794–8.

5. Health AIo, Welfare. Cancer in Australia 2019; 2019.
6. Bridge JA, Hogendoorn PCW, Mertens F, Fletcher CD. WHO classification of tumours of soft tissue and bone. Lyon: International Agency for Research on Cancer; 2013.
7. Rubin BP, Antonescu CR, Gannon FH, Hunt JL, Inwards CY, Klein MJ, et al. Protocol for the examination of specimens from patients with tumors of bone. Arch Pathol Lab Med. 2010;134(4):e1–7.
8. Hogendoorn PC, Group EEW, Athanasou N, Bielack S, De Alava E, Dei Tos AP, et al. Bone sarcomas: ESMO Clinical Practice Guidelines for diagnosis, treatment and follow-up. Ann Oncol. 2010;21(Suppl 5):v204–13.
9. Mangham DC, Athanasou NA. Guidelines for histopathological specimen examination and diagnostic reporting of primary bone tumours. Clin Sarcoma Res. 2011;1(1):6.
10. Edge SB, Compton CC. The American Joint Committee on Cancer: the 7th edition of the AJCC cancer staging manual and the future of TNM. Ann Surg Oncol. 2010;17(6):1471–4.
11. Smith GM, Johnson GD, Grimer RJ, Wilson S. Trends in presentation of bone and soft tissue sarcomas over 25 years: little evidence of earlier diagnosis. Ann R Coll Surg Engl. 2011;93(7):542–7.
12. Wittig JC, Bickels J, Priebat D, Jelinek J, Kellar-Graney K, Shmookler B, et al. Osteosarcoma: a multidisciplinary approach to diagnosis and treatment. Am Fam Physician. 2002;65(6):1123–32.
13. Nascimento D, Suchard G, Hatem M, de Abreu A. The role of magnetic resonance imaging in the evaluation of bone tumours and tumour-like lesions. Insights Imaging. 2014;5(4):419–40.
14. Messerschmitt PJ, Garcia RM, Abdul-Karim FW, Greenfield EM, Getty PJ. Osteosarcoma. J Am Acad Orthop Surg. 2009;17(8):515–27.
15. Koscick RL, Petersilge CA, Makley JT, Abdul-Karim FW. CT-guided fine needle aspiration and needle core biopsy of skeletal lesions. Complementary diagnostic techniques. Acta Cytol. 1998;42(3):697–702.
16. Kaur I, Handa U, Kundu R, Garg SK, Mohan H. Role of fine-needle aspiration cytology and core needle biopsy in diagnosing musculoskeletal neoplasms. J Cytol. 2016;33(1):7–12.
17. Cardoso PF, Esteves J, Oliveira V, Rodrigues-Pinto R. Comparison of fine needle aspiration and core needle biopsy in the diagnosis of bone tumours. Acta Orthop Belg. 2018;84(1):30–7.
18. Pohlig F, Kirchhoff C, Lenze U, Schauwecker J, Burgkart R, Rechl H, et al. Percutaneous core needle biopsy versus open biopsy in diagnostics of bone and soft tissue sarcoma: a retrospective study. Eur J Med Res. 2012;17:29.
19. Layfield LJ, Schmidt RL, Sangle N, Crim JR. Diagnostic accuracy and clinical utility of biopsy in musculoskeletal lesions: a comparison of fine-needle aspiration, core, and open biopsy techniques. Diagn Cytopathol. 2014;42(6):476–86.
20. Larrea-Oyarbide N, Valmaseda-Castellon E, Berini-Aytes L, Gay-Escoda C. Osteomas of the craniofacial region. Review of 106 cases. J Oral Pathol Med. 2008;37(1):38–42.
21. Sayan NB, Ucok C, Karasu HA, Gunhan O. Peripheral osteoma of the oral and maxillofacial region: a study of 35 new cases. J Oral Maxillofac Surg. 2002;60(11):1299–301.
22. Onerci M, Hosal S, Korkmaz H. Nasal osteoma: a case report. J Oral Maxillofac Surg. 1993;51(4):423–5.
23. Greenspan A. Benign bone-forming lesions: osteoma, osteoid osteoma, and osteoblastoma. Clinical, imaging, pathologic, and differential considerations. Skelet Radiol. 1993;22(7):485–500.
24. Loizaga JM, Calvo M, Lopez Barea F, Martinez Tello FJ, Perez Villanueva J. Osteoblastoma and osteoid osteoma. Clinical and morphological features of 162 cases. Pathol Res Pract. 1993;189(1):33–41.
25. Dahlin DC. Bone tumors: general aspects and data on 6,221 cases. Springfield: Charles C. Thomas Publisher; 1978.
26. Healey JH, Ghelman B. Osteoid osteoma and osteoblastoma. Current concepts and recent advances. Clin Orthop Relat Res. 1986;204:76–85.
27. Mankin HJ. Osteoid osteoma and osteoblastoma: two related bone tumors. In: GREAT educator series: pathophysiology of orthopaedic diseases, vol. 2. Rosemont: American Academy of Orthopaedic Surgeons; 2009. p. 79–85.

28. Byers PD. Solitary benign osteoblastic lesions of bone. Osteoid osteoma and benign osteoblastoma. Cancer. 1968;22(1):43–57.
29. Lucas DR, Unni KK, McLeod RA, O'Connor MI, Sim FH. Osteoblastoma: clinicopathologic study of 306 cases. Hum Pathol. 1994;25(2):117–34.
30. Frassica FJ, Waltrip RL, Sponseller PD, Ma LD, McCarthy EF Jr. Clinicopathologic features and treatment of osteoid osteoma and osteoblastoma in children and adolescents. Orthop Clin North Am. 1996;27(3):559–74.
31. Mirabello L, Troisi RJ, Savage SA. International osteosarcoma incidence patterns in children and adolescents, middle ages and elderly persons. Int J Cancer. 2009;125(1):229–34.
32. Sergi C, Zwerschke W. Osteogenic sarcoma (osteosarcoma) in the elderly: tumor delineation and predisposing conditions. Exp Gerontol. 2008;43(12):1039–43.
33. Mirabello L, Troisi RJ, Savage SA. Osteosarcoma incidence and survival rates from 1973 to 2004: data from the Surveillance, Epidemiology, and End Results Program. Cancer. 2009;115(7):1531–43.
34. Hansen MF, Koufos A, Gallie BL, Phillips RA, Fodstad O, Brogger A, et al. Osteosarcoma and retinoblastoma: a shared chromosomal mechanism revealing recessive predisposition. Proc Natl Acad Sci U S A. 1985;82(18):6216–20.
35. Li FP, Fraumeni JF Jr, Mulvihill JJ, Blattner WA, Dreyfus MG, Tucker MA, et al. A cancer family syndrome in twenty-four kindreds. Cancer Res. 1988;48(18):5358–62.
36. Wang LL, Gannavarapu A, Kozinetz CA, Levy ML, Lewis RA, Chintagumpala MM, et al. Association between osteosarcoma and deleterious mutations in the RECQL4 gene in Rothmund-Thomson syndrome. J Natl Cancer Inst. 2003;95(9):669–74.
37. Ottaviani G, Jaffe N. The etiology of osteosarcoma. Cancer Treat Res. 2009;152:15–32.
38. Le Vu B, de Vathaire F, Shamsaldin A, Hawkins MM, Grimaud E, Hardiman C, et al. Radiation dose, chemotherapy and risk of osteosarcoma after solid tumours during childhood. Int J Cancer. 1998;77(3):370–7.
39. Dahlin DC, Coventry MB. Osteogenic sarcoma. A study of six hundred cases. J Bone Joint Surg Am. 1967;49(1):101–10.
40. Dahlin DC, Unni KK. Bone tumors: general aspects and data on 8,547 cases. Springfield: Charles C. Thomas; 1986.
41. Iannaci G, Luise R, Sapere P, Costanzo R, Rossiello R. Extraskeletal osteosarcoma: a very rare case report of primary tumor of the colon–rectum and review of the literature. Pathol Res Pract. 2013;209(6):393–6.
42. Moore DD, Luu HH. Osteosarcoma. Orthopaedic oncology. New York: Springer; 2014. p. 65–92.
43. Fletcher CD, Unni KK, Mertens F. Pathology and genetics of tumours of soft tissue and bone. Lyon: IARC; 2002.
44. Hauben E, Weeden S, Pringle J, Van Marck E, Hogendoorn PCW. Does the histological subtype of high-grade central osteosarcoma influence the response to treatment with chemotherapy and does it affect overall survival? A study on 570 patients of two consecutive trials of the European Osteosarcoma Intergroup. Eur J Cancer. 2002;38(9):1218–25.
45. Klein MJ, Siegal GP. Osteosarcoma: anatomic and histologic variants. Am J Clin Pathol. 2006;125(4):555–81.
46. Unni KK, Inwards CY. Dahlin's bone tumors: general aspects and data on 10,165 cases. Philadelphia: Lippincott Williams & Wilkins; 2010.
47. Mervak TR, Unni KK, Pritchard DJ, McLeod RA. Telangiectatic osteosarcoma. Clin Orthop Relat Res. 1991;270:135–9.
48. Matsuno T, Unni KK, McLeod RA, Dahlin DC. Telangiectatic osteogenic sarcoma. Cancer. 1976;38(6):2538–47.
49. Ayala AG, Ro JY, Raymond AK, Jaffe N, Chawla S, Carrasco H, et al. Small cell osteosarcoma. A clinicopathologic study of 27 cases. Cancer. 1989;64(10):2162–73.
50. Bertoni F, Present D, Bacchini P, Pignatti G, Picci P, Campanacci M. The Istituto Rizzoli experience with small cell osteosarcoma. Cancer. 1989;64(12):2591–9.
51. Nakajima H, Sim FH, Bond JR, Unni KK. Small cell osteosarcoma of bone. Review of 72 cases. Cancer. 1997;79(11):2095–106.

52. Martin SE, Dwyer A, Kissane JM, Costa J. Small-cell osteosarcoma. Cancer. 1982;50(5):990–6.
53. Yarmish G, Klein MJ, Landa J, Lefkowitz RA, Hwang S. Imaging characteristics of primary osteosarcoma: nonconventional subtypes. Radiographics. 2010;30(6):1653–72.
54. Devaney K, Vinh TN, Sweet DE. Small cell osteosarcoma of bone: an immunohistochemical study with differential diagnostic considerations. Hum Pathol. 1993;24(11):1211–25.
55. Devoe K, Weidner N. Immunohistochemistry of small round-cell tumors. Semin Diagn Pathol. 2000;17(3):216–24.
56. Machado I, Alberghini M, Giner F, Corrigan M, O'Sullivan M, Noguera R, et al. Histopathological characterization of small cell osteosarcoma with immunohistochemistry and molecular genetic support. A study of 10 cases. Histopathology. 2010;57(1):162–7.
57. Folpe AL, Hill CE, Parham DM, O'Shea PA, Weiss SW. Immunohistochemical detection of FLI-1 protein expression: a study of 132 round cell tumors with emphasis on CD99-positive mimics of Ewing's sarcoma/primitive neuroectodermal tumor. Am J Surg Pathol. 2000;24(12):1657–62.
58. Lee AF, Hayes MM, Lebrun D, Espinosa I, Nielsen GP, Rosenberg AE, et al. FLI-1 distinguishes Ewing sarcoma from small cell osteosarcoma and mesenchymal chondrosarcoma. Appl Immunohistochem Mol Morphol. 2011;19(3):233–8.
59. Bertoni F, Bacchini P, Fabbri N, Mercuri M, Picci P, Ruggieri P, et al. Osteosarcoma. Low-grade intraosseous-type osteosarcoma, histologically resembling parosteal osteosarcoma, fibrous dysplasia, and desmoplastic fibroma. Cancer. 1993;71(2):338–45.
60. Kurt AM, Unni KK, McLeod RA, Pritchard DJ. Low-grade intraosseous osteosarcoma. Cancer. 1990;65(6):1418–28.
61. Schwab JH, Antonescu CR, Athanasian EA, Boland PJ, Healey JH, Morris CD. A comparison of intramedullary and juxtacortical low-grade osteogenic sarcoma. Clin Orthop Relat Res. 2008;466(6):1318–22.
62. Andresen KJ, Sundaram M, Unni KK, Sim FH. Imaging features of low-grade central osteosarcoma of the long bones and pelvis. Skelet Radiol. 2004;33(7):373–9.
63. Unni KK, Dahlin DC, McLeod RA, Pritchard DJ. Intraosseous well-differentiated osteosarcoma. Cancer. 1977;40(3):1337–47.
64. Tarkkanen M, Bohling T, Gamberi G, Ragazzini P, Benassi MS, Kivioja A, et al. Comparative genomic hybridization of low-grade central osteosarcoma. Mod Pathol. 1998;11(5):421–6.
65. Gisselsson D, Palsson E, Hoglund M, Domanski H, Mertens F, Pandis N, et al. Differentially amplified chromosome 12 sequences in low- and high-grade osteosarcoma. Genes Chromosomes Cancer. 2002;33(2):133–40.
66. Ragazzini P, Gamberi G, Benassi MS, Orlando C, Sestini R, Ferrari C, et al. Analysis of SAS gene and CDK4 and MDM2 proteins in low-grade osteosarcoma. Cancer Detect Prev. 1999;23(2):129–36.
67. Yoshida A, Ushiku T, Motoi T, Shibata T, Beppu Y, Fukayama M, et al. Immunohistochemical analysis of MDM2 and CDK4 distinguishes low-grade osteosarcoma from benign mimics. Mod Pathol. 2010;23(9):1279–88.
68. Dujardin F, Binh MB, Bouvier C, Gomez-Brouchet A, Larousserie F, Muret A, et al. MDM2 and CDK4 immunohistochemistry is a valuable tool in the differential diagnosis of low-grade osteosarcomas and other primary fibro-osseous lesions of the bone. Mod Pathol. 2011;24(5):624–37.
69. Okada K, Frassica FJ, Sim FH, Beabout JW, Bond JR, Unni KK. Parosteal osteosarcoma. A clinicopathological study. J Bone Joint Surg Am. 1994;76(3):366–78.
70. Hang JF, Chen PC. Parosteal osteosarcoma. Arch Pathol Lab Med. 2014;138(5):694–9.
71. Bertoni F, Bacchini P, Staals EL, Davidovitz P. Dedifferentiated parosteal osteosarcoma: the experience of the Rizzoli Institute. Cancer. 2005;103(11):2373–82.
72. Sheth DS, Yasko AW, Raymond AK, Ayala AG, Carrasco CH, Benjamin RS, et al. Conventional and dedifferentiated parosteal osteosarcoma. Diagnosis, treatment, and outcome. Cancer. 1996;78(10):2136–45.

73. Duhamel LA, Ye H, Halai D, Idowu BD, Presneau N, Tirabosco R, et al. Frequency of Mouse Double Minute 2 (MDM2) and Mouse Double Minute 4 (MDM4) amplification in parosteal and conventional osteosarcoma subtypes. Histopathology. 2012;60(2):357–9.
74. Cesari M, Alberghini M, Vanel D, Palmerini E, Staals EL, Longhi A, et al. Periosteal osteosarcoma: a single-institution experience. Cancer. 2011;117(8):1731–5.
75. Grimer RJ, Bielack S, Flege S, Cannon SR, Foleras G, Andreeff I, et al. Periosteal osteosarcoma--a European review of outcome. Eur J Cancer. 2005;41(18):2806–11.
76. Murphey MD, Jelinek JS, Temple HT, Flemming DJ, Gannon FH. Imaging of periosteal osteosarcoma: radiologic-pathologic comparison. Radiology. 2004;233(1):129–38.
77. Unni KK, Dahlin DC, Beabout JW. Periosteal osteogenic sarcoma. Cancer. 1976;37(5):2476–85.
78. Okada K, Unni KK, Swee RG, Sim FH. High grade surface osteosarcoma: a clinicopathologic study of 46 cases. Cancer. 1999;85(5):1044–54.
79. Staals EL, Bacchini P, Bertoni F. High-grade surface osteosarcoma: a review of 25 cases from the Rizzoli Institute. Cancer. 2008;112(7):1592–9.
80. Qasem SA, DeYoung BR, editors. Cartilage-forming tumors. Seminars in diagnostic pathology. Amsterdam: Elsevier; 2014.
81. Unni K, Inwards C, Bridge J, Kindblom L, Wold LJ. Tumors of the bones and joints (Atlas of Tumor Pathology series IV). Washington, DC: American Registry of Pathology; 2005. p. 324–30.
82. Douis H, Saifuddin A. The imaging of cartilaginous bone tumours. I. Benign lesions. Skelet Radiol. 2012;41(10):1195–212.
83. Bauer TW, Dorfman HD, Latham JT Jr. Periosteal chondroma. A clinicopathologic study of 23 cases. Am J Surg Pathol. 1982;6(7):631–7.
84. Weiner SD. Enchondroma and chondrosarcoma of bone: clinical, radiologic, and histologic differentiation. Instr Course Lect. 2004;53:645–9.
85. Romeo S, Hogendoorn PC, Dei Tos AP. Benign cartilaginous tumors of bone: from morphology to somatic and germ-line genetics. Adv Anat Pathol. 2009;16(5):307–15.
86. Gherlinzoni F, Rock M, Picci P. Chondromyxoid fibroma. The experience at the Istituto Ortopedico Rizzoli. J Bone Joint Surg Am. 1983;65(2):198–204.
87. Wu CT, Inwards CY, O'Laughlin S, Rock MG, Beabout JW, Unni KK. Chondromyxoid fibroma of bone: a clinicopathologic review of 278 cases. Hum Pathol. 1998;29(5):438–46.
88. Lersundi A, Mankin HJ, Mourikis A, Hornicek FJ. Chondromyxoid fibroma: a rarely encountered and puzzling tumor. Clin Orthop Relat Res. 2005;439:171–5.
89. Lee FY, Mankin HJ, Fondren G, Gebhardt MC, Springfield DS, Rosenberg AE, et al. Chondrosarcoma of bone: an assessment of outcome. J Bone Joint Surg Am. 1999;81(3):326–38.
90. Evans HL, Ayala AG, Romsdahl MM. Prognostic factors in chondrosarcoma of bone: a clinicopathologic analysis with emphasis on histologic grading. Cancer. 1977;40(2):818–31.
91. Bjornsson J, McLeod RA, Unni KK, Ilstrup DM, Pritchard DJ. Primary chondrosarcoma of long bones and limb girdles. Cancer. 1998;83(10):2105–19.
92. Skeletal Lesions Interobserver Correlation among Expert Diagnosticians (SLICED) Study Group. Reliability of histopathologic and radiologic grading of cartilaginous neoplasms in long bones. J Bone Joint Surg Am. 2007;89(10):2113–23.
93. Eefting D, Schrage YM, Geirnaerdt MJ, Le Cessie S, Taminiau AH, Bovee JV, et al. Assessment of interobserver variability and histologic parameters to improve reliability in classification and grading of central cartilaginous tumors. Am J Surg Pathol. 2009;33(1):50–7.
94. Unni KK. Cartilaginous lesions of bone. J Orthop Sci. 2001;6(5):457–72.
95. Amary MF, Bacsi K, Maggiani F, Damato S, Halai D, Berisha F, et al. IDH1 and IDH2 mutations are frequent events in central chondrosarcoma and central and periosteal chondromas but not in other mesenchymal tumours. J Pathol. 2011;224(3):334–43.
96. Marco RA, Gitelis S, Brebach GT, Healey JH. Cartilage tumors: evaluation and treatment. J Am Acad Orthop Surg. 2000;8(5):292–304.

97. Pansuriya TC, van Eijk R, d'Adamo P, van Ruler MA, Kuijjer ML, Oosting J, et al. Somatic mosaic IDH1 and IDH2 mutations are associated with enchondroma and spindle cell hemangioma in Ollier disease and Maffucci syndrome. Nat Genet. 2011;43(12):1256–61.
98. Dahlin DC, Beabout JW. Dedifferentiation of low-grade chondrosarcomas. Cancer. 1971;28(2):461–6.
99. McFarland GB Jr, McKinley LM, Reed RJ. Dedifferentiation of low grade chondrosarcomas. Clin Orthop Relat Res. 1977;122:157–64.
100. Anract P, Tomeno B, Forest M. [Dedifferentiated chondrosarcoma. A study of 13 clinical cases and review of the literature]. Rev Chir Orthop Reparatrice Appar Mot. 1994;80(8):669–80.
101. Dickey ID, Rose PS, Fuchs B, Wold LE, Okuno SH, Sim FH, et al. Dedifferentiated chondrosarcoma: the role of chemotherapy with updated outcomes. J Bone Joint Surg Am. 2004;86(11):2412–8.
102. Bruns J, Fiedler W, Werner M, Delling G. Dedifferentiated chondrosarcoma--a fatal disease. J Cancer Res Clin Oncol. 2005;131(6):333–9.
103. Wehrli BM, Huang W, De Crombrugghe B, Ayala AG, Czerniak B. Sox9, a master regulator of chondrogenesis, distinguishes mesenchymal chondrosarcoma from other small blue round cell tumors. Hum Pathol. 2003;34(3):263–9.
104. Aigner T, Dertinger S, Belke J, Kirchner T. Chondrocytic cell differentiation in clear cell chondrosarcoma. Hum Pathol. 1996;27(12):1301–5.
105. Folpe AL. Fibrosarcoma: a review and update. Histopathology. 2014;64(1):12–25.
106. Bahrami A, Folpe AL. Adult-type fibrosarcoma: a reevaluation of 163 putative cases diagnosed at a single institution over a 48-year period. Am J Surg Pathol. 2010;34(10):1504–13.
107. Campanacci M, Baldini N, Boriani S, Sudanese A. Giant-cell tumor of bone. J Bone Joint Surg Am. 1987;69(1):106–14.
108. Thomas DM, Skubitz KM. Giant cell tumour of bone. Curr Opin Oncol. 2009;21(4):338–44.
109. Raskin KA, Schwab JH, Mankin HJ, Springfield DS, Hornicek FJ. Giant cell tumor of bone. J Am Acad Orthop Surg. 2013;21(2):118–26.
110. Turcotte RE. Giant cell tumor of bone. Orthop Clin North Am. 2006;37(1):35–51.
111. Blackley HR, Wunder JS, Davis AM, White LM, Kandel R, Bell RS. Treatment of giant-cell tumors of long bones with curettage and bone-grafting. J Bone Joint Surg Am. 1999;81(6):811–20.
112. Goldenberg RR, Campbell CJ, Bonfiglio M. Giant-cell tumor of bone. An analysis of two hundred and eighteen cases. J Bone Joint Surg Am. 1970;52(4):619–64.
113. Lausten GS, Jensen PK, Schiodt T, Lund B. Local recurrences in giant cell tumour of bone. Long-term follow up of 31 cases. Int Orthop. 1996;20(3):172–6.
114. Malek F, Krueger P, Hatmi ZN, Malayeri AA, Faezipour H, O'Donnell RJ. Local control of long bone giant cell tumour using curettage, burring and bone grafting without adjuvant therapy. Int Orthop. 2006;30(6):495–8.
115. Masui F, Ushigome S, Fujii K. Giant cell tumor of bone: a clinicopathologic study of prognostic factors. Pathol Int. 1998;48(9):723–9.
116. Siebenrock KA, Unni KK, Rock MG. Giant-cell tumour of bone metastasising to the lungs. A long-term follow-up. J Bone Joint Surg Br. 1998;80(1):43–7.
117. Miller IJ, Blank A, Yin SM, McNickle A, Gray R, Gitelis S. A case of recurrent giant cell tumor of bone with malignant transformation and benign pulmonary metastases. Diagn Pathol. 2010;5:62.
118. Okamoto Y, Mathew S, Daw NC, Neel MD, McCarville MB, Dome JS, et al. Giant cell tumor of bone with pulmonary metastases. Med Pediatr Oncol. 2003;41(5):454–9.
119. Dominkus M, Ruggieri P, Bertoni F, Briccoli A, Picci P, Rocca M, et al. Histologically verified lung metastases in benign giant cell tumours--14 cases from a single institution. Int Orthop. 2006;30(6):499–504.
120. Atkins GJ, Haynes DR, Graves SE, Evdokiou A, Hay S, Bouralexis S, et al. Expression of osteoclast differentiation signals by stromal elements of giant cell tumors. J Bone Miner Res. 2000;15(4):640–9.

121. Goldring SR, Roelke MS, Petrison KK, Bhan AK. Human giant cell tumors of bone identification and characterization of cell types. J Clin Invest. 1987;79(2):483–91.
122. Huang L, Xu J, Wood DJ, Zheng MH. Gene expression of osteoprotegerin ligand, osteoprotegerin, and receptor activator of NF-κB in giant cell tumor of bone: possible involvement in tumor cell-induced osteoclast-like cell formation. Am J Pathol. 2000;156(3):761–7.
123. Morgan T, Atkins GJ, Trivett MK, Johnson SA, Kansara M, Schlicht SL, et al. Molecular profiling of giant cell tumor of bone and the osteoclastic localization of ligand for receptor activator of nuclear factor κB. Am J Pathol. 2005;167(1):117–28.
124. Roux S, Amazit L, Meduri G, Guiochon-Mantel A, Milgrom E, Mariette X. RANK (receptor activator of nuclear factor kappa B) and RANK ligand are expressed in giant cell tumors of bone. Am J Clin Pathol. 2002;117(2):210–6.
125. Skubitz KM, Cheng EY, Clohisy DR, Thompson RC, Skubitz AP. Gene expression in giant-celltumors. J Lab Clin Med. 2004;144(4):193–200.
126. Hofbauer LC, Khosla S, Dunstan CR, Lacey DL, Boyle WJ, Riggs BL. The roles of osteoprotegerin and osteoprotegerin ligand in the paracrine regulation of bone resorption. J Bone Miner Res. 2000;15(1):2–12.
127. Lacey DL, Timms E, Tan HL, Kelley MJ, Dunstan CR, Burgess T, et al. Osteoprotegerin ligand is a cytokine that regulates osteoclast differentiation and activation. Cell. 1998;93(2):165–76.
128. Nakagawa N, Kinosaki M, Yamaguchi K, Shima N, Yasuda H, Yano K, et al. RANK is the essential signaling receptor for osteoclast differentiation factor in osteoclastogenesis. Biochem Biophys Res Commun. 1998;253(2):395–400.
129. Gurney JG, Davis S, Severson RK, Fang JY, Ross JA, Robison LL. Trends in cancer incidence among children in the US. Cancer. 1996;78(3):532–41.
130. Flanagan AM, Lindsay D. A diagnostic approach to bone tumours. Pathology. 2017;49(7):675–87.
131. Bleyer A, O'Leary M, Barr R, Ries LAJ. Cancer epidemiology in older adolescents and young adults 15 to 29 years of age, including SEER incidence and survival: 1975–2000; 2006.
132. Cotterill SJ, Ahrens S, Paulussen M, Jurgens HF, Voute PA, Gadner H, et al. Prognostic factors in Ewing's tumor of bone: analysis of 975 patients from the European Intergroup Cooperative Ewing's Sarcoma Study Group. J Clin Oncol. 2000;18(17):3108–14.
133. Applebaum MA, Worch J, Matthay KK, Goldsby R, Neuhaus J, West DC, et al. Clinical features and outcomes in patients with extraskeletal Ewing sarcoma. Cancer. 2011;117(13):3027–32.
134. Choi EY, Gardner JM, Lucas DR, McHugh JB, Patel RM. Ewing sarcoma. Semin Diagn Pathol. 2014;31(1):39–47.
135. Llombart-Bosch A, Machado I, Navarro S, Bertoni F, Bacchini P, Alberghini M, et al. Histological heterogeneity of Ewing's sarcoma/PNET: an immunohistochemical analysis of 415 genetically confirmed cases with clinical support. Virchows Arch. 2009;455(5):397–411.
136. Ba L, Tan H, Xiao H, Guan Y, Gao J, Gao X. Radiologic and clinicopathologic findings of peripheral primitive neuroectodermal tumors. Acta Radiol. 2015;56(7):820–8.
137. Xiao H, Bao F, Tan H, Wang B, Liu W, Gao J, et al. CT and clinical findings of peripheral primitive neuroectodermal tumour in children. Br J Radiol. 2016;89(1060):20140450.
138. Folpe AL, Goldblum JR, Rubin BP, Shehata BM, Liu W, Dei Tos AP, et al. Morphologic and immunophenotypic diversity in Ewing family tumors: a study of 66 genetically confirmed cases. Am J Surg Pathol. 2005;29(8):1025–33.
139. Nascimento AG, Unii KK, Pritchard DJ, Cooper KL, Dahlin DC. A clinicopathologic study of 20 cases of large-cell (atypical) Ewing's sarcoma of bone. Am J Surg Pathol. 1980;4(1):29–36.
140. Machado I, Noguera R, Mateos EA, Calabuig-Farinas S, Lopez FI, Martinez A, et al. The many faces of atypical Ewing's sarcoma. A true entity mimicking sarcomas, carcinomas and lymphomas. Virchows Arch. 2011;458(3):281–90.
141. Ozdemirli M, Fanburg-Smith JC, Hartmann DP, Azumi N, Miettinen M. Differentiating lymphoblastic lymphoma and Ewing's sarcoma: lymphocyte markers and gene rearrangement. Mod Pathol. 2001;14(11):1175–82.

142. Granter SR, Renshaw AA, Fletcher CD, Bhan AK, Rosenberg AE. CD99 reactivity in mesenchymal chondrosarcoma. Hum Pathol. 1996;27(12):1273–6.
143. Lae ME, Roche PC, Jin L, Lloyd RV, Nascimento AG. Desmoplastic small round cell tumor: a clinicopathologic, immunohistochemical, and molecular study of 32 tumors. Am J Surg Pathol. 2002;26(7):823–35.
144. Rossi S, Orvieto E, Furlanetto A, Laurino L, Ninfo V, Dei Tos AP. Utility of the immunohistochemical detection of FLI-1 expression in round cell and vascular neoplasm using a monoclonal antibody. Mod Pathol. 2004;17(5):547–52.
145. Lin O, Filippa DA, Teruya-Feldstein J. Immunohistochemical evaluation of FLI-1 in acute lymphoblastic lymphoma (ALL): a potential diagnostic pitfall. Appl Immunohistochem Mol Morphol. 2009;17(5):409–12.
146. Wang WL, Patel NR, Caragea M, Hogendoorn PC, Lopez-Terrada D, Hornick JL, et al. Expression of ERG, an Ets family transcription factor, identifies ERG-rearranged Ewing sarcoma. Mod Pathol. 2012;25(10):1378–83.
147. Turc-Carel C, Aurias A, Mugneret F, Lizard S, Sidaner I, Volk C, et al. Chromosomes in Ewing's sarcoma. I. An evaluation of 85 cases of remarkable consistency of t(11;22)(q24;q12). Cancer Genet Cytogenet. 1988;32(2):229–38.
148. Delattre O, Zucman J, Plougastel B, Desmaze C, Melot T, Peter M, et al. Gene fusion with an ETS DNA-binding domain caused by chromosome translocation in human tumours. Nature. 1992;359(6391):162–5.
149. Zucman J, Delattre O, Desmaze C, Plougastel B, Joubert I, Melot T, et al. Cloning and characterization of the Ewing's sarcoma and peripheral neuroepithelioma t(11;22) translocation breakpoints. Genes Chromosomes Cancer. 1992;5(4):271–7.
150. Sorensen PH, Lessnick SL, Lopez-Terrada D, Liu XF, Triche TJ, Denny CT. A second Ewing's sarcoma translocation, t(21;22), fuses the EWS gene to another ETS-family transcription factor, ERG. Nat Genet. 1994;6(2):146–51.
151. Jeon IS, Davis JN, Braun BS, Sublett JE, Roussel MF, Denny CT, et al. A variant Ewing's sarcoma translocation (7;22) fuses the EWS gene to the ETS gene ETV1. Oncogene. 1995;10(6):1229–34.
152. Peter M, Couturier J, Pacquement H, Michon J, Thomas G, Magdelenat H, et al. A new member of the ETS family fused to EWS in Ewing tumors. Oncogene. 1997;14(10):1159–64.
153. Ptaszynski K, Szumera-Cieckiewicz A, Pekul M, Nowecki Z. Differential diagnosis of small round cell tumours (SRCT), fluorescence in situ hybridization (FISH) and immunohistochemical (IHC) study. Pol J Pathol. 2009;60(4):151–62.
154. Machado I, Navarro L, Pellin A, Navarro S, Agaimy A, Tardio JC, et al. Defining Ewing and Ewing-like small round cell tumors (SRCT): the need for molecular techniques in their categorization and differential diagnosis. A study of 200 cases. Ann Diagn Pathol. 2016;22:25–32.
155. Chen QR, Vansant G, Oades K, Pickering M, Wei JS, Song YK, et al. Diagnosis of the small round blue cell tumors using multiplex polymerase chain reaction. J Mol Diagn. 2007;9(1):80–8.
156. Lewis TB, Coffin CM, Bernard PS. Differentiating Ewing's sarcoma from other round blue cell tumors using a RT-PCR translocation panel on formalin-fixed paraffin-embedded tissues. Mod Pathol. 2007;20(3):397–404.
157. Dispenzieri A. POEMS syndrome: 2011 update on diagnosis, risk-stratification, and management. Am J Hematol. 2011;86(7):591–601.
158. Palumbo A, Anderson K. Multiple myeloma. N Engl J Med. 2011;364(11):1046–60.
159. Kyle RA, Gertz MA, Witzig TE, Lust JA, Lacy MQ, Dispenzieri A, et al. Review of 1027 patients with newly diagnosed multiple myeloma. Mayo Clin Proc. 2003;78(1):21–33.
160. Kaya H, Peressini B, Jawed I, Martincic D, Elaimy AL, Lamoreaux WT, et al. Impact of age, race and decade of treatment on overall survival in a critical population analysis of 40,000 multiple myeloma patients. Int J Hematol. 2012;95(1):64–70.
161. Grogan T, Spier C. The B cell immunoproliferative disorders, including multiple myeloma and amyloidosis. Neoplastic hematopathology. Baltimore: Williams and Wilkins; 1992. p. 1235–65.

162. Kyle RA, Rajkumar SV. Multiple myeloma. N Engl J Med. 2004;351(18):1860–73.
163. Rajkumar SV, Dimopoulos MA, Palumbo A, Blade J, Merlini G, Mateos M-V, et al. International Myeloma Working Group updated criteria for the diagnosis of multiple myeloma. Lancet Oncol. 2014;15(12):e538–e48.
164. Chilosi M, Adami F, Lestani M, Montagna L, Cimarosto L, Semenzato G, et al. CD138/syndecan-1: a useful immunohistochemical marker of normal and neoplastic plasma cells on routine trephine bone marrow biopsies. Mod Pathol. 1999;12(12):1101–6.
165. Costes V, Magen V, Legouffe E, Durand L, Baldet P, Rossi JF, et al. The Mi15 monoclonal antibody (anti-syndecan-1) is a reliable marker for quantifying plasma cells in paraffin-embedded bone marrow biopsy specimens. Hum Pathol. 1999;30(12):1405–11.
166. O'Connell FP, Pinkus JL, Pinkus GS. CD138 (syndecan-1), a plasma cell marker immunohistochemical profile in hematopoietic and nonhematopoietic neoplasms. Am J Clin Pathol. 2004;121(2):254–63.
167. Harada H, Kawano MM, Huang N, Harada Y, Iwato K, Tanabe O, et al. Phenotypic difference of normal plasma cells from mature myeloma cells. Blood. 1993;81(10):2658–63.
168. Terstappen LW, Johnsen S, Segers-Nolten IM, Loken MR. Identification and characterization of plasma cells in normal human bone marrow by high-resolution flow cytometry. Blood. 1990;76(9):1739–47.
169. Falini B, Fizzotti M, Pucciarini A, Bigerna B, Marafioti T, Gambacorta M, et al. A monoclonal antibody (MUM1p) detects expression of the MUM1/IRF4 protein in a subset of germinal center B cells, plasma cells, and activated T cells. Blood. 2000;95(6):2084–92.
170. Rajkumar SV, Fonseca R, Dispenzieri A, Lacy MQ, Lust JA, Witzig TE, et al. Methods for estimation of bone marrow plasma cell involvement in myeloma: predictive value for response and survival in patients undergoing autologous stem cell transplantation. Am J Hematol. 2001;68(4):269–75.
171. Al-Quran SZ, Yang L, Magill JM, Braylan RC, Douglas-Nikitin VK. Assessment of bone marrow plasma cell infiltrates in multiple myeloma: the added value of CD138 immunohistochemistry. Hum Pathol. 2007;38(12):1779–87.
172. Ng AP, Wei A, Bhurani D, Chapple P, Feleppa F, Juneja S. The sensitivity of CD138 immunostaining of bone marrow trephine specimens for quantifying marrow involvement in MGUS and myeloma, including samples with a low percentage of plasma cells. Haematologica. 2006;91(7):972–5.
173. Frebet E, Abraham J, Genevieve F, Lepelley P, Daliphard S, Bardet V, et al. A GEIL flow cytometry consensus proposal for quantification of plasma cells: application to differential diagnosis between MGUS and myeloma. Cytometry B Clin Cytom. 2011;80(3):176–85.
174. Greipp PR, San Miguel J, Durie BG, Crowley JJ, Barlogie B, Blade J, et al. International staging system for multiple myeloma. J Clin Oncol. 2005;23(15):3412–20.
175. Palumbo A, Avet-Loiseau H, Oliva S, Lokhorst HM, Goldschmidt H, Rosinol L, et al. Revised International Staging System for Multiple Myeloma: a report from International Myeloma Working Group. J Clin Oncol. 2015;33(26):2863–9.
176. International Myeloma Working Group. Criteria for the classification of monoclonal gammopathies, multiple myeloma and related disorders: a report of the International Myeloma Working Group. Br J Haematol. 2003;121(5):749–57.
177. Soutar R, Lucraft H, Jackson G, Reece A, Bird J, Low E, et al. Guidelines on the diagnosis and management of solitary plasmacytoma of bone and solitary extramedullary plasmacytoma. Clin Oncol (R Coll Radiol). 2004;16(6):405–13.
178. Horsman JM, Thomas J, Hough R, Hancock BW. Primary bone lymphoma: a retrospective analysis. Int J Oncol. 2006;28(6):1571–5.
179. Kitsoulis P, Vlychou M, Papoudou-Bai A, Karatzias G, Charchanti A, Agnantis NJ, et al. Primary lymphomas of bone. Anticancer Res. 2006;26(1A):325–37.
180. Ostrowski ML, Unni KK, Banks PM, Shives TC, Evans RG, O'Connell MJ, et al. Malignant lymphoma of bone. Cancer. 1986;58(12):2646–55.
181. Messina C, Christie D, Zucca E, Gospodarowicz M, Ferreri AJ. Primary and secondary bone lymphomas. Cancer Treat Rev. 2015;41(3):235–46.

182. Alencar A, Pitcher D, Byrne G Jr, Lossos IS. Primary bone lymphoma–the University of Miami experience. Leuk Lymphoma. 2010;51(1):39–49.
183. Gianelli U, Patriarca C, Moro A, Ponzoni M, Giardini R, Massimino M, et al. Lymphomas of the bone: a pathological and clinical study of 54 cases. Int J Surg Pathol. 2002;10(4):257–66.
184. Glotzbecker MP, Kersun LS, Choi JK, Wills BP, Schaffer AA, Dormans JP. Primary non-Hodgkin's lymphoma of bone in children. J Bone Joint Surg Am. 2006;88(3):583–94.
185. Heyning FH, Hogendoorn PC, Kramer MH, Hermans J, Kluin-Nelemans JC, Noordijk EM, et al. Primary non-Hodgkin's lymphoma of bone: a clinicopathological investigation of 60 cases. Leukemia. 1999;13(12):2094–8.
186. Lieberman PH, Jones CR, Steinman RM, Erlandson RA, Smith J, Gee T, et al. Langerhans cell (eosinophilic) granulomatosis. A clinicopathologic study encompassing 50 years. Am J Surg Pathol. 1996;20(5):519–52.
187. Wester SM, Beabout JW, Unni KK, Dahlin DC. Langerhans' cell granulomatosis (histiocytosis X) of bone in adults. Am J Surg Pathol. 1982;6(5):413–26.
188. Tani M, Ishii N, Kumagai M, Ban M, Sasase A, Mishima Y. Malignant Langerhans cell tumour. Br J Dermatol. 1992;126(4):398–403.
189. Pileri S, Grogan T, Harris N, Banks P, Campo E, Chan J, et al. Tumours of histiocytes and accessory dendritic cells: an immunohistochemical approach to classification from the International Lymphoma Study Group based on 61 cases. Histopathology. 2002;41(1):1–29.
190. Jaffe R, Weiss LM, Facchetti F. Tumours derived from Langerhans cells. In: Swerdlow SH, Campo E, Harris NL, Jaffe ES, Pileri SA, Stein H, et al., editors. WHO classification of tumours of haematopoietic and lymphoid tissues. Lyon: IARC; 2008. p. 358–60.
191. Emile JF, Wechsler J, Brousse N, Boulland ML, Cologon R, Fraitag S, et al. Langerhans' cell histiocytosis. Definitive diagnosis with the use of monoclonal antibody O10 on routinely paraffin-embedded samples. Am J Surg Pathol. 1995;19(6):636–41.
192. Ioachim HL, Medeiros LJ. Ioachim's lymph node pathology. Philadelphia: Lippincott Williams & Wilkins; 2009.
193. Ahmed A, Crowson N, Magro CM. A comprehensive assessment of cutaneous Rosai-Dorfman disease. Ann Diagn Pathol. 2019;40:166–73.
194. Kenn W, Eck M, Allolio B, Jakob F, Illg A, Marx A, et al. Erdheim-Chester disease: evidence for a disease entity different from Langerhans cell histiocytosis? Three cases with detailed radiological and immunohistochemical analysis. Hum Pathol. 2000;31(6):734–9.
195. Haroche J, Arnaud L, Cohen-Aubart F, Hervier B, Charlotte F, Emile J-F, et al. Erdheim-Chester disease. Rheum Dis Clin N Am. 2013;39(2):299–311.

Soft Tissue Tumour Pathology

7

Vanessa Tran and John Slavin

7.1 General Approach to Soft Tissue Tumours

The pathologist's approach to a soft tissue tumour firstly involves understanding the clinical and radiological situation. Knowledge of such features, in conjunction with pathological assessment, allows for consideration of the likely differential diagnoses. Factors that are considered include the age of the patient (Table 7.1) and the size and location of the (Table 7.2) It is also useful to know which tissue layer the tumour has arisen within—if it is superficial, lies within the subcutaneous fat, is deep to the deep fascia or is located intramuscularly. It is also important to obtain the patient's past medical history, as some tumours have associations or may be part of a syndrome. Neurofibromatosis-1 (NF-1), for example, is a genetic syndrome that is associated with development of neurofibromas and malignant peripheral nerve sheath tumours (MPNST) [1–3]. Familial adenomatous polyposis (FAP) is another syndrome, caused by a germline mutation in the adenomatous polyposis coli (APC) gene, that is associated with intra-abdominal desmoid fibromatosis [4–6]. Desmoid fibromatosis is also associated with pregnancy and often occurs within the abdominal wall in this patient population [7–9].

7.2 Handling Biopsy Specimens

Initial sampling of tumours by core biopsy can provide enough tissue for diagnosis, which includes the use of ancillary tests such as immunohistochemistry (IHC), flow cytometry, molecular testing and cultures of micro-organisms. Fresh tissue is

V. Tran (✉)
Department of Surgery, University of Melbourne, Melbourne, VIC, Australia

J. Slavin
Department of Anatomical Pathology, St. Vincent's Hospital Melbourne, Melbourne, VIC, Australia
e-mail: john.slavin@svha.org.au

P. F. M. Choong (ed.), *Sarcoma*, https://doi.org/10.1007/978-981-15-9414-4_7

Table 7.1 Summary of common soft tissue tumours based on age of patient [183]

Age	Soft tissue tumour
Infants (<3 years)	Infantile fibrosarcoma Inclusion body fibromatosis Fibrous hamartoma of infancy Lipoblastoma Myofibroma
Paediatric	Embryonal rhabdomyosarcoma Extrarenal rhabdoid tumour
Adolescence and young adults (<30 years)	Synovial sarcoma Alveolar rhabdomyosarcoma Alveolar soft part sarcoma Epithelioid sarcoma Epithelioid haemangioendothelioma Desmoplastic small round cell tumour Low-grade fibromyxoid sarcoma Myxoid liposarcoma Inflammatory myofibroblastic sarcoma Nodular fasciitis
Adults (<40 years)	Clear cell sarcoma Dermatofibrosarcoma protuberans Epithelioid haemangioendothelioma Fibroma of tendon sheath Myositis ossificans
Adults (middle age)	Intramuscular myxoma Spindle cell lipoma Liposarcoma well-differentiated and dedifferentiated types Extraskeletal myxoid chondrosarcoma Solitary fibrous tumour
Elderly/older adults	Atypical fibroxanthoma Myofibrosarcoma Undifferentiated pleomorphic sarcoma

required for cultures and flow cytometry, as well as some molecular analyses. Once the tissue has been triaged, cores are fixed in formalin, processed and embedded in paraffin wax. Tissue is then cut and stained with haematoxylin and eosin (H&E). The tissue should be used sparingly to preserve remaining tissue for IHC or molecular testing. In some centres, fine needle aspiration (FNA) cytology is used. The problems encountered for both core samples and FNA include difficulty sampling the tumour, obtaining insufficient amount of tissue for testing and sampling areas of necrosis or haemorrhage. Tumours that are heterogeneous or have areas of dedifferentiation can also lead to diagnostic inaccuracies. Neural tumours and retroperitoneal liposarcomas, for example, often have variable areas. Sometimes, a definitive diagnosis cannot be reached from the core sample, and some reports are limited to descriptive information, such as "low-grade myxoid tumour, probably benign". In these circumstances, the type of re-biopsy required, whether a repeat core or local excision, needs to be carefully considered. The core biopsy tract is often excised, and the path of the biopsy needs consideration to avoid uninvolved tissue

Table 7.2 Summary of common soft tissue tumours that arise in sites and locations of the body [183]

Anatomical site	Soft tissue tumour
Distal tumours (fingers, toes, palm)	Fibromatosis Fibroma of tendon sheath Glomus tumour Soft tissue chondroma Epithelioid sarcoma
Limbs	Myxoid liposarcoma Well-differentiated liposarcoma Synovial sarcoma
Girdle and trunk	Fibromatosis Elastofibroma (scapular) Spindle cell lipoma (back of neck) Dermatofibrosarcoma protuberans
Head and neck	Embryonal rhabdomyosarcoma Synovial sarcoma Alveolar soft part sarcoma
Retroperitoneum	Well-differentiated and dedifferentiated liposarcoma Schwannoma Perivascular epithelioid cell tumour (PEComa)
Intra-abdominal (mesentery, peritoneum)	Fibromatosis Desmoplastic small round cell tumour Inflammatory myofibroblastic tumour Gastrointestinal stromal tumour

compartments. Advantages of core biopsies include the ability to perform it as an outpatient procedure, the low risk of morbidity and its ability to diagnose other tumour types, including carcinoma, melanoma, lymphoma and infections.

7.3 Classification of Soft Tissue Tumours

Soft tissue tumours are diverse in their classification, and their behaviour is predicted by the diagnostic classification and tumour grade. Given that each tumour subtype is unique in its clinical behaviour, prognosis and treatment, accurate diagnosis is essential. Soft tissue tumour behaviour can first be differentiated into benign, intermediate or malignant types. Benign tumours often lack the ability to invade surrounding tissues and respond favourable to treatment. Those with intermediate biologic potential may be locally aggressive and carry a minimal risk for metastasis, while malignant neoplasms are both locally aggressive and have metastatic potential.

Classification of soft tissue tumours is based on the lineage of the tumour by recognising the type of normal, differentiated mesenchymal tissue that the tumour exhibits. This can be achieved by observing the appearance of the tumour on H&E sections but may often require further immunohistochemical profiling and, in some cases, molecular testing. Tumours can be subdivided into large groups based on differentiation and morphology (Table 7.3). Within each group, there are benign,

Table 7.3 Summary of classification of tumours based on line of differentiation [183]

Class	Soft tissue tumour
Adipose	Angiolipoma Spindle cell lipoma Liposarcoma (further subtypes)
Fibroblastic/ myofibroblastic	Fibroma tendon sheath Desmoid-type fibromatosis Solitary fibrous tumour Myxofibrosarcoma
So-called fibrohistiocytic	Langerhans cell histiocytosis Histiocytic sarcoma
Pericytic (perivascular)	Glomus tumour Myofibroma Angiomyoma
Smooth muscle tumours	Leiomyoma Leiomyosarcoma
Skeletal muscle tumours	Rhabdomyoma Rhabdomyosarcoma
Vascular tumours	Papillary endothelial hyperplasia Haemangioma (subtypes)
Epithelioid tumours	Haemangioendothelioma Angiosarcoma
Chondro-osseous tumours	Synovial chondromatosis Extraskeletal mesenchymal chondrosarcoma
Gastrointestinal stromal tumours	Gastrointestinal stromal tumour
Nerve sheath tumours	Schwannoma Neurofibroma Granular cell tumour Malignant peripheral nerve sheath tumour
Tumours of uncertain differentiation	Myxoma Myoepithelioma Synovial sarcoma Epithelioid sarcoma Clear cell sarcoma Alveolar soft part sarcoma Extraskeletal myxoid sarcoma Ewing's sarcoma
Undifferentiated/ unclassified tumours	Undifferentiated pleomorphic sarcoma Undifferentiated sarcomas with molecular changes (CIC-DUX4 translocation or BCOR-CCNB3 fusion-positive sarcoma)

intermediate and malignant subtypes, in addition to many morphologic variants with diverse appearances. These include pleomorphic appearances, spindle cells, epithelioid cells, round cells, biphasic and mixed patterns, myxoid changes, sclerosis and inflammatory changes. In cases where a line of differentiation is difficult to determine, immunohistochemistry can be useful in determining the protein expression of the tumour cells that can indicate their lineage.

7.4 Immunohistochemistry (IHC)

Immunoprofiles are not only useful in identifying the lineage of a tumour but also in supporting the diagnosis of rare tumours or tumours that have occurred in unusual situations or sites. The technique employs manufactured antibodies that bind to and identify the proteins (antigens) expressed by cells. Technical aspects of this method will influence its ability to detect an antigen in tumour tissue. Firstly, there needs to be enough representative tissue that is well processed. Identifiable tumour tissue needs to be present in the sample. In addition, controls are required to confirm that the test has worked. There are a wide variety of antibodies available, and these are used in a panel to distinguish between histologically similar tumours with different immunoprofiles.

Pleomorphic carcinoma, melanoma and pleomorphic sarcoma are three distinct types of tumours that can appear histologically similar under the microscope. They can be distinguished, however, based on their differing immunoprofiles. Epithelial markers, such as keratin, are expressed in majority of carcinomas [10], whereas markers S100 and Melan A are found in melanoma. In the case of pleomorphic sarcoma, on the other hand, no specific expression should be seen.

One limitation with IHC is the overlap in tumour immunoprofiles, and the markers used have variable specificity and sensitivity. In addition, there can be patchy expression of the antigen within the tumour, so a negative result may be due to a sampling issue. Interpretation of IHC stains requires knowledge of the staining pattern of the antibody and the expected result for each disease.

In some tumours, there is a characteristic staining pattern and localisation that can be detected. In Ewing's sarcoma, for example, IHC for CD99 characteristically shows strong, diffusely positive staining of the cell membrane [11, 12], whereas in solitary fibrous tumours, staining of STAT6 demonstrates strong nuclear expression [13, 14]. In smooth muscle tumours, on the other hand, staining for smooth muscle actin (SMA) is seen in the cytoplasm of cells [15, 16]. Another immunohistochemical marker, INI1 (SMARCB1), is expressed in the nucleus of normal cells but is often absent in tumours such as malignant rhabdoid tumours and epithelioid sarcoma [17].

7.4.1 Epithelial Markers

Keratins are widely expressed in epithelial cells and are encountered in some soft tissue tumours. These markers are necessary in the diagnosis of epithelioid sarcoma [18], synovial sarcoma [19–22] and desmoplastic round cell tumour [23, 24]. Positivity is also often encountered in tumours including epithelioid angiosarcoma [25], leiomyosarcoma [26] and rhabdomyosarcoma [27].

7.4.2 Myogenic Markers

Various muscular markers are useful in identifying smooth muscle and skeletal muscle tumours. Smooth muscle markers include smooth muscle actin (SMA) and muscle-specific actin (HHF35). SMA is almost invariably positive in smooth muscle tumours, benign and malignant [28–30]. It is also seen in myofibroblastic, myoepithelial and glomus tumours [28]. HHF35, on the other hand, is a monoclonal antibody against muscle actin that stains rhabdomyosarcomas [31]. Desmin is another myogenic marker that is positive in both smooth and skeletal muscle lineages, as well as myofibroblastic lesions and desmoplastic small round cell tumours [23, 32, 33]. In order to support smooth muscle differentiation, h-caldesmon can be used as it is negative for myofibroblastic and skeletal muscle tumours [34]. Skeletal muscle markers include myogenin and MyoD1, which are skeletal muscle-specific transcription factors that show nuclear positivity in rhabdomyosarcoma [35].

7.4.3 Endothelial (Vascular) Markers

CD31 and CD34 are useful markers in identifying vascular tumours. CD34 is normally expressed in vascular endothelial cells, although stains many soft tissue tumours, such as vascular tumours, dermatofibrosarcoma protuberans (DFSP), solitary fibrous tumour, peripheral nerve sheath tumours (PNSTs) and epithelioid sarcoma [36]. CD31 is a more specific and sensitive endothelial marker than CD34. Its positivity is indicative of malignant vascular tumours, such as epithelioid haemangioma, angiosarcoma and Kaposi's sarcoma [37, 38]. More recently, the ETS family transcription factors, ERG and FLI-1, have been shown to stain vascular tumours [39, 40]. D2-40 is a novel marker for lymphatic endothelium that stains positively in Kaposi's sarcoma and other vascular lesions [41, 42].

7.4.4 Neural Crest/Melanoma Markers

Neural crest markers are best used in panels as these markers are non-specific and positive in various tumours, including PNST, clear cell sarcoma and melanoma. S100, for example, is positive in schwannomas but also stains other peripheral nerve tumours, including neurofibroma, granular cell tumour and malignant PNST tumours [43–45]. In addition, they have demonstrated positivity in melanoma [46], clear cell sarcoma [47, 48], extraskeletal myxoid chondrosarcoma [49, 50] and myoepithelioma [44, 51, 52]. Other markers, Melan-A, MiTF and HMB45 all demonstrate positivity in melanoma, PEComa and clear cell sarcoma [53–56]. SOX10 stains melanoma, benign and malignant PNSTs and myoepithelioma, while H3K27me3 shows loss of nuclear staining in malignant peripheral nerve sheath tumours [57]. Despite their non-specific staining, the use of a panel of neural crest markers can be diagnostically valuable.

7.4.5 Other Useful Markers

There are also a number of other markers that are useful in the diagnosis of soft tissue tumours. TLE1 is a marker that shows strong, diffuse nuclear expression in synovial sarcoma [58, 59]. It demonstrates reasonable specificity for synovial sarcoma; however it is also seen in other tumours, such as solitary fibrous tumour and malignant peripheral nerve sheath tumour [60]. STAT6 is a highly specific marker for solitary fibrous tumour [61]. In the diagnosis of gastrointestinal tumours, DOG1 and cKIT are useful markers [62–65].

7.5 Grading Sarcoma

In conjunction with histologic classification, tumours are graded to predict the outcome and risk of metastases in soft tissue sarcomas. The most commonly used grading system is the French Federation of Cancer Centers Sarcoma Group (FNCLCC) grading system. This scores three histologic factors—(1) degree of cellular differentiation, (2) mitotic rate and (3) percentage of necrosis. Each factor is scored and the total determines the grade (Table 7.4).

7.6 Problems and Limitations of Grading

There are multiple limitations to grading soft tissue tumours. Firstly, the heterogeneity of some tumours can lead to sampling errors, and core biopsies may not be representative of the whole tumour. Cellular differentiation and mitotic areas can

Table 7.4 Summary of criteria and scoring matrix for FNCLCC grading system [184]

Differentiation scores	
Score 1	Well-differentiated tumours resembling normal mesenchymal tissue
Score 2	The histologic type is certain
Score 3	Embryonal and undifferentiated sarcomas, synovial sarcoma and sarcomas of uncertain differentiation
Mitotic rate scores (mitoses per 10 high-power fields)	
Score 1	0–9 mitoses
Score 2	10–19 mitoses
Score 3	>19 mitoses
Tumour necrosis score	
Score 1	No necrosis
Score 2	Necrosis <50% of total tumour volume
Score 3	Necrosis ≥50% of total tumour volume
Histologic grade	
Grade 1	**Total score: 2–3**
Grade 2	**Total score: 4–5**
Grade 3	**Total score: 6–8**

vary throughout a tumour and may therefore not be accurately captured through core sampling. Necrotic areas may also be under-represented as these areas tend to be avoided to target viable tumour that carries diagnostic value. Resection specimens that have received preoperative radiotherapy or chemotherapy often show altered histology that cannot be accurately graded.

In some tumours, histologic classification defines the grade of the tumour. For example, infantile fibrosarcoma, well-differentiated liposarcoma and standard dermatofibrosarcoma protuberans are, by definition, Grade 1. Angiosarcoma, Ewing's sarcoma, embryonal and alveolar rhabdomyosarcoma, malignant rhabdoid tumours and mesenchymal chondrosarcoma, on the other hand, are high-grade tumours. In some tumours, grading adds little value. Examples of these include alveolar soft part sarcoma, epithelioid sarcoma, clear cell sarcoma and extraskeletal myxoid chondrosarcoma.

7.7 Sarcoma Staging

The American Joint Committee on Cancer (AJCC) uses the Tumour Node Metastasis (TNM) classification for soft tissue sarcomas of the trunk, extremities and retroperitoneum, with separate criteria for other sites. Recently, the AJCC has added Grade to produce Anatomic Stage/Prognostic groups (Tables 7.5 and 7.6).

7.8 Diagnostic Approach to Soft Tissue Tumours with Overlap Patterns

The histologic pattern of different soft tissue tumours can often overlap and be source of confusion in diagnosis. When assessing the pathology of a tumour, the first step is to identify the pattern of the tumour to create a list of differentials.

Table 7.5 Summary of criteria for TNM classification for primary tumour [185]

T category	
Tx	Primary tumour cannot be assessed
T0	No evidence of primary tumour
T1	Tumour 5 cm or less
T2	Tumour greater than 5 cm and less than or equal to 10 cm
T3	Tumour greater than 10 cm and less than or equal to 15 cm
T4	Tumour greater than 15 cm
Regional nodes	
N0	No regional lymph node metastasis
N1	Regional lymph node metastasis
Distant metastasis	
M0	No distant metastasis
M1	Distant metastasis

Table 7.6 Summary of criteria for AJCC Prognostic Stage Group [186]

T	N	M	G (grade)	Stage Group
T1	N0	M0	G1, GX	IA
T2, T3, T4	N0	M0	G1, GX	IB
T1	N0	M0	G2, G3	II
T2	N0	M0	G2, G3	IIIA
T3, T4	N0	M0	G2, G3	IIIB
Any T	N1	M0	Any G	IV
Any T	N0	M1	Any G	IV

GX Grade cannot be assessed

Common overlap patterns include spindle cell, epithelioid, round cell, pleomorphic, biphasic/mixed and myxoid tumours. After the histological features are determined, further ancillary tests can be applied to inform the diagnosis. This section will discuss each morphological pattern and their associated differentials.

7.9 Spindle Cell Pattern

Spindle cell lesions can be of both mesenchymal and non-mesenchymal lineage. Non-mesenchymal lesions include spindle cell carcinoma and melanoma. Mesenchymal tumours with a spindle cell pattern are very common and can be further subdivided into reactive, benign or malignant proliferations. Examples of spindle cell tumours are smooth muscle tumours, nerve sheath tumours, nodular fasciitis, solitary fibrous tumour, synovial sarcoma, dermatofibrosarcoma protuberans and fibromatosis. Given the vast and diverse differentials within the spindle cell group of tumours, other histological factors must be assessed to determine the correct diagnosis. This includes consideration of the architectural arrangement of the cells, the growth pattern, associated vascular pattern, background stroma or matrix, mitoses and necrosis [66].

Typically, smooth muscle tumours will have eosinophilic cytoplasm and blunt-ended cigar-shaped nuclei with variable nuclear atypia (Fig. 7.1). The cells are arranged in bundles or fascicles and are often perpendicular to one another. The tumours can be well-circumscribed or infiltrative and can show associated myxoid, hyaline and calcific change. Assessing mitoses and necrosis is important in distinguishing leiomyoma from leiomyosarcoma [66].

Cutaneous leiomyomas (CLMs) can be associated with hereditary leiomyomatosis and renal cell cancer (HLRCC) syndrome and, in this context, may appear as multiple lesions [67, 68]. Deep, non-uterine soft tissue leiomyosarcoma can arise from femoral or retroperitoneal vessels, such as the inferior vena cava [69, 70].

Schwannoma is a well-circumscribed, encapsulated mass arising eccentrically from a nerve. Histologically, it exhibits plump spindle cells arranged in variable cellular fascicles with hypercellular areas (Antoni A) and hypocellular areas (Antoni B). These cells have indistinct cytoplasmic borders and focal nuclear atypical with some pseudonuclear inclusions [71]. The atypia can be marked in

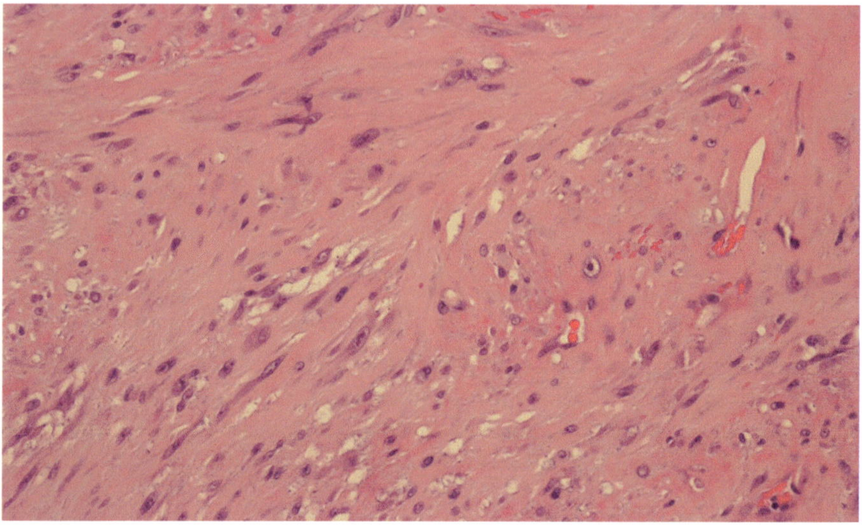

Fig. 7.1 Leiomyosarcoma containing spindle cells with "cigar-shaped" nuclei and strap-like eosinophilic cytoplasm

"ancient" schwannomas, which are tumours that show extensive degenerative changes [72]. Nuclear palisading can also often be seen [71]. Thick-walled, hyalinised vessels with areas of haemosiderin deposition and focal chronic inflammation are often present in the stroma. Schwannomas can be painful and present at any age, often located in the upper and lower extremities, retroperitoneum, posterior mediastinum and head and neck regions [66]. Most schwannomas are sporadic, though some are associated with neurofibromatosis and schwannomatosis [73, 74].

Dermatofibrosarcoma protuberans (DFSP) is an infiltrative, ill-defined, spindle cell proliferation involving the dermis and subcutaneous fat. It extends along fibrous septa within the subcutis, entrapping fat and infiltrating skeletal muscle. The uniform cells are arranged in a storiform pattern and have mild nuclear enlargement and atypia [66, 75]. In some DFSP, intracytoplasmic melanin can be seen [76]. The stroma is usually collagenous, sometimes with myxoid change [77]. IHC staining shows the cells are strongly and diffusely positive for CD34 [78]. There can be progression to a higher grade with fibrosarcomatous transformation, where there is increased cellularity, fascicular or herringbone pattern, more pronounced nuclear atypia, increased mitotic activity and the presence of necrosis [79]. DFSP occurs on the trunk and extremities as a slow-growing nodular mass in young to middle-aged adults [80]. Local recurrences are common and can be multicentric if the lesion is not completely and widely excised [81–83]. Due to the infiltrative growth pattern of the lesion, the full extent of disease can often be difficult to assess, as its spread along fibrous septa cannot be easily visualised or palpated. Metastasis in conventional DFSP is rare; however fibrosarcomatous transformation is associated with increased metastatic risk. DFSP harbours a characteristic t(17;22) translocation that results in a COL1A-PDGFB fusion [84, 85]. This makes the tumour sensitive to the tyrosine kinase receptor inhibitor, imatinib [86, 87].

Fibromatosis has an infiltrative growth pattern comprised of bland, uniform, elongated spindle cells with thin, elongated, tapering nuclei. The cells are arranged in sweeping fascicles and set in collagenous stroma. There is a vague nodularity, and in certain places, prominent small vessels stand out [66]. IHC demonstrates nuclear positivity with beta-catenin and some cytoplasmic SMA positivity [88, 89]. Sporadic deep fibromatoses have somatic mutations in CTNNB1 gene [90]. Germline mutations in the APC gene are seen in FAP/Gardner syndrome [91]. Fibromatosis presents in both superficial (palmar or plantar) or deep sites, where they can involve the abdominal wall (rectus abdominis muscle), extra-abdominal (shoulder, pelvis, chest wall, proximal limbs, axilla and head and neck) and intra-abdominal sites (mesentery and pelvis) [66]. They are locally aggressive with variable rate of growth. Up to 5% of tumours can be multicentric, often within the same region or limb, but do not metastasise [92–94].

Solitary fibrous tumours (SFT) are comprised of a variable mix of spindle cells and collagenous stroma. The cells are rounded to spindle shaped with scant cytoplasm and uniform appearance. The nuclei are uniform and oval and have vesicular chromatin. The cells are arranged in small clusters and short fascicles with non-specific, "patternless" architecture. Thin-walled vessels have a staghorn branching appearance, with other thicker-walled vessels showing hyalinised walls [66, 95]. IHC demonstrates CD34 and STAT6 positivity [13, 14]. SFT commonly carries a NAB2-STAT6 gene fusion resulting in upregulation of STAT6 [96]. SFT is a slow-growing mass of the deep tissue in the extremities, retroperitoneum, pleura and visceral organs [97, 98]. Prognostic factors include age, size greater than 15 cm, mitotic index greater than 4 per 10 high-power fields (HPF) and necrosis [66, 99]. Dedifferentiation areas can show loss of CD34 staining [100].

Synovial sarcoma is a monotonous spindle cell proliferation with variable epithelial differentiation. The tumour may be monophasic with a predominance of spindle cells, biphasic with prominent epithelial appearance or poorly differentiated cellular proliferation with small round to spindle-shaped cells [101]. The cells have indistinct cytoplasm and uniform crowding and overlapping nuclei in short fascicles (Fig. 7.2). Wiry or hyalinised collagenous stroma with calcification is relatively commonly seen. Ectatic thin-walled vessels with staghorn branching pattern are common. IHC staining for cytokeratin subtypes CK7 and CK19 is almost exclusive to synovial sarcoma, though not expressed in all cases [102]. EMA is positive in epithelial areas and expressed in almost all synovial sarcoma but lacks specificity [101, 103]. CD34 and desmin are typically negative [104]. S100 can be positive in some cases, which may confuse the diagnosis for MPNST [22, 105, 106]. TLE1 showing strong diffuse nuclear expression is seen in virtually all synovial sarcoma but is also seen in some malignant nerve sheath tumours and solitary fibrous tumours [58, 60, 107]. A characteristic balanced translocation t(x;18) results in a SS18-SSX fusion oncogene [108, 109], with some variation in SS18's partner, being SSX1, SSX2 or other unusual variants [110–112]. Detection methods include cytogenetic karyotyping, FISH or reverse polymerase chain reaction (RT-PCR) [109, 113, 114].

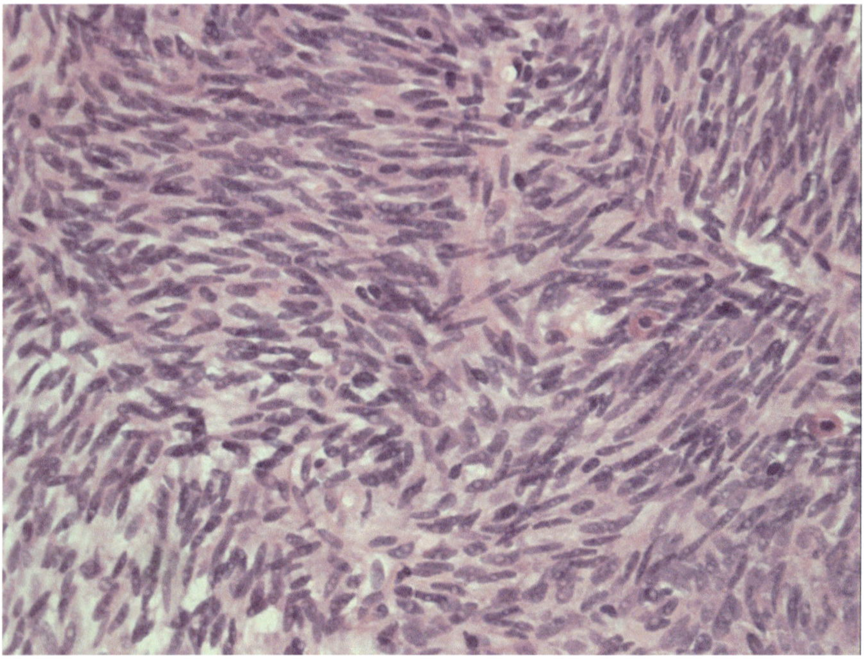

Fig. 7.2 Synovial sarcoma with uniform, monotonous spindle cells arranged in short fascicles

Synovial sarcoma often presents as a slow-growing, sometimes painful, mass, usually located in deep soft tissue of the extremities, often the popliteal fossa close to a neurovascular bundle, the pleura or the head and neck region [115]. Metastases, which can occur years to decades later, typically appear in the lung, bone and rarely lymph nodes [115].

7.10 Epithelioid Mesenchymal Tumours

Soft tissue tumours with large polygonal or small cells may resemble carcinoma, melanoma or large lymphoma, and these therefore need to be excluded. In addition, there are epithelioid variants of mesenchymal tumours, including leiomyosarcoma, fibrosarcoma, GIST and vascular and neural tumours.

Epithelioid sarcoma (ES) is composed of epithelioid cells with abundant eosinophilic cytoplasm, vesicular nuclei with small nucleoli and a collagenous stroma. The cells are arranged in small aggregates and form nodules, often with areas of central necrosis, which give a pseudo-granulomatous appearance. Vascular and perineural infiltration is often seen. There is low mitotic activity and calcification may be present. IHC shows cells to be reactive to keratins and EMA. CD34 is positive in up to 50% of cases. The SMARCB1 (INI1) tumour suppressor gene is inactivated in ES, and IHC for INI1 shows loss of nuclear staining. Conventional ES presents as a firm slow-growing nodule in the skin (hands, wrist and forearm) of young adults. A proximal variant, involving the pelvis or axilla, occurs in an older age group and carries a worse prognosis. Local recurrence is common and may be seen more proximally in the affected limb and is reduced by wide excision. ES can have a protracted course over many years.

Alveolar soft part sarcoma (ASPS) shows large epithelioid cells with abundant cytoplasm that may be eosinophilic, granular or clear. The cells can be arranged in nests, which can be solid, or the cells are discohesive and form the alveolar pattern. The nests are surrounded by thin wall vessels. PAS-positive, diastase-resistant intracytoplasmic granules and crystals can be demonstrated. IHC staining is used to rule out other differentials; however TFE3 is often positive in ASPS. ASPS has a characteristic unbalanced t(X;17) translocation with TLE3 fusing with ASPSCR1.

7.11 Round Cell Mesenchymal Tumours

Round cell malignancies include both mesenchymal and non-mesenchymal tumours. Non-mesenchymal tumours include lymphoma, melanoma and some carcinomas (Merkel cell and small cell carcinoma). Mesenchymal round cell tumours include rhabdomyosarcoma, neuroblastoma, desmoplastic small round cell tumour, poorly differentiated synovial sarcoma, Ewing's sarcoma and undifferentiated round cell sarcomas (previously called Ewing-like/atypical Ewing), CIC-rearranged sarcoma and BCOR-rearranged sarcoma [66]. Round cell areas can be seen in myxoid liposarcoma and mesenchymal chondrosarcoma. There is a major role for IHC and molecular typing in this category of tumours [116, 117]. These tumours often occur in children and younger adults and therefore have different treatment protocols [66].

Rhabdomyosarcoma is the most common soft tissue sarcoma in children [118, 119]. Subtypes include alveolar, embryonal, spindle cell/sclerosing and pleomorphic [120]. Alveolar rhabdomyosarcoma (ARMS) shows highly cellular nests and sheets of round cells with fibrous septa and loss of cellular cohesion that form alveolar spaces. Some cells have elongated strap-like shape with the appearance of rhabdomyoblasts. Wreath-like multinucleated giant cells can also be seen. Mitoses are prominent and necrosis may be seen. IHC demonstrates desmin positivity [121, 122]. Newer markers, myogenin and MyoD1, show nuclear positivity and are highly specific for RMS [35, 123–125]. Approximately 80% of ARMS have chromosomal translocations t(2;13) and t(1;13) resulting in FOX01 fusion with either PAX3 or PAX7. FOX01-PAX3 fusion has shown worse prognosis than a PAX7 fusion [126]. These tumours occur as a rapidly enlarging mass in adolescents/young adults in the deep soft tissue of extremities, paraspinal areas and head and neck. Embryonal rhabdomyosarcomas (ERMS) are more common than ARMS and occur in the younger age group, most commonly in the first decade of life. It is often located in the urogenital tract or head and neck sites.

7.12 Myxoid Tumours

Myxoid tumours of the soft tissue are a broad, heterogeneous group of tumours that are characterised by their abundance of extracellular matrix. These tumours range from benign lesions, such as myxoma, angiomyxoma and myoepithelioma, to malignant tumours, such as extraskeletal myxoid chondrosarcoma, low-grade fibromyxoid sarcoma and myxofibrosarcoma. The significant overlap in morphological features can often present a diagnostic challenge for pathologists. In addition, there are some non-myxoid tumours that can sometimes show a myxoid stroma under the microscope, such as PNSTs, DFSP, synovial sarcoma and SFT. Due to the wide-ranging clinical behaviours and different treatment courses, accurate diagnosis is essential in ensuring appropriate management. Thus, the incorporation of ancillary techniques such as IHC and cytogenetics can provide valuable information.

Low-grade fibromyxoid sarcoma (LGFMS) is a rather innocuous-appearing tumour that carries a deceptive risk of local recurrence and metastasis [127, 128]. It typically appears as a painless, large mass in the deep soft tissues of young to middle-aged patients [127–129]. The tumour is often a well-circumscribed lesion that demonstrates spindle cells of uniform appearance without nuclear atypia and few mitoses. A subset of these lesions show areas of palisading epithelioid cells surrounding a core of dense collagen core, forming characteristic "giant rosettes" [129, 130]. Immunohistochemically, MUC4 is a useful marker given its high sensitivity and specificity for LGFMS [131]. Majority of all cases harbour a characteristic t(7;16)(q34;p11) translocation resulting in the FUS-CREB3L2 fusion product [132].

Myxofibrosarcoma is a malignant myxoid tumour that commonly arises in the upper and lower limbs of elderly patients, with a slight male preponderance [133–136]. It has also been described in the trunk and head and neck regions and, less commonly, the skin, breast, heart and paratesticular areas [136]. It most commonly presents as a painless, slowly enlarging mass, most often within the subcutaneous tissue. Macroscopically, it appears as a multinodular grey-white mass with infiltrative margins [137]. Histological examination demonstrates a background of myxoid stroma containing few spindle or pleomorphic cells with small, hyperchromatic nuclei. Pseudolipoblasts may be encountered [66, 137]. Blood vessels take a characteristic thin-walled curvilinear shape, which can be useful for diagnosis [133, 134]. IHC is of limited use in diagnosing myxofibrosarcoma but may be useful to exclude other tumour types [66].

7.13 Adipocytic Tumours

Adipocytic tumours comprise a large group of heterogeneous tumours that display various pathological appearances and distinct clinical behaviours. These tumours can often present diagnostic challenges due to their overlapping features on histology. Benign fatty tumours include areas of fat necrosis, angiolipoma, hibernoma (brown fat), spindle cell lipoma, intramuscular lipoma and lipoblastoma. Angiolipomas often appear as multiple lesions and may be painful, particularly on palpation [138, 139]. Spindle cell lipomas often present on the upper back and neck of middle-aged males [140–142], while lipoblastomas typically present on the extremities of infants [143–145]. Liposarcomas are malignant adipocytic lesions that generally present as a large mass within the deeper tissue planes in adult patients. They tend to occur in the extremities, retroperitoneum and spermatic cord [146, 147]. There are various subtypes of liposarcomas, which have different pathological appearances and clinical behaviours. Adipose tissue may also be a component of other tumours such as angiomyolipoma, solitary fibrous tumour and angiomyofibroblastoma, adding to the complexity in diagnosing these lesions.

Well-differentiated liposarcomas (WDLPS) are one of the most common soft tissue neoplasms [148, 149]. Histologically, these lesions often demonstrate mature adipocytes with variable cell size and atypical, enlarged, hyperchromatic nuclei. There are often thickened fibrous septa that contain atypical spindle cells with enlarged hyperchromatic nuclei. Lipoblasts can sometimes be encountered, though their presence is not essential for diagnosis. Sclerosing liposarcoma shows abundant collagenous tissue [148]. Oftentimes, however, the tumours display lipoma-like features or lack cytologic atypia which makes the distinction of WDLPS from lipoma difficult. In these situations, ancillary molecular techniques are useful. WDLPS have characteristic ring or giant marker chromosome, which consistently harbour amplified sequences of the murine double minute 2 (MDM2) gene [150–152]. The gold-standard detection method for MDM2 amplification is FISH, and this can help to distinguish WDLPS from lipoma in ambiguous cases [85, 153–156]. WDLPS are low-grade tumours which carry a risk of local recurrence but lack metastatic potential [157]. However, there is also risk of dedifferentiation, particularly in retroperitoneal WDLPS [158–160].

Dedifferentiated liposarcoma (DDLPS) occurs when a WDLPS contains a spindle cell non-lipogenic sarcomatous component (Fig. 7.3). The dedifferentiated areas will show MDM2 amplification, which helps to distinguish DDLPS from other sarcoma types [161]. DDLPS has a 40–60% risk of local recurrence and, unlike WDLPS, has shown to metastasise in 15–20% of cases [159, 162].

Myxoid liposarcomas, which also include round cell liposarcomas, occur in the deep tissues of the extremities in young to middle-aged adults [163, 164]. The typical histological appearance shows myxoid stroma with mucin pools and thin branching capillary vessels described as "chicken wire" pattern. There is variable cellularity with hypocellular bland spindle cells, accompanied by uni- or bi-vacuolated lipoblasts. The presence of a round cell component, which demonstrates hypercellular sheets of undifferentiated round cells, represents a higher-grade tumour. When this comprises more than 5% of the total tumour, this confers a worse prognosis [165]. Metastatic disease has a unique non-pulmonary pattern and is common within the bone and soft tissues, including the retroperitoneum [166]. Immunohistochemically, the tumours can be S100 positive [167]. In 90% of cases, they demonstrate a characteristic t(12;16) translocation involving the DDIT3 and FUS genes [167–169].

Pleomorphic liposarcomas are aggressive neoplasms, which appear in the deep soft tissues of the extremities and retroperitoneum, typically in an older patient cohort [170–172]. Histological appearance is of a high grade, markedly pleomorphic tumour

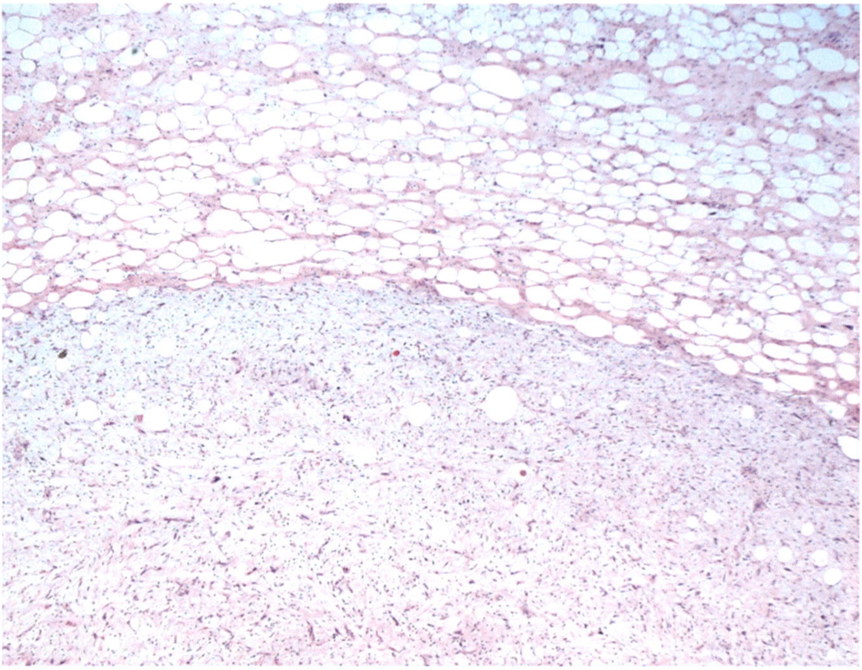

Fig. 7.3 Dedifferentiated liposarcoma showing a characteristic non-lipogenic, markedly atypical sarcomatous component (above) directly next to well-differentiated, fatty areas with mildly enlarged, hyperchromatic nuclei

with lipoblasts that have markedly atypical and bizarre nuclei. Unlike DDLPS, these tumours lack a well-differentiated component. Immunohistochemically, the lipoblasts are often S100 positive [171, 173]. The chromosomes demonstrate complex, non-specific changes [174]. Pleomorphic liposarcomas have an infiltrative growth pattern that is commonly associated with local recurrence and metastasis to the lungs, with an overall 5-year survival of approximately 50–60% [171, 172].

7.14 Undifferentiated Tumours

Undifferentiated or unclassified tumours encompass a subset of tumours that display markedly atypical cells in the absence of any obvious line of differentiation on histology. A prominent example of these tumours is undifferentiated pleomorphic sarcoma (UPS), a highly aggressive tumour that accounts for 5–10% of all sarcomas arising in adults [175–177]. Previously, UPS belonged to larger entity called malignant fibrous histiocytoma (MFH), a diagnosis previously given to poorly differentiated mesenchymal tumours that could not be otherwise classified [178]. With the addition of ancillary testing, it is now understood that MFH encompassed a heterogeneous group of both mesenchymal and non-mesenchymal tumours, which shared similar histological features [175]. Nowadays, UPS is typically the diagnosis of exclusion for undifferentiated mesenchymal tumours, following immunohistochemical interrogation for other sarcoma entities [175, 176].

UPS arise in the deep soft tissue compartments, most commonly in the lower limbs, upper limbs and trunk [177, 179, 180]. While a small proportion were thought to arise in the retroperitoneum, it has been shown that most undifferentiated tumours of the retroperitoneum are, in fact, DDLPS [181]. Histologically, UPS contain a heterogeneous collection of atypical cells, varying from spindle-shaped to epithelioid or round cells, arranged in a storiform, fascicular or nested pattern (Fig. 7.4). The nuclei are often pleomorphic and demonstrate both typical and atypical mitotic activity. An inflammatory infiltrate is common, along with the presence of multinucleated, osteoclastic giant cells. IHC is essential in ruling out histologic mimics, such as other high-grade sarcomas, including myxofibrosarcoma, pleomorphic leiomyosarcoma, pleomorphic liposarcoma or DDLPS [175, 176]. Cytogenetic testing of UPS and its mimics, with the exception of DDLPS, adds minimal diagnostic value as these tumours all demonstrate a non-specific, complex karyotype [182]. In the diagnosis of undifferentiated tumours, adequate tissue sampling is essential to overcome tumour heterogeneity and ensure accurate diagnosis.

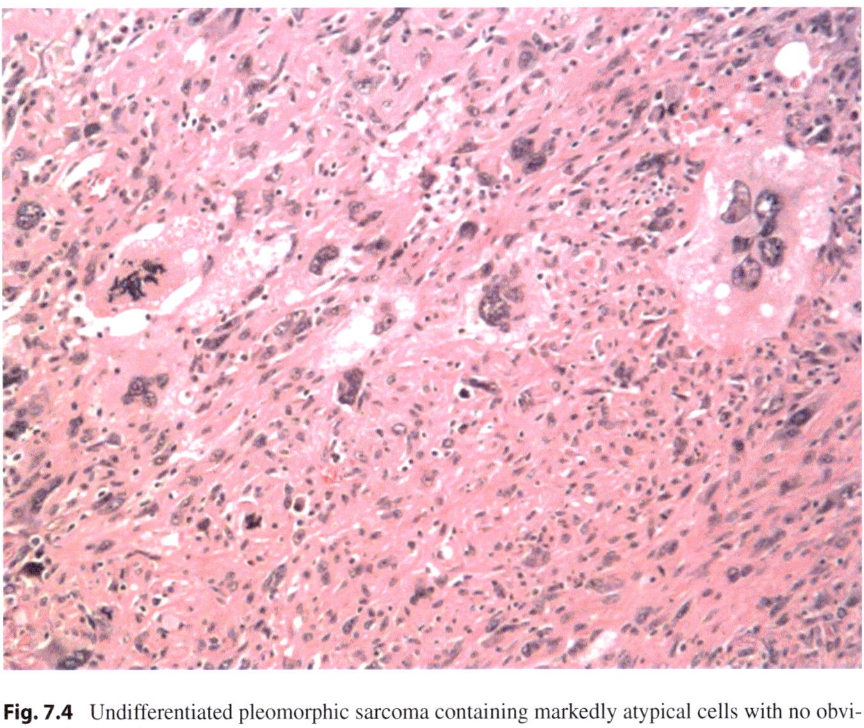

Fig. 7.4 Undifferentiated pleomorphic sarcoma containing markedly atypical cells with no obvious differentiating features

References

1. Bata BM, Hodge DO, Mohney BG. Neurofibromatosis type 1: a population-based study. J Pediatr Ophthalmol Strabismus. 2019;56(4):243–7.
2. Malbari F, Spira M, Knight PB, Zhu C, Roth M, Gill J, et al. Malignant peripheral nerve sheath tumors in neurofibromatosis: impact of family history. J Pediatr Hematol Oncol. 2018;40(6):e359–e63.
3. Higham CS, Dombi E, Rogiers A, Bhaumik S, Pans S, Connor SEJ, et al. The characteristics of 76 atypical neurofibromas as precursors to neurofibromatosis 1 associated malignant peripheral nerve sheath tumors. Neuro-Oncology. 2018;20(6):818–25.
4. Marchis MLD, Tonelli F, Quaresmini D, Lovero D, Della-Morte D, Silvestris F, et al. Desmoid tumors in familial adenomatous polyposis. Anticancer Res. 2017;37(7):3357–66.
5. Slowik V, Attard T, Dai H, Shah R, Septer S. Desmoid tumors complicating familial adenomatous polyposis: a meta-analysis mutation spectrum of affected individuals. BMC Gastroenterol. 2015;15:84.
6. van Houdt WJ, Wei IH, Kuk D, Qin LX, Jadeja B, Villano A, et al. Yield of colonoscopy in identification of newly diagnosed desmoid-type fibromatosis with underlying familial adenomatous polyposis. Ann Surg Oncol. 2019;26(3):765–71.
7. Gansar GF, Markowitz IP, Cerise EJ. Thirty years of experience with desmoid tumors at Charity Hospital. Am Surg. 1987;53(6):318–9.
8. Johner A, Tiwari P, Zetler P, Wiseman SM. Abdominal wall desmoid tumors associated with pregnancy: current concepts. Expert Rev Anticancer Ther. 2009;9(11):1675–82.
9. Fiore M, Coppola S, Cannell AJ, Colombo C, Bertagnolli MM, George S, et al. Desmoid-type fibromatosis and pregnancy: a multi-institutional analysis of recurrence and obstetric risk. Ann Surg. 2014;259(5):973–8.
10. Chu P, Wu E, Weiss LM. Cytokeratin 7 and cytokeratin 20 expression in epithelial neoplasms: a survey of 435 cases. Mod Pathol. 2000;13(9):962–72.
11. Folpe AL, Goldblum JR, Rubin BP, Shehata BM, Liu W, Dei Tos AP, et al. Morphologic and immunophenotypic diversity in Ewing family tumors: a study of 66 genetically confirmed cases. Am J Surg Pathol. 2005;29(8):1025–33.
12. Llombart-Bosch A, Machado I, Navarro S, Bertoni F, Bacchini P, Alberghini M, et al. Histological heterogeneity of Ewing's sarcoma/PNET: an immunohistochemical analysis of 415 genetically confirmed cases with clinical support. Virchows Arch. 2009;455(5):397–411.
13. Doyle LA, Vivero M, Fletcher CD, Mertens F, Hornick JL. Nuclear expression of STAT6 distinguishes solitary fibrous tumor from histologic mimics. Mod Pathol. 2014;27(3):390–5.
14. Yoshida A, Tsuta K, Ohno M, Yoshida M, Narita Y, Kawai A, et al. STAT6 immunohistochemistry is helpful in the diagnosis of solitary fibrous tumors. Am J Surg Pathol. 2014;38(4):552–9.
15. Rangdaeng S, Truong LD. Comparative immunohistochemical staining for desmin and muscle-specific actin. A study of 576 cases. Am J Clin Pathol. 1991;96(1):32–45.
16. Wijnaendts LC, van der Linden JC, van Unnik AJ, Delemarre JF, Voute PA, Meijer CJ. The expression pattern of contractile and intermediate filament proteins in developing skeletal muscle and rhabdomyosarcoma of childhood: diagnostic and prognostic utility. J Pathol. 1994;174(4):283–92.
17. Hollmann TJ, Hornick JL. INI1-deficient tumors: diagnostic features and molecular genetics. Am J Surg Pathol. 2011;35(10):e47–63.
18. Miettinen M, Fanburg-Smith JC, Virolainen M, Shmookler BM, Fetsch JF. Epithelioid sarcoma: an immunohistochemical analysis of 112 classical and variant cases and a discussion of the differential diagnosis. Hum Pathol. 1999;30(8):934–42.
19. Wrba F, Fertl H, Amann G, Tell E, Krepler R. Epithelial markers in synovial sarcoma. An immunohistochemical study on paraffin embedded tissues. Virchows Arch A Pathol Anat Histopathol. 1989;415(3):253–8.

20. Ordonez NG, Mahfouz SM, Mackay B. Synovial sarcoma: an immunohistochemical and ultrastructural study. Hum Pathol. 1990;21(7):733–49.
21. Lopes JM, Bjerkehagen B, Holm R, Bruland O, Sobrinho-Simoes M, Nesland JM. Immunohistochemical profile of synovial sarcoma with emphasis on the epithelial-type differentiation. A study of 49 primary tumours, recurrences and metastases. Pathol Res Pract. 1994;190(2):168–77.
22. Folpe AL, Schmidt RA, Chapman D, Gown AM. Poorly differentiated synovial sarcoma: immunohistochemical distinction from primitive neuroectodermal tumors and high-grade malignant peripheral nerve sheath tumors. Am J Surg Pathol. 1998;22(6):673–82.
23. Ordonez NG. Desmoplastic small round cell tumor: II: an ultrastructural and immunohistochemical study with emphasis on new immunohistochemical markers. Am J Surg Pathol. 1998;22(11):1314–27.
24. Gerald WL, Ladanyi M, de Alava E, Cuatrecasas M, Kushner BH, LaQuaglia MP, et al. Clinical, pathologic, and molecular spectrum of tumors associated with t(11;22)(p13;q12): desmoplastic small round-cell tumor and its variants. J Clin Oncol. 1998;16(9):3028–36.
25. Miettinen M, Fetsch JF. Distribution of keratins in normal endothelial cells and a spectrum of vascular tumors: implications in tumor diagnosis. Hum Pathol. 2000;31(9):1062–7.
26. Miettinen M. Immunoreactivity for cytokeratin and epithelial membrane antigen in leiomyosarcoma. Arch Pathol Lab Med. 1988;112(6):637–40.
27. Miettinen M, Rapola J. Immunohistochemical spectrum of rhabdomyosarcoma and rhabdomyosarcoma-like tumors. Expression of cytokeratin and the 68-kD neurofilament protein. Am J Surg Pathol. 1989;13(2):120–32.
28. Miettinen J, Helin H, Pakarinen M, Jalanko H, Lauronen J. Histopathology and biomarkers in prediction of renal function in children after kidney transplantation. Transpl Immunol. 2014;31(2):105–11.
29. Jones H, Steart PV, Du Boulay CE, Roche WR. Alpha-smooth muscle actin as a marker for soft tissue tumours: a comparison with desmin. J Pathol. 1990;162(1):29–33.
30. Miettinen M. Antibody specific to muscle actins in the diagnosis and classification of soft tissue tumors. Am J Pathol. 1988;130(1):205–15.
31. Schmidt RA, Cone R, Haas JE, Gown AM. Diagnosis of rhabdomyosarcomas with HHF35, a monoclonal antibody directed against muscle actins. Am J Pathol. 1988;131(1):19–28.
32. Truong LD, Rangdaeng S, Cagle P, Ro JY, Hawkins H, Font RL. The diagnostic utility of desmin. A study of 584 cases and review of the literature. Am J Clin Pathol. 1990;93(3):305–14.
33. Folpe AL, Weiss SW, Fletcher CD, Gown AM. Tenosynovial giant cell tumors: evidence for a desmin-positive dendritic cell subpopulation. Mod Pathol. 1998;11(10):939–44.
34. Ceballos KM, Nielsen GP, Selig MK, O'Connell JX. Is anti-h-caldesmon useful for distinguishing smooth muscle and myofibroblastic tumors? An immunohistochemical study. Am J Clin Pathol. 2000;114(5):746–53.
35. Cessna MH, Zhou H, Perkins SL, Tripp SR, Layfield L, Daines C, et al. Are myogenin and myoD1 expression specific for rhabdomyosarcoma? A study of 150 cases, with emphasis on spindle cell mimics. Am J Surg Pathol. 2001;25(9):1150–7.
36. Coindre JM. Immunohistochemistry in the diagnosis of soft tissue tumours. Histopathology. 2003;43(1):1–16.
37. Kuzu I, Bicknell R, Harris AL, Jones M, Gatter KC, Mason DY. Heterogeneity of vascular endothelial cells with relevance to diagnosis of vascular tumours. J Clin Pathol. 1992;45(2):143–8.
38. Miettinen M, Lindenmayer AE, Chaubal A. Endothelial cell markers CD31, CD34, and BNH9 antibody to H- and Y-antigens--evaluation of their specificity and sensitivity in the diagnosis of vascular tumors and comparison with von Willebrand factor. Mod Pathol. 1994;7(1):82–90.
39. Folpe AL, Chand EM, Goldblum JR, Weiss SW. Expression of Fli-1, a nuclear transcription factor, distinguishes vascular neoplasms from potential mimics. Am J Surg Pathol. 2001;25(8):1061–6.

40. Miettinen M, Wang ZF, Paetau A, Tan SH, Dobi A, Srivastava S, et al. ERG transcription factor as an immunohistochemical marker for vascular endothelial tumors and prostatic carcinoma. Am J Surg Pathol. 2011;35(3):432–41.
41. Kahn HJ, Bailey D, Marks A. Monoclonal antibody D2-40, a new marker of lymphatic endothelium, reacts with Kaposi's sarcoma and a subset of angiosarcomas. Mod Pathol. 2002;15(4):434–40.
42. Fukunaga M. Expression of D2-40 in lymphatic endothelium of normal tissues and in vascular tumours. Histopathology. 2005;46(4):396–402.
43. Kahn HJ, Marks A, Thom H, Baumal R. Role of antibody to S100 protein in diagnostic pathology. Am J Clin Pathol. 1983;79(3):341–7.
44. Weiss SW, Langloss JM, Enzinger FM. Value of S-100 protein in the diagnosis of soft tissue tumors with particular reference to benign and malignant Schwann cell tumors. Lab Investig. 1983;49(3):299–308.
45. Schmitt FC, Bacchi CE. S-100 protein: is it useful as a tumour marker in diagnostic immunocytochemistry? Histopathology. 1989;15(3):281–8.
46. Springall DR, Gu J, Cocchia D, Michetti F, Levene A, Levene MM, et al. The value of S-100 immunostaining as a diagnostic tool in human malignant melanomas. A comparative study using S-100 and neuron-specific enolase antibodies. Virchows Arch A Pathol Anat Histopathol. 1983;400(3):331–43.
47. Chinoy RF, Jadav J. Clear cell sarcomas of the tendon sheath. An experience of 22 cases seen over 16 years. Indian J Cancer. 1989;26(3):164–74.
48. Feasel PC, Cheah AL, Fritchie K, Winn B, Piliang M, Billings SD. Primary clear cell sarcoma of the head and neck: a case series with review of the literature. J Cutan Pathol. 2016;43(10):838–46.
49. Meis-Kindblom JM, Bergh P, Gunterberg B, Kindblom LG. Extraskeletal myxoid chondrosarcoma: a reappraisal of its morphologic spectrum and prognostic factors based on 117 cases. Am J Surg Pathol. 1999;23(6):636–50.
50. Okamoto S, Hisaoka M, Ishida T, Imamura T, Kanda H, Shimajiri S, et al. Extraskeletal myxoid chondrosarcoma: a clinicopathologic, immunohistochemical, and molecular analysis of 18 cases. Hum Pathol. 2001;32(10):1116–24.
51. Matsunou H, Shimoda T, Kakimoto S, Yamashita H, Ishikawa E, Mukai M. Histopathologic and immunohistochemical study of malignant tumors of peripheral nerve sheath (malignant schwannoma). Cancer. 1985;56(9):2269–79.
52. Wick MR, Swanson PE, Scheithauer BW, Manivel JC. Malignant peripheral nerve sheath tumor. An immunohistochemical study of 62 cases. Am J Clin Pathol. 1987;87(4):425–33.
53. Ohsie SJ, Sarantopoulos GP, Cochran AJ, Binder SW. Immunohistochemical characteristics of melanoma. J Cutan Pathol. 2008;35(5):433–44.
54. Hornick JL, Fletcher CD. PEComa: what do we know so far? Histopathology. 2006;48(1):75–82.
55. Busam KJ, Jungbluth AA. Melan-A, a new melanocytic differentiation marker. Adv Anat Pathol. 1999;6(1):12–8.
56. Kindblom LG, Lodding P, Angervall L. Clear-cell sarcoma of tendons and aponeuroses. An immunohistochemical and electron microscopic analysis indicating neural crest origin. Virchows Arch A Pathol Anat Histopathol. 1983;401(1):109–28.
57. Schaefer IM, Fletcher CD, Hornick JL. Loss of H3K27 trimethylation distinguishes malignant peripheral nerve sheath tumors from histologic mimics. Mod Pathol. 2016;29(1):4–13.
58. Terry J, Saito T, Subramanian S, Ruttan C, Antonescu CR, Goldblum JR, et al. TLE1 as a diagnostic immunohistochemical marker for synovial sarcoma emerging from gene expression profiling studies. Am J Surg Pathol. 2007;31(2):240–6.
59. Knosel T, Heretsch S, Altendorf-Hofmann A, Richter P, Katenkamp K, Katenkamp D, et al. TLE1 is a robust diagnostic biomarker for synovial sarcomas and correlates with t(X;18): analysis of 319 cases. Eur J Cancer. 2010;46(6):1170–6.

60. Kosemehmetoglu K, Vrana JA, Folpe AL. TLE1 expression is not specific for synovial sarcoma: a whole section study of 163 soft tissue and bone neoplasms. Mod Pathol. 2009;22(7):872–8.
61. Robinson DR, Wu YM, Kalyana-Sundaram S, Cao X, Lonigro RJ, Sung YS, et al. Identification of recurrent NAB2-STAT6 gene fusions in solitary fibrous tumor by integrative sequencing. Nat Genet. 2013;45(2):180–5.
62. Hirota S, Isozaki K, Moriyama Y, Hashimoto K, Nishida T, Ishiguro S, et al. Gain-of-function mutations of c-kit in human gastrointestinal stromal tumors. Science. 1998;279(5350):577–80.
63. Sarlomo-Rikala M, Kovatich AJ, Barusevicius A, Miettinen M. CD117: a sensitive marker for gastrointestinal stromal tumors that is more specific than CD34. Mod Pathol. 1998;11(8):728–34.
64. Miettinen M, Wang ZF, Lasota J. DOG1 antibody in the differential diagnosis of gastrointestinal stromal tumors: a study of 1840 cases. Am J Surg Pathol. 2009;33(9):1401–8.
65. Novelli M, Rossi S, Rodriguez-Justo M, Taniere P, Seddon B, Toffolatti L, et al. DOG1 and CD117 are the antibodies of choice in the diagnosis of gastrointestinal stromal tumours. Histopathology. 2010;57(2):259–70.
66. Hornick JL. Practical soft tissue pathology: a diagnostic approach e-book: a volume in the pattern recognition series. Amsterdam: Elsevier Health Sciences; 2017.
67. Alam NA, Barclay E, Rowan AJ, Tyrer JP, Calonje E, Manek S, et al. Clinical features of multiple cutaneous and uterine leiomyomatosis: an underdiagnosed tumor syndrome. Arch Dermatol. 2005;141(2):199–206.
68. Patel VM, Handler MZ, Schwartz RA, Lambert WC. Hereditary leiomyomatosis and renal cell cancer syndrome: an update and review. J Am Acad Dermatol. 2017;77(1):149–58.
69. Alkhalili E, Greenbaum A, Langsfeld M, Marek J, Rana MA, Glew R, et al. Leiomyosarcoma of the inferior vena cava: a case series and review of the literature. Ann Vasc Surg. 2016;33:245–51.
70. Wachtel H, Gupta M, Bartlett EK, Jackson BM, Kelz RR, Karakousis GC, et al. Outcomes after resection of leiomyosarcomas of the inferior vena cava: a pooled data analysis of 377 cases. Surg Oncol. 2015;24(1):21–7.
71. Scheithauer BW, Woodruff JM, Erlandson RA. Tumors of the peripheral nervous system. Silver Spring: Amer Registry of Pathology; 1999.
72. Hilton DA, Hanemann CO. Schwannomas and their pathogenesis. Brain Pathol. 2014;24(3):205–20.
73. Plotkin SR, Wick A. Neurofibromatosis and schwannomatosis. Semin Neurol. 2018;38(1):73–85.
74. Gonzalvo A, Fowler A, Cook RJ, Little NS, Wheeler H, McDonald KL, et al. Schwannomatosis, sporadic schwannomatosis, and familial schwannomatosis: a surgical series with long-term follow-up. Clinical article. J Neurosurg. 2011;114(3):756–62.
75. Laskin WB. Dermatofibrosarcoma protuberans. CA Cancer J Clin. 1992;42(2):116–25.
76. Fletcher CD, Theaker JM, Flanagan A, Krausz T. Pigmented dermatofibrosarcoma protuberans (Bednar tumour): melanocytic colonization or neuroectodermal differentiation? A clinicopathological and immunohistochemical study. Histopathology. 1988;13(6):631–43.
77. Thway K, Noujaim J, Jones RL, Fisher C. Dermatofibrosarcoma protuberans: pathology, genetics, and potential therapeutic strategies. Ann Diagn Pathol. 2016;25:64–71.
78. Song JS, Kim EJ, Park CS, Cho KJ. Dermatofibrosarcoma protuberans: an immunomarker study of 57 cases that included putative mesenchymal stem cell markers. Appl Immunohistochem Mol Morphol. 2017;25(8):586–91.
79. Connelly JH, Evans HL. Dermatofibrosarcoma protuberans. A clinicopathologic review with emphasis on fibrosarcomatous areas. Am J Surg Pathol. 1992;16(10):921–5.
80. Monnier D, Vidal C, Martin L, Danzon A, Pelletier F, Puzenat E, et al. Dermatofibrosarcoma protuberans: a population-based cancer registry descriptive study of 66 consecutive cases diagnosed between 1982 and 2002. J Eur Acad Dermatol Venereol. 2006;20(10):1237–42.
81. Gloster HM Jr. Dermatofibrosarcoma protuberans. J Am Acad Dermatol. 1996;35(3 Pt 1):355–74; quiz 75–6.

82. Chang CK, Jacobs IA, Salti GI. Outcomes of surgery for dermatofibrosarcoma protuberans. Eur J Surg Oncol. 2004;30(3):341–5.
83. Fiore M, Miceli R, Mussi C, Lo Vullo S, Mariani L, Lozza L, et al. Dermatofibrosarcoma protuberans treated at a single institution: a surgical disease with a high cure rate. J Clin Oncol. 2005;23(30):7669–75.
84. Pedeutour F, Simon MP, Minoletti F, Barcelo G, Terrier-Lacombe MJ, Combemale P, et al. Translocation, t(17;22)(q22;q13), in dermatofibrosarcoma protuberans: a new tumor-associated chromosome rearrangement. Cytogenet Cell Genet. 1996;72(2–3):171–4.
85. Sirvent N, Maire G, Pedeutour F. Genetics of dermatofibrosarcoma protuberans family of tumors: from ring chromosomes to tyrosine kinase inhibitor treatment. Genes Chromosomes Cancer. 2003;37(1):1–19.
86. McArthur GA, Demetri GD, van Oosterom A, Heinrich MC, Debiec-Rychter M, Corless CL, et al. Molecular and clinical analysis of locally advanced dermatofibrosarcoma protuberans treated with imatinib: Imatinib Target Exploration Consortium Study B2225. J Clin Oncol. 2005;23(4):866–73.
87. Noujaim J, Thway K, Fisher C, Jones RL. Dermatofibrosarcoma protuberans: from translocation to targeted therapy. Cancer Biol Med. 2015;12(4):375–84.
88. Montgomery E, Lee JH, Abraham SC, Wu TT. Superficial fibromatoses are genetically distinct from deep fibromatoses. Mod Pathol. 2001;14(7):695–701.
89. Carlson JW, Fletcher CD. Immunohistochemistry for beta-catenin in the differential diagnosis of spindle cell lesions: analysis of a series and review of the literature. Histopathology. 2007;51(4):509–14.
90. Le Guellec S, Soubeyran I, Rochaix P, Filleron T, Neuville A, Hostein I, et al. CTNNB1 mutation analysis is a useful tool for the diagnosis of desmoid tumors: a study of 260 desmoid tumors and 191 potential morphologic mimics. Mod Pathol. 2012;25(12):1551–8.
91. Lips DJ, Barker N, Clevers H, Hennipman A. The role of APC and beta-catenin in the aetiology of aggressive fibromatosis (desmoid tumors). Eur J Surg Oncol. 2009;35(1):3–10.
92. Sundaram M, Duffrin H, McGuire MH, Vas W. Synchronous multicentric desmoid tumors (aggressive fibromatosis) of the extremities. Skelet Radiol. 1988;17(1):16–9.
93. Watanabe K, Ogura G, Tajino T, Suzuki T. Extra-abdominal desmoid fibromatosis: two familial cases with synchronous and metachronous multicentric hyalinizing nodules. Histopathology. 2002;41(2):118–21.
94. Kohli K, Kawatra V, Khurana N, Jain S. Multicentric synchronous recurrent aggressive fibromatosis. J Cytol. 2012;29(1):57–9.
95. Fletcher CD. Diagnostic histopathology of tumors: 2-volume set with CD-ROMs. Amsterdam: Elsevier Health Sciences; 2007.
96. Schweizer L, Koelsche C, Sahm F, Piro RM, Capper D, Reuss DE, et al. Meningeal hemangiopericytoma and solitary fibrous tumors carry the NAB2-STAT6 fusion and can be diagnosed by nuclear expression of STAT6 protein. Acta Neuropathol. 2013;125(5):651–8.
97. Chan JK. Solitary fibrous tumour--everywhere, and a diagnosis in vogue. Histopathology. 1997;31(6):568–76.
98. Brunnemann RB, Ro JY, Ordonez NG, Mooney J, El-Naggar AK, Ayala AG. Extrapleural solitary fibrous tumor: a clinicopathologic study of 24 cases. Mod Pathol. 1999;12(11):1034–42.
99. Demicco EG, Park MS, Araujo DM, Fox PS, Bassett RL, Pollock RE, et al. Solitary fibrous tumor: a clinicopathological study of 110 cases and proposed risk assessment model. Mod Pathol. 2012;25(9):1298–306.
100. Mosquera JM, Fletcher CD. Expanding the spectrum of malignant progression in solitary fibrous tumors: a study of 8 cases with a discrete anaplastic component--is this dedifferentiated SFT? Am J Surg Pathol. 2009;33(9):1314–21.
101. Fisher C. Synovial sarcoma: ultrastructural and immunohistochemical features of epithelial differentiation in monophasic and biphasic tumors. Hum Pathol. 1986;17(10):996–1008.
102. Miettinen M. Keratin subsets in spindle cell sarcomas. Keratins are widespread but synovial sarcoma contains a distinctive keratin polypeptide pattern and desmoplakins. Am J Pathol. 1991;138(2):505–13.

103. Corson JM, Weiss LM, Banks-Schlegel SP, Pinkus GS. Keratin proteins and carcinoembryonic antigen in synovial sarcomas: an immunohistochemical study of 24 cases. Hum Pathol. 1984;15(7):615–21.
104. Pelmus M, Guillou L, Hostein I, Sierankowski G, Lussan C, Coindre JM. Monophasic fibrous and poorly differentiated synovial sarcoma: immunohistochemical reassessment of 60 t(X;18)(SYT-SSX)-positive cases. Am J Surg Pathol. 2002;26(11):1434–40.
105. Smith TA, Machen SK, Fisher C, Goldblum JR. Usefulness of cytokeratin subsets for distinguishing monophasic synovial sarcoma from malignant peripheral nerve sheath tumor. Am J Clin Pathol. 1999;112(5):641–8.
106. van de Rijn M, Barr FG, Xiong QB, Hedges M, Shipley J, Fisher C. Poorly differentiated synovial sarcoma: an analysis of clinical, pathologic, and molecular genetic features. Am J Surg Pathol. 1999;23(1):106–12.
107. Foo WC, Cruise MW, Wick MR, Hornick JL. Immunohistochemical staining for TLE1 distinguishes synovial sarcoma from histologic mimics. Am J Clin Pathol. 2011;135(6):839–44.
108. Reeves BR, Smith S, Fisher C, Warren W, Knight J, Martin C, et al. Characterization of the translocation between chromosomes X and 18 in human synovial sarcomas. Oncogene. 1989;4(3):373–8.
109. Knight J, Reeves B, Smith S, Clark J, Fisher C, Fletcher C, et al. Cytogenetic and molecular analysis of synovial sarcoma. Int J Oncol. 1992;1(7):747–52.
110. Clark J, Rocques PJ, Crew AJ, Gill S, Shipley J, Chan AM, et al. Identification of novel genes, SYT and SSX, involved in the t(X;18)(p11.2;q11.2) translocation found in human synovial sarcoma. Nat Genet. 1994;7(4):502–8.
111. Skytting B, Nilsson G, Brodin B, Xie Y, Lundeberg J, Uhlen M, et al. A novel fusion gene, SYT-SSX4, in synovial sarcoma. J Natl Cancer Inst. 1999;91(11):974–5.
112. Storlazzi CT, Mertens F, Mandahl N, Gisselsson D, Isaksson M, Gustafson P, et al. A novel fusion gene, SS18L1/SSX1, in synovial sarcoma. Genes Chromosomes Cancer. 2003;37(2):195–200.
113. Terry J, Barry TS, Horsman DE, Hsu FD, Gown AM, Huntsman DG, et al. Fluorescence in situ hybridization for the detection of t(X;18)(p11.2;q11.2) in a synovial sarcoma tissue microarray using a breakapart-style probe. Diagn Mol Pathol. 2005;14(2):77–82.
114. Guillou L, Coindre J, Gallagher G, Terrier P, Gebhard S, de Saint Aubain Somerhausen N, et al. Detection of the synovial sarcoma translocation t(X;18) (SYT;SSX) in paraffin-embedded tissues using reverse transcriptase-polymerase chain reaction: a reliable and powerful diagnostic tool for pathologists. A molecular analysis of 221 mesenchymal tumors fixed in different fixatives. Hum Pathol. 2001;32(1):105–12.
115. Fisher C. Synovial sarcoma. Ann Diagn Pathol. 1998;2(6):401–21.
116. Hornick JL. Novel uses of immunohistochemistry in the diagnosis and classification of soft tissue tumors. Mod Pathol. 2014;27(Suppl 1):S47–63.
117. Marino-Enriquez A. Advances in the molecular analysis of soft tissue tumors and clinical implications. Surg Pathol Clin. 2015;8(3):525–37.
118. Hawkins DS, Spunt SL, Skapek SX, Committee COGSTS. Children's Oncology Group's 2013 blueprint for research: soft tissue sarcomas. Pediatr Blood Cancer. 2013;60(6):1001–8.
119. Malempati S, Hawkins DS. Rhabdomyosarcoma: review of the Children's Oncology Group (COG) Soft-Tissue Sarcoma Committee experience and rationale for current COG studies. Pediatr Blood Cancer. 2012;59(1):5–10.
120. Skapek SX, Ferrari A, Gupta AA, Lupo PJ, Butler E, Shipley J, et al. Rhabdomyosarcoma. Nat Rev Dis Primers. 2019;5(1):1.
121. Seidal T, Kindblom LG, Angervall L. Myoglobin, desmin and vimentin in ultrastructurally proven rhabdomyomas and rhabdomyosarcomas. An immunohistochemical study utilizing a series of monoclonal and polyclonal antibodies. Appl Pathol. 1987;5(4):201–19.
122. Fisher C. Immunohistochemistry in diagnosis of soft tissue tumours. Histopathology. 2011;58(7):1001–12.
123. Dias P, Parham DM, Shapiro DN, Webber BL, Houghton PJ. Myogenic regulatory protein (MyoD1) expression in childhood solid tumors: diagnostic utility in rhabdomyosarcoma. Am J Pathol. 1990;137(6):1283–91.

124. Kumar S, Perlman E, Harris CA, Raffeld M, Tsokos M. Myogenin is a specific marker for rhabdomyosarcoma: an immunohistochemical study in paraffin-embedded tissues. Mod Pathol. 2000;13(9):988–93.
125. Cui S, Hano H, Harada T, Takai S, Masui F, Ushigome S. Evaluation of new monoclonal anti-MyoD1 and anti-myogenin antibodies for the diagnosis of rhabdomyosarcoma. Pathol Int. 1999;49(1):62–8.
126. Sorensen PH, Lynch JC, Qualman SJ, Tirabosco R, Lim JF, Maurer HM, et al. PAX3-FKHR and PAX7-FKHR gene fusions are prognostic indicators in alveolar rhabdomyosarcoma: a report from the children's oncology group. J Clin Oncol. 2002;20(11):2672–9.
127. Evans HL. Low-grade fibromyxoid sarcoma. A report of two metastasizing neoplasms having a deceptively benign appearance. Am J Clin Pathol. 1987;88(5):615–9.
128. Evans HL. Low-grade fibromyxoid sarcoma. A report of 12 cases. Am J Surg Pathol. 1993;17(6):595–600.
129. Folpe AL, Lane KL, Paull G, Weiss SW. Low-grade fibromyxoid sarcoma and hyalinizing spindle cell tumor with giant rosettes: a clinicopathologic study of 73 cases supporting their identity and assessing the impact of high-grade areas. Am J Surg Pathol. 2000;24(10):1353–60.
130. Lane KL, Shannon RJ, Weiss SW. Hyalinizing spindle cell tumor with giant rosettes: a distinctive tumor closely resembling low-grade fibromyxoid sarcoma. Am J Surg Pathol. 1997;21(12):1481–8.
131. Doyle LA, Moller E, Dal Cin P, Fletcher CD, Mertens F, Hornick JL. MUC4 is a highly sensitive and specific marker for low-grade fibromyxoid sarcoma. Am J Surg Pathol. 2011;35(5):733–41.
132. Reid R, de Silva MV, Paterson L, Ryan E, Fisher C. Low-grade fibromyxoid sarcoma and hyalinizing spindle cell tumor with giant rosettes share a common t(7;16)(q34;p11) translocation. Am J Surg Pathol. 2003;27(9):1229–36.
133. Angervall L, Kindblom LG, Merck C. Myxofibrosarcoma. A study of 30 cases. Acta Pathol Microbiol Scand A. 1977;85A(2):127–40.
134. Mentzel T, Calonje E, Wadden C, Camplejohn RS, Beham A, Smith MA, et al. Myxofibrosarcoma. Clinicopathologic analysis of 75 cases with emphasis on the low-grade variant. Am J Surg Pathol. 1996;20(4):391–405.
135. Huang HY, Lal P, Qin J, Brennan MF, Antonescu CR. Low-grade myxofibrosarcoma: a clinicopathologic analysis of 49 cases treated at a single institution with simultaneous assessment of the efficacy of 3-tier and 4-tier grading systems. Hum Pathol. 2004;35(5):612–21.
136. Merck C, Angervall L, Kindblom LG, Oden A. Myxofibrosarcoma. A malignant soft tissue tumor of fibroblastic-histiocytic origin. A clinicopathologic and prognostic study of 110 cases using multivariate analysis. Acta Pathol Microbiol Immunol Scand Suppl. 1983;282:1–40.
137. Graadt van Roggen JF, Hogendoorn PC, Fletcher CD. Myxoid tumours of soft tissue. Histopathology. 1999;35(4):291–312.
138. Howard WR, Helwig EB. Angiolipoma. Arch Dermatol. 1960;82:924–31.
139. Dixon AY, McGregor DH, Lee SH. Angiolipomas: an ultrastructural and clinicopathological study. Hum Pathol. 1981;12(8):739–47.
140. Enzinger FM, Harvey DA. Spindle cell lipoma. Cancer. 1975;36(5):1852–9.
141. Angervall L, Dahl I, Kindblom LG, Save S. Spindle cell lipoma. Acta Pathol Microbiol Scand A. 1976;84(6):477–87.
142. Fletcher CD, Martin-Bates E. Spindle cell lipoma: a clinicopathological study with some original observations. Histopathology. 1987;11(8):803–17.
143. Chung EB, Enzinger FM. Benign lipoblastomatosis. An analysis of 35 cases. Cancer. 1973;32(2):482–92.
144. Mentzel T, Calonje E, Fletcher CD. Lipoblastoma and lipoblastomatosis: a clinicopathological study of 14 cases. Histopathology. 1993;23(6):527–33.
145. Collins MH, Chatten J. Lipoblastoma/lipoblastomatosis: a clinicopathologic study of 25 tumors. Am J Surg Pathol. 1997;21(10):1131–7.
146. Kindblom LG, Angervall L, Svendsen P. Liposarcoma a clinicopathologic, radiographic and prognostic study. Acta Pathol Microbiol Scand Suppl. 1975;253:1–71.

147. Hashimoto H, Enjoji M. Liposarcoma. A clinicopathologic subtyping of 52 cases. Acta Pathol Jpn. 1982;32(6):933–48.
148. Laurino L, Furlanetto A, Orvieto E, Dei Tos AP. Well-differentiated liposarcoma (atypical lipomatous tumors). Semin Diagn Pathol. 2001;18(4):258–62.
149. Thway K. Well-differentiated liposarcoma and dedifferentiated liposarcoma: an updated review. Semin Diagn Pathol. 2019;36(2):112–21.
150. Dal Cin P, Kools P, Sciot R, De Wever I, Van Damme B, Van de Ven W, et al. Cytogenetic and fluorescence in situ hybridization investigation of ring chromosomes characterizing a specific pathologic subgroup of adipose tissue tumors. Cancer Genet Cytogenet. 1993;68(2):85–90.
151. Rosai J, Akerman M, Dal Cin P, DeWever I, Fletcher CD, Mandahl N, et al. Combined morphologic and karyotypic study of 59 atypical lipomatous tumors. Evaluation of their relationship and differential diagnosis with other adipose tissue tumors (a report of the CHAMP Study Group). Am J Surg Pathol. 1996;20(10):1182–9.
152. Nilbert M, Rydholm A, Willen H, Mitelman F, Mandahl N. MDM2 gene amplification correlates with ring chromosome in soft tissue tumors. Genes Chromosomes Cancer. 1994;9(4):261–5.
153. Weaver J, Downs-Kelly E, Goldblum JR, Turner S, Kulkarni S, Tubbs RR, et al. Fluorescence in situ hybridization for MDM2 gene amplification as a diagnostic tool in lipomatous neoplasms. Mod Pathol. 2008;21(8):943–9.
154. Kimura H, Dobashi Y, Nojima T, Nakamura H, Yamamoto N, Tsuchiya H, et al. Utility of fluorescence in situ hybridization to detect MDM2 amplification in liposarcomas and their morphological mimics. Int J Clin Exp Pathol. 2013;6(7):1306–16.
155. Creytens D, van Gorp J, Ferdinande L, Speel EJ, Libbrecht L. Detection of MDM2/CDK4 amplification in lipomatous soft tissue tumors from formalin-fixed, paraffin-embedded tissue: comparison of multiplex ligation-dependent probe amplification (MLPA) and fluorescence in situ hybridization (FISH). Appl Immunohistochem Mol Morphol. 2015;23(2):126–33.
156. Thway K, Wang J, Swansbury J, Min T, Fisher C. Fluorescence in situ hybridization for MDM2 amplification as a routine ancillary diagnostic tool for suspected well-differentiated and dedifferentiated liposarcomas: experience at a tertiary center. Sarcoma. 2015;2015:812089.
157. Coindre JM, Pedeutour F, Aurias A. Well-differentiated and dedifferentiated liposarcomas. Virchows Arch. 2010;456(2):167–79.
158. Evans HL. Liposarcoma: a study of 55 cases with a reassessment of its classification. Am J Surg Pathol. 1979;3(6):507–23.
159. Henricks WH, Chu YC, Goldblum JR, Weiss SW. Dedifferentiated liposarcoma: a clinicopathological analysis of 155 cases with a proposal for an expanded definition of dedifferentiation. Am J Surg Pathol. 1997;21(3):271–81.
160. Azumi N, Curtis J, Kempson RL, Hendrickson MR. Atypical and malignant neoplasms showing lipomatous differentiation. A study of 111 cases. Am J Surg Pathol. 1987;11(3):161–83.
161. Sirvent N, Coindre JM, Maire G, Hostein I, Keslair F, Guillou L, et al. Detection of MDM2-CDK4 amplification by fluorescence in situ hybridization in 200 paraffin-embedded tumor samples: utility in diagnosing adipocytic lesions and comparison with immunohistochemistry and real-time PCR. Am J Surg Pathol. 2007;31(10):1476–89.
162. McCormick D, Mentzel T, Beham A, Fletcher CD. Dedifferentiated liposarcoma. Clinicopathologic analysis of 32 cases suggesting a better prognostic subgroup among pleomorphic sarcomas. Am J Surg Pathol. 1994;18(12):1213–23.
163. Kilpatrick SE, Doyon J, Choong PF, Sim FH, Nascimento AG. The clinicopathologic spectrum of myxoid and round cell liposarcoma. A study of 95 cases. Cancer. 1996;77(8):1450–8.
164. Orvieto E, Furlanetto A, Laurino L, Dei Tos AP. Myxoid and round cell liposarcoma: a spectrum of myxoid adipocytic neoplasia. Semin Diagn Pathol. 2001;18(4):267–73.
165. Antonescu CR, Tschernyavsky SJ, Decuseara R, Leung DH, Woodruff JM, Brennan MF, et al. Prognostic impact of P53 status, TLS-CHOP fusion transcript structure, and histological grade in myxoid liposarcoma: a molecular and clinicopathologic study of 82 cases. Clin Cancer Res. 2001;7(12):3977–87.

166. Estourgie SH, Nielsen GP, Ott MJ. Metastatic patterns of extremity myxoid liposarcoma and their outcome. J Surg Oncol. 2002;80(2):89–93.
167. Gibas Z, Miettinen M, Limon J, Nedoszytko B, Mrozek K, Roszkiewicz A, et al. Cytogenetic and immunohistochemical profile of myxoid liposarcoma. Am J Clin Pathol. 1995;103(1):20–6.
168. Rabbitts TH, Forster A, Larson R, Nathan P. Fusion of the dominant negative transcription regulator CHOP with a novel gene FUS by translocation t(12;16) in malignant liposarcoma. Nat Genet. 1993;4(2):175–80.
169. Crozat A, Aman P, Mandahl N, Ron D. Fusion of CHOP to a novel RNA-binding protein in human myxoid liposarcoma. Nature. 1993;363(6430):640–4.
170. Oliveira AM, Nascimento AG. Pleomorphic liposarcoma. Semin Diagn Pathol. 2001;18(4):274–85.
171. Gebhard S, Coindre JM, Michels JJ, Terrier P, Bertrand G, Trassard M, et al. Pleomorphic liposarcoma: clinicopathologic, immunohistochemical, and follow-up analysis of 63 cases: a study from the French Federation of Cancer Centers Sarcoma Group. Am J Surg Pathol. 2002;26(5):601–16.
172. Hornick JL, Bosenberg MW, Mentzel T, McMenamin ME, Oliveira AM, Fletcher CD. Pleomorphic liposarcoma: clinicopathologic analysis of 57 cases. Am J Surg Pathol. 2004;28(10):1257–67.
173. Wang L, Ren W, Zhou X, Sheng W, Wang J. Pleomorphic liposarcoma: a clinicopathological, immunohistochemical and molecular cytogenetic study of 32 additional cases. Pathol Int. 2013;63(11):523–31.
174. Anderson WJ, Jo VY. Pleomorphic liposarcoma: updates and current differential diagnosis. Semin Diagn Pathol. 2019;36(2):122–8.
175. Fletcher CD. Pleomorphic malignant fibrous histiocytoma: fact or fiction? A critical reappraisal based on 159 tumors diagnosed as pleomorphic sarcoma. Am J Surg Pathol. 1992;16(3):213–28.
176. Fletcher CDM, Gustafson P, Rydholm A, Willén H, Åkerman M. Clinicopathologic re-evaluation of 100 malignant fibrous histiocytomas: prognostic relevance of subclassification. J Clin Oncol. 2001;19(12):3045–50.
177. Vodanovich DA, Spelman T, May D, Slavin J, Choong PFM. Predicting the prognosis of undifferentiated pleomorphic soft tissue sarcoma: a 20-year experience of 266 cases. ANZ J Surg. 2019;89(9):1045–50.
178. Weiss SW, Enzinger FM. Malignant fibrous histiocytoma: an analysis of 200 cases. Cancer. 1978;41(6):2250–66.
179. Gibbs JF, Huang PP, Lee RJ, McGrath B, Brooks J, McKinley B, et al. Malignant fibrous histiocytoma: an institutional review. Cancer Investig. 2001;19(1):23–7.
180. Peiper M, Zurakowski D, Knoefel WT, Izbicki JR. Malignant fibrous histiocytoma of the extremities and trunk: an institutional review. Surgery. 2004;135(1):59–66.
181. Coindre JM, Mariani O, Chibon F, Mairal A, De Saint Aubain Somerhausen N, Favre-Guillevin E, et al. Most malignant fibrous histiocytomas developed in the retroperitoneum are dedifferentiated liposarcomas: a review of 25 cases initially diagnosed as malignant fibrous histiocytoma. Mod Pathol. 2003;16(3):256–62.
182. Mertens F, Fletcher CD, Dal Cin P, De Wever I, Mandahl N, Mitelman F, et al. Cytogenetic analysis of 46 pleomorphic soft tissue sarcomas and correlation with morphologic and clinical features: a report of the CHAMP Study Group. Chromosomes and MorPhology. Genes Chromosomes Cancer. 1998;22(1):16–25.
183. Lindberg MR. Diagnostic pathology: soft tissue tumors. Amsterdam: Elsevier Health Sciences; 2015.
184. Trojani M, Contesso G, Coindre JM, Rouesse J, Bui NB, de Mascarel A, et al. Soft-tissue sarcomas of adults; study of pathological prognostic variables and definition of a histopathological grading system. Int J Cancer. 1984;33(1):37–42.
185. Brierley JD, Gospodarowicz MK, Wittekind C. TNM classification of malignant tumours. New York: Wiley; 2017.
186. Amin MB, Edge SB. AJCC cancer staging manual. New York: Springer; 2017.

Immunohistochemistry in Bone and Soft Tissue Tumours

8

Vanessa Tran and John Slavin

8.1 Introduction

Immunohistochemistry (IHC) is an indispensable tool in the diagnosis of sarcomas. Sarcomas are a vast, diverse and complex group of neoplasms arising from mesenchymal origin. They present a diagnostic challenge as they are rare and have many overlapping appearances under the microscope. Accurate diagnosis of sarcomas is necessary for deciding management and prognostication of the disease. Historically, the categorisation of sarcomas has been based on their presumed line of differentiation [1, 2]. In some cases, the histomorphology is straightforward and distinct; however, in other cases, the histogenesis can be ambiguous, and further investigation is required to assist with the diagnosis [3]. To compound this, benign mesenchymal lesions and non-sarcomatous tumours are frequently encountered as differential diagnoses to sarcomas and thus present an additional diagnostic challenge [4]. The use of ancillary pathological techniques, therefore, is essential in the evaluation of mesenchymal tumour samples. IHC is a microscopy-based method that utilises immunological and biochemical principles to detect protein expression in tumour cells. Since its discovery in 1942, IHC has progressively improved through development of new antibodies. Nowadays, it has established itself as a valuable adjunctive step in the pathological diagnosis of surgical specimens of bone and soft tissue tumours.

V. Tran (✉)
Department of Surgery, University of Melbourne, Melbourne, VIC, Australia

J. Slavin
Department of Anatomical Pathology, St. Vincent's Hospital Melbourne, Melbourne, VIC, Australia
e-mail: john.slavin@svha.org.au

P. F. M. Choong (ed.), *Sarcoma*, https://doi.org/10.1007/978-981-15-9414-4_8

8.2 History of IHC: "Putting Tail Lights on Antibodies"

While IHC was discovered by Dr. Albert Coons in 1942, the story of its development is vast and involves the contribution of many scientists. Its inception can be traced back to the late 1800s, when Dr. Emil von Behring first described antibodies in the context of passive immunisation against diphtheria and tetanus and successfully treated his first patient [5]. It was through this work that earned him the first Nobel Prize in physiology and medicine in 1901 [6]. Following this, many other scientists contributed to research into antigen-antibody interactions, including Professor Paul Ehrlich, who further characterised the antigen-antibody interaction [7]; Dr. Kraus, who developed the precipitin test, a technique for detecting antigen-antibody complexes in solution [8]; and Dr. John Marrack, who attached dye to antibodies in order to visualise these complexes [9].

One important catalyst in the development of IHC occurred in the early 1920s, when Michael Heidelberger and Oswald Avery produced coloured antigen-antibody complexes to demonstrate that antigens were polysaccharides [10]. Then, by attaching a purple azo dye to antigens, Heidelberger and another associate, Forrest Kendall, were able to produce coloured antigen-antibody complex precipitates [11].

In 1942, Dr. Albert Coons developed fluorescein-labelled antibodies that could be detected by light microscopy and, thus, discovered the technique of IHC [12]. Immunofluorescence, however, was unable to be detected by electron microscopy, so subsequent developments aimed to address this limitation. In 1959, Dr. S. J. Singer detected antigens by electron microscopy by using ferritin-antibody [13]. Later, Graham and Karnovsky pioneered a new immunoenzyme labelling method by tagging antibodies with enzymes [14]. Through this work, Elizabeth Leduc, Stratis Avrameas and, separately, Paul Nakane, developed new immunoperoxidase techniques, which allowed detection of antigens and both light and electron microscopy levels [15, 16]. This technique was further modified by Ludwig Sternberger with the peroxidase-antiperoxidase (PAP) technique, thus improving sensitivity and efficacy [17]. In 1971, W. Page Faulk and G. Malcolm Taylor used colloidal gold as a label to detect antigens by electron microscopy [18]. Jurgen Roth, Moise Bendayan and Lelio Orci contributed further improvements to this protocol over the next decade through introduction of protein A-coated colloidal gold and thus developed the technique that is widely used today [19].

8.3 Procedure, Technical Considerations and Possible Limitations

The general concept of IHC involves using antibodies attached with a chromogenic enzyme to highlight and visualise a specific antigen of interest. The process of IHC is heavily protocolised to ensure strict standardisation and reproducibility of results [20]. The process of IHC is lengthy and complex, with each step contributing to its overall accuracy. The quality assurance of IHC is comprised on many critical components, including tissue handling, fixation, processing, sectioning, testing and interpretation of results [21].

The IHC protocol can be broadly simplified to three main players: (1) the tissue sample in question, (2) the antibodies to be used for testing and (3) the method of detection and analysis. The careful consideration of each of these main components determines the reliability of the IHC test. Each factor, their technical considerations and possible limitations will be discussed in further detail below.

8.3.1 Preparing the Tissue Sample

The first critical task is ensuring that enough viable tumour tissue is obtained in order to perform all necessary histology and ancillary tests. It is essential that the surgeon captures sufficient cells representative of the tumour to make an accurate diagnosis. This can be challenging when performing a biopsy. It has been shown that open biopsy has the greatest diagnostic accuracy when compared with fine needle aspiration and core biopsy [22]. Open biopsy, however, is more invasive, has higher risk of contamination and carries higher costs, so core biopsy is most often preferred as the next most accurate technique [23].

The pre-analytical phase of IHC is critical for accurate analysis. This includes tissue handling, fixation, paraffinisation, sectioning, storage and antigen retrieval, and each of these steps influences the quality of the result later. Firstly, the time from resection to fixation of a tissue sample can affect the detection of proteins by IHC due to the length of ischaemic time that the tissue undergoes [24]. During this period of time, the tissue undergoes ‘cold ischaemia’, in which proteins, RNA and DNA are degraded as a result of anoxic damage [25]. Studies of various cancer types have shown differences in IHC results when there is a delay in fixation [26–28]. Fixation itself is another area of potential variability or error. Factors including the duration, formula of the formalin solution and the tissue to fixative ratio all influence the quality of IHC [24, 29]. The tissue, once fixed, then undergoes further processing that includes washing and removal of excess fixative, dehydration and clearing and paraffin impregnation. These paraffin blocks are sectioned into thin slices and stored. Thickness of the sections may also influence IHC results and increase intensity of immunostaining. Tears sustained during the cutting process may cause artefact or loss of protein staining [25]. Storage of these sections also has impact on IHC, with studies demonstrating a loss of p53 staining with prolonged storage of sections [30, 31].

8.3.2 Selecting Useful Antibodies

In order to perform IHC, pathologists firstly need to select a panel of suitable antibodies that will help guide the diagnosis. The selection, application and interpretation of useful antibodies are discussed in further detail in this chapter. There are also some antibodies that have been shown to be non-specific and, as a result, do not provide diagnostic relevance. Vimentin, for example, is a marker that is widely expressed in almost all tumour types, mesenchymal and non-mesenchymal and therefore not recommended for use [3, 32, 33]. Similarly, histiocytic markers alpha-1-antitrypsin and alpha-1-antichymotrypsin demonstrate widespread expression and have been replaced by the more specific CD68 [4, 33]. Myoglobin was previously used for detection of rhabdomyosarcoma, however is only expressed in approximately 60% of cases [34, 35]. Nowadays, myogenin is used in its place as a marker in rhabdomyosarcoma.

At the manufacturer level, it is necessary to enforce strict protocols for quality control in order to ensure standardisation of all reagents. There are also various technical considerations regarding storage of antibody reagents. Improper storage, for example, can be responsible for greater than 50% of IHC failures [36].

8.3.3 Detecting and Analysing the Reaction

Once the antigen-antibody reaction has taken place, there needs to be an adequate system to visualise and analyse the IHC results in a reproducible and reliable fashion. This part of the process can be broadly broken up into two broad steps: (1) detection of immunoreactivity and (2) clinical interpretation of results.

Detection systems are necessary to visualise whether an antigen-antibody reaction has taken place, since antibodies alone cannot be seen under light or electron microscopy. In order to do this, labels are attached to the antibodies. Common detection systems include direct-conjugate-labelled antibody method, indirect procedure, avidin-biotin complex method, streptavidin-biotin systems, phosphatase anti-phosphatase label system, polymer-based detection and tyramine amplification system [37]. These are all various techniques used to attach a chromogenic label to the antibodies. Polymeric- and tyramine-based amplification methods are beneficial in that they greatly improve sensitivity; however, they are also associated with more complex protocols that result in worse standardisation and reproducibility [21]. In order to better highlight the immunoreaction, counter staining can also be performed to provide further contrast to the antibody labels. Haematoxylin is the most common counterstain used for IHC, although eosin, methylene blue, methylene green and toluidine blue can also be used [21, 37].

In order to accurately interpret the results, pathologists also need to understand the relative sensitivities and specificities of the reagents. It must be emphasised that, while IHC is a powerful diagnostic tool, there is no single antibody or antibody combination that is completely unique to tumour type [38]. The interpretation of these markers in the context of bone and soft tissue tumours will be discussed in detail in this chapter.

8.4 Immunohistochemical Markers

8.4.1 Broad-Spectrum Markers

In sarcoma diagnosis, a panel of antibodies is routinely used in the initial instance to analyse a tissue sample. These markers can either confirm a diagnosis or characterise cell phenotypes to further guide immunohistochemical or molecular testing. Frequently used cell-typic markers include cytokeratins, epithelial membrane antigen (EMA), S100 protein, desmin, smooth muscle actin (SMA) and CD34. These antibodies are largely non-specific, which means that they are expressed in multiple sarcoma subtypes. The interpretation of these markers, therefore, is most useful in combination with the wider clinical, radiological and histopathological picture.

8.4.1.1 Cytokeratins

Keratins are a family of proteins expressed in normal epithelial tissue. As such, the detection of keratins, in particular low-molecular-weight keratins, may indicate epithelial differentiation of soft tissue tumours [33]. There are 20 described keratin protein types, of which 8 have basic or higher isoelectric points (Type I; KRT 1–8) and the remainder has acidic or lower isoelectric points (Type II; KRT 9–20) [39]. AE1/AE3 are broad-spectrum immunohistochemical antibodies that are most commonly used to detect keratins in surgical pathology. AE1 contains antibodies to Type I keratins (KRT 10, 14–16 and 19), while AE3 recognises Type II keratins (1–8) [40]. This antibody cocktail is used as a first-line immunohistochemical investigation for spindle cell, pleomorphic, round cell and epithelioid tumours. They are also extremely useful in the differentiation between sarcoma and its carcinoma mimics [41].

8.4.1.2 Epithelial Membrane Antigen

EMA is a transmembrane glycoprotein that is widely expressed in normal epithelial tissue and their neoplastic counterparts. In addition to carcinomas, some soft tissue tumours demonstrate recurrent EMA expression. These tumours typically include epithelioid sarcoma [42], synovial sarcoma [43–46] and myoepithelioma [47, 48] but are widely absent in many other soft tissue tumours [49].

8.4.1.3 S100 Protein

The S100 protein describes a multigene family of 21 proteins that demonstrate close structural similarity but widely varying function that includes participation in proliferation, migration, inflammation and differentiation [50–52]. It is commonly positive in a range of soft tissue tumours, including melanomas, benign peripheral nerve sheath tumours (PNST), clear cell sarcoma and myoepitheliomas.

8.4.1.4 Desmin

Desmin, a muscular marker, is an intermediate filament that is normally expressed in skeletal muscle and smooth muscle cells [53, 54]. In surgical pathology, its main utility resides in the identification of rhabdomyosarcomas and leiomyosarcomas, as well as their benign counterparts [53, 55]. Desmin is, however, positive in a number of other sarcomas, including desmoplastic small round tumours [56, 57], myofibroblastic tumours [53, 54, 58] and tenosynovial giant cell tumours [59]. Its interpretation is best made alongside other myogenic markers, including SMA and more specific markers myogenin and MyoD1, in the differentiation and diagnosis of muscular tumours.

8.4.1.5 Smooth Muscle Actin

SMA is another muscular marker that is expressed in normal smooth muscle cells. It is a useful marker in diagnosis of smooth muscle tumours and myofibroblastic tumours. It is also expressed in normal myofibroblasts, myoepithelial cells and smooth muscle-related pericytes and glomus cells and, therefore, positive in the tumours of the respective lineages [60].

8.4.1.6 CD34

CD34 is a transmembrane glycoprotein that is widely expressed in many soft tissue tumours, particularly spindle cell and epithelioid cell tumours [4]. Its expression is encountered consistently in malignant vascular tumours [61, 62], solitary fibrous tumour (SFT), dermatofibrosarcoma protuberans and spindle cell lipomas. Variable expression is seen in GISTs, epithelioid sarcoma and MPNST.

8.4.1.7 CD99

CD99, also known as MIC2, is a transmembrane glycoprotein normally expressed on the cell surface of T lymphocytes [63]. In surgical pathology, it is a non-specific marker that is useful in the classification of round cell tumours. It is particularly useful in the identification of Ewing's sarcoma/PNET, in which it demonstrates strong membranous staining [64–66].

8.4.2 Novel Markers

The advent of molecular techniques has allowed the genetic characterisation of soft tissue tumours and discovery of recurrent mutations including reciprocal translocations, amplifications and point mutations. An understanding of these genetic aberrations and their respective protein products have allowed pathologists to develop targeted immunohistochemical surrogates for the identification of genetic mutations in tumours samples that can aid in its diagnosis.

8.4.2.1 FLI-1

In translocations, these surrogate markers do not detect the fusion itself but rather identifies the resultant overexpression of specific proteins [67].

Ewing's sarcoma/primitive neuroectodermal tumours (PNET) are a class of small, blue, round cell tumours that share a similar histomorphology with tumours such as neuroblastoma, rhabdomyosarcoma and poorly differentiated synovial sarcomas [68]. A specific t(11;22) translocation is found in approximately 90% of all Ewing's sarcoma/PNET, resulting in an EWSR1-FLI-1 fusion product [69–71]. The sc-356 immunohistochemical stain is a polyclonal antibody to the carboxy-terminal of FLI that has demonstrated 71% sensitivity and 92% specificity for Ewing's sarcoma/PNET in previous studies [68, 72].

8.4.2.2 MDM2 and CDK4

Atypical lipomatous tumours/well-differentiated liposarcomas (ALT/WDLPS) and dedifferentiated liposarcomas (DDLPS) are two separate types of fatty tumours that are both characterised by complex genomes, resulting in supernumerary ring and giant marker chromosomes and the amplification of 12q13–15 gene locus [73, 74]. MDM2 and CDK4 are two genes within this locus, and their amplified protein products can be detected by IHC [75, 76].

8.5 Application and Interpretation of IHC

IHC has a well-established role in the diagnosis of bone and soft tissue tumours. The frequent overlapping histological features of sarcomas require the use of ancillary techniques, such as IHC, to help further distinguish tissue characteristics. As described in Fig. 8.1, IHC plays three key roles in the differential diagnosis of bone and soft tissue tumours: (a) in establishing any rare or atypical benign mesenchymal lesions that may resemble malignant tumours; (b) the identification of malignant lesions of non-mesenchymal origin; and (c) the characterisation of specific sarcoma subtypes, in particularly distinguishing one sarcoma type from histologic mimics. Ultimately, accurate diagnosis of mesenchymal neoplasms is essential in providing prognostic information for patients and guiding appropriate therapeutic care.

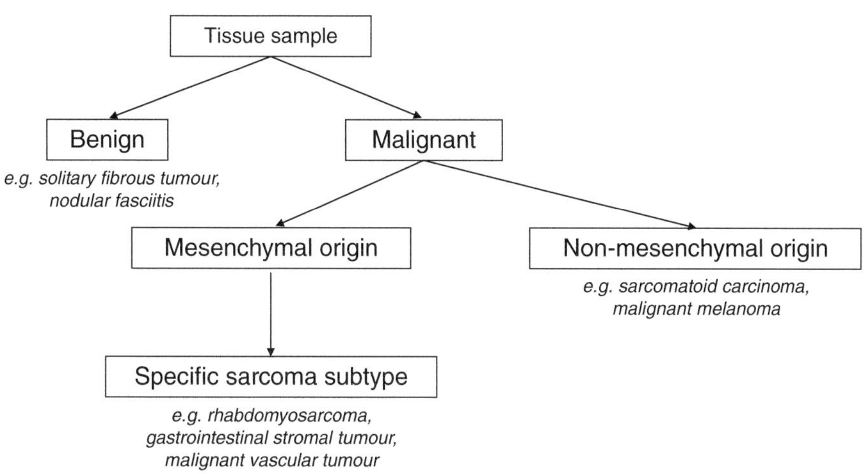

Fig. 8.1 A schematic overview of the application of immunohistochemistry (IHC) in the diagnostic process of sarcomas

8.5.1 Identification of Benign Tumours

While IHC alone cannot definitively differentiate all benign and malignant tumours [38], it can be extremely useful in identifying atypical benign lesions that share similar histological appearances with a malignancy. Clarification of whether a tumour is benign or malignant may influence the course of treatment, for example, the type of excision (marginal vs wide local excision) or the addition of neoadjuvant therapy. Tumours that may mimic malignancies include SFT and benign PNST.

8.5.1.1 Solitary Fibrous Tumour

SFT is a benign soft tissue tumour of spindle cell morphology. Its histologic features can be difficult to distinguish from various other soft tissue tumours, including mesothelioma or other spindle cell tumours [4, 77]. IHC reveals CD34 and Bcl-2 positivity in most cases, and these markers are therefore highly sensitive for SFT [78, 79]. Negative staining for both markers would strongly suggest an alternative diagnosis [80]. IHC for STAT6 can be used as a surrogate marker of the NAB2-STAT6 fusion product highly characteristic for SFT [81]. STAT6 is therefore a highly specific marker for SFT and is useful in distinguishing from histologic mimics [82, 83]. Other valuable markers in the diagnosis of SFT include CD99 and beta-catenin [78, 84].

8.5.1.2 Nodular Fasciitis

Nodular fasciitis (NF) typically presents as a rapidly growing, poorly circumscribed mass that reveals dense cellularity and high mitotic activity on pathological examination. It is not uncommon for NF to be misdiagnosed as sarcoma, such as dermatofibrosarcoma protuberans, low-grade myofibroblastic sarcoma or malignant peripheral nerve sheath tumour (MPNST), thus warranting IHC for definitive diagnosis [85–87]. IHC demonstrates positive staining for SMA in almost all cases with consistent negativity for desmin, h-caldesmon, S100 and beta-catenin [88, 89].

8.5.2 Exclusion of Non-mesenchymal/ Non-sarcomatous Tumours

Once a benign lesion has been ruled out and the tumour has been classified as malignant, the pathologist must exclude the diagnosis of a non-mesenchymal tumour. There are various non-sarcomatous lesions that may resemble sarcomas due to their overlapping histological features. Common examples include sarcomatoid carcinoma, melanoma, lymphoma and mesothelioma.

8.5.2.1 Sarcomatoid Carcinoma

Histologically, sarcomatoid carcinomas may be confused with undifferentiated spindle cell or pleomorphic sarcomas [60]. It is most often associated with primary breast carcinoma, renal cell carcinoma and mucosal or cutaneous squamous cell carcinoma, although it can present at any site [41]. In these cases, it is important to use IHC to identify areas of epithelial differentiation, which will support a diagnosis of carcinoma [90]. Broad-spectrum keratins, such as AE1/AE3 and pan-cytokeratin and EMA, are expressed in almost all sarcomatoid carcinoma, allowing distinction from histologically similar sarcomas [91–94].

8.5.2.2 Malignant Melanoma

Malignant melanoma can prove a diagnostic challenge for pathologists as they often mimic sarcomas, even in their immunohistochemical profile. Primary malignant melanoma, for example, can appear histologically like MPNST and clear cell sarcomas. Both MPNST and malignant melanoma have been shown to express S100 [95–99], as has clear cell sarcoma [100–102]. In this situation, the pattern of staining carries significance in delineating these entities. S100 expression is more commonly diffuse in melanoma, compared with MPNST, in which it is usually focal or multifocal. In clear cell sarcoma, staining for HMB45 is generally more intense or diffuse than S100, which is not the case in melanoma [41].

8.5.3 For Diagnosis of Mesenchymal Tumours

In some sarcomas, IHC forms a crucial part of diagnosis, where the immunohistochemical profile of a tissue sample may be diagnostic or highly suggestive of a sarcoma subtype. Examples discussed further below are rhabdomyosarcoma, gastrointestinal stromal tumours (GIST) and malignant vascular tumours.

8.5.3.1 Rhabdomyosarcomas

Rhabdomyosarcomas encompass multiple subtypes, of which embryonal rhabdomyosarcoma (ERMS) and alveolar rhabdomyosarcoma (ARMS) are the most common. Desmin, alongside more lineage-specific markers MyoD1 and myogenin, is useful for diagnosis [103, 104]. These markers are positive in almost 100% of ERMS and ARMS and up to 90% of all rhabdomyosarcomas [53, 103, 105, 106]. The expression pattern of myogenin is also of significance in these tumours. For instance, myogenin staining is often stronger and more uniform in ARMS than ERMS [107]. A diffuse expression of myogenin has also been correlated with poor survival in paediatric patients with rhabdomyosarcoma [108].

8.5.3.2 Gastrointestinal Stromal Tumours

Identification and diagnosis of gastrointestinal stromal tumours (GIST) is crucial for patient outcomes as there is a highly effective treatment available [109]. KIT (CD117) is a receptor tyrosine kinase that is activated in 85–90% of GISTs through a gain-of-function mutation [110–113]. This results in the constitutive activation of KIT receptor tyrosine kinase in a ligand-independent manner [114]. Immunohistochemical detection of CD117, therefore, is highly supportive of a GIST diagnosis. This finding is particularly significant given the availability of targeted therapies such as imatinib, an inhibitor of KIT-tyrosine kinase [115, 116]. It is important to note, however, that CD117 can be positive in other tumours including Ewing sarcoma [117–119] and angiosarcoma [120–122], so the immunohistochemical results must be interpreted in the context of clinical and radiological findings. The small subset of GISTs that are KIT-negative is often positive for DOG1, also called anoctamin-1 (Ano-1). DOG1/Ano-1 is considered the antibody of choice in addition to CD117 in the immunohistochemical testing for GISTs [123], with similar sensitivities and specificities between DOG1/Ano-1 and CD117 [124].

8.5.3.3 Malignant Vascular Tumours

Malignant vascular tumours encompass a broad class of tumours including angiosarcoma, epithelioid and spindle vascular tumours and Kaposi sarcoma. IHC plays a valuable role in diagnosing malignant vascular tumours because due to their wide spectrum of histopathological patterns that are not easily identifiable on histology alone. In assessing these tumours, CD31, CD34 and Fli-1 are useful immunohistochemical markers. CD31 is considered the gold-standard marker in the diagnosis of malignant vascular tumours, as it demonstrates positivity in angiosarcomas, Kaposi sarcomas and epithelioid haemangioepitheliomas [61, 125, 126]. ERG is also a highly sensitive vascular marker in the diagnosis of angiosarcoma [126]. CD34 is often positive in angiosarcoma and Kaposi sarcoma but variably expressed in epithelioid vascular tumours [61, 127]. A more recent marker, Fli-1, also demonstrates good sensitivity for spindle and epithelioid tumours [128]. Additionally, Kaposi sarcoma is an atypical vascular lesion that is uniquely defined by the presence of human herpes virus-8 (HHV-8), which can be detected by IHC [129, 130].

References

1. Fletcher CD. The evolving classification of soft tissue tumours—an update based on the new 2013 WHO classification. Histopathology. 2014;64(1):2–11.
2. Jo VY, Fletcher CD. WHO classification of soft tissue tumours: an update based on the 2013 (4th) edition. Pathology. 2014;46(2):95–104.
3. Wei S, Henderson-Jackson E, Qian X, Bui MM. Soft tissue tumor immunohistochemistry update: illustrative examples of diagnostic pearls to avoid pitfalls. Arch Pathol Lab Med. 2017;141(8):1072–91.
4. Coindre JM. Immunohistochemistry in the diagnosis of soft tissue tumours. Histopathology. 2003;43(1):1–16.
5. Behring Ev. Über das zustandekommen der diphtherie-immunität und der tetanus-immunität bei thieren; 1890.
6. Kaufmann SH. Remembering Emil von Behring: from tetanus treatment to antibody cooperation with phagocytes. MBio. 2017;8(1):e00117-17.
7. Kasten FH. Paul Ehrlich: pathfinder in cell biology. 1. Chronicle of his life and accomplishments in immunology, cancer research, and chemotherapy. Biotech Histochem. 1996;71(1):2–37.
8. Kraus R. Uber spezifische Reaktionen in keimfreien Filtraten aus Cholera, Typhus and Pestbouillonkulturen, erzeugt durch homologues Serum. Wien Klin Wochschr. 1897;10:736–8.
9. Marrack JR. Derived antigens as a means of studying the relation of specific combination to chemical structure: (section of therapeutics and pharmacology). Proc R Soc Med. 1934;27(8):1063–5.

10. Heidelberger M, Avery OT. The soluble specific substance of pneumococcus. J Exp Med. 1923;38(1):73–9.
11. Heidelberger M, Kendall FE. A quantitative study of the precipitin reaction between type III pneumococcus polysaccharide and purified homologous antibody. J Exp Med. 1929;50(6):809–23.
12. Coons AH, Creech HJ, Jones RN. Immunological properties of an antibody containing a fluorescent group. Proc Soc Exp Biol Med. 1941;47(2):200–2.
13. Singer SJ. Preparation of an electron-dense antibody conjugate. Nature. 1959;183(4674):1523–4.
14. Graham RC Jr, Karnovsky MJ. The early stages of absorption of injected horseradish peroxidase in the proximal tubules of mouse kidney: ultrastructural cytochemistry by a new technique. J Histochem Cytochem. 1966;14(4):291–302.
15. Leduc EH, Avrameas S, Bouteille M. Ultrastructural localization of antibody in differentiating plasma cells. J Exp Med. 1968;127(1):109–18.
16. Nakane PK, Pierce GB Jr. Enzyme-labeled antibodies for the light and electron microscopic localization of tissue antigens. J Cell Biol. 1967;33(2):307–18.
17. Sternberger LA, Hardy PH Jr, Cuculis JJ, Meyer HG. The unlabeled antibody enzyme method of immunohistochemistry: preparation and properties of soluble antigen-antibody complex (horseradish peroxidase-antihorseradish peroxidase) and its use in identification of spirochetes. J Histochem Cytochem. 1970;18(5):315–33.
18. Faulk WP, Taylor GM. An immunocolloid method for the electron microscope. Immunochemistry. 1971;8(11):1081–3.
19. Roth J, Bendayan M, Orci L. Ultrastructural localization of intracellular antigens by the use of protein A-gold complex. J Histochem Cytochem. 1978;26(12):1074–81.
20. Hewitt S, Robinowitz M, Bogen S, Gown A, Kalra K, Otis C, et al. Quality assurance for design control and implementation of immunohistochemistry assays: approved guideline. Wayne: Clinical Lab Standards Institute; 2011.
21. Dabbs DJ. Diagnostic Immunohistochemistry E-Book: theranostic and genomic applications, expert consult: online and print. Amsterdam: Elsevier Health Sciences; 2013.
22. Layfield LJ, Schmidt RL, Sangle N, Crim JR. Diagnostic accuracy and clinical utility of biopsy in musculoskeletal lesions: a comparison of fine-needle aspiration, core, and open biopsy techniques. Diagn Cytopathol. 2014;42(6):476–86.
23. Traina F, Errani C, Toscano A, Pungetti C, Fabbri D, Mazzotti A, et al. Current concepts in the biopsy of musculoskeletal tumors: AAOS exhibit selection. J Bone Joint Surg Am. 2015;97(2):e7.
24. Engel KB, Moore HM. Effects of preanalytical variables on the detection of proteins by immunohistochemistry in formalin-fixed, paraffin-embedded tissue. Arch Pathol Lab Med. 2011;135(5):537–43.
25. Taylor CR, Shi S-R, Barr N, Wu N. Techniques of immunohistochemistry: principles, pitfalls, and standardization. Diagn immunohistochem. 2013;2:1–42.
26. Khoury T, Sait S, Hwang H, Chandrasekhar R, Wilding G, Tan D, et al. Delay to formalin fixation effect on breast biomarkers. Mod Pathol. 2009;22(11):1457–67.
27. Di Tommaso L, Kapucuoglu N, Losi L, Trere D, Eusebi V. Impact of delayed fixation on evaluation of cell proliferation in intracranial malignant tumors. Appl Immunohistochem Mol Morphol. 1999;7(3):209.
28. Qiu J, Kulkarni S, Chandrasekhar R, Rees M, Hyde K, Wilding G, et al. Effect of delayed formalin fixation on estrogen and progesterone receptors in breast cancer: a study of three different clones. Am J Clin Pathol. 2010;134(5):813–9.
29. Grizzle WE. Special symposium: fixation and tissue processing models. Biotech Histochem. 2009;84(5):185–93.
30. Prioleau J, Schnitt SJ. p53 antigen loss in stored paraffin slides. N Engl J Med. 1995;332(22):1521–2.
31. Wester K, Wahlund E, Sundstrom C, Ranefall P, Bengtsson E, Russell PJ, et al. Paraffin section storage and immunohistochemistry. Effects of time, temperature, fixation, and retrieval

protocol with emphasis on p53 protein and MIB1 antigen. Appl Immunohistochem Mol Morphol. 2000;8(1):61–70.
32. Chan JK. Advances in immunohistochemistry: impact on surgical pathology practice. Semin Diagn Pathol. 2000;17(3):170–7.
33. Miettinen M. Immunohistochemistry of soft tissue tumours—review with emphasis on 10 markers. Histopathology. 2014;64(1):101–18.
34. Kodet R. Rhabdomyosarcoma in childhood. An immunohistological analysis with myoglobin, desmin and vimentin. Pathol Res Pract. 1989;185(2):207–13.
35. Leader M, Patel J, Collins M, Henry K. Myoglobin: an evaluation of its role as a marker of rhabdomyosarcomas. Br J Cancer. 1989;59(1):106–9.
36. Johnson CW. Issues in immunohistochemistry. Toxicol Pathol. 1999;27(2):246–8.
37. Kim SW, Roh J, Park CS. Immunohistochemistry for pathologists: protocols, pitfalls, and tips. J Pathol Transl Med. 2016;50(6):411–8.
38. Goldblum JR, Weiss SW, Folpe AL. Enzinger and Weiss's soft tissue tumors E-book: expert consult: online and print. Amsterdam: Elsevier Health Sciences; 2013.
39. Moll R, Franke WW, Schiller DL, Geiger B, Krepler R. The catalog of human cytokeratins: patterns of expression in normal epithelia, tumors and cultured cells. Cell. 1982;31(1):11–24.
40. Cooper D, Schermer A, Sun TT. Classification of human epithelia and their neoplasms using monoclonal antibodies to keratins: strategies, applications, and limitations. Lab Investig. 1985;52(3):243–56.
41. Doyle LA. Non-mesenchymal mimics of sarcoma. Surg Pathol Clin. 2015;8(3):493–513.
42. Miettinen M, Fanburg-Smith JC, Virolainen M, Shmookler BM, Fetsch JF. Epithelioid sarcoma: an immunohistochemical analysis of 112 classical and variant cases and a discussion of the differential diagnosis. Hum Pathol. 1999;30(8):934–42.
43. Wrba F, Fertl H, Amann G, Tell E, Krepler R. Epithelial markers in synovial sarcoma. An immunohistochemical study on paraffin embedded tissues. Virchows Arch A Pathol Anat Histopathol. 1989;415(3):253–8.
44. Ordonez NG, Mahfouz SM, Mackay B. Synovial sarcoma: an immunohistochemical and ultrastructural study. Hum Pathol. 1990;21(7):733–49.
45. Lopes JM, Bjerkehagen B, Holm R, Bruland O, Sobrinho-Simoes M, Nesland JM. Immunohistochemical profile of synovial sarcoma with emphasis on the epithelial-type differentiation. A study of 49 primary tumours, recurrences and metastases. Pathol Res Pract. 1994;190(2):168–77.
46. van de Rijn M, Barr FG, Xiong QB, Hedges M, Shipley J, Fisher C. Poorly differentiated synovial sarcoma: an analysis of clinical, pathologic, and molecular genetic features. Am J Surg Pathol. 1999;23(1):106–12.
47. Kilpatrick SE, Hitchcock MG, Kraus MD, Calonje E, Fletcher CD. Mixed tumors and myoepitheliomas of soft tissue: a clinicopathologic study of 19 cases with a unifying concept. Am J Surg Pathol. 1997;21(1):13–22.
48. Michal M, Miettinen M. Myoepitheliomas of the skin and soft tissues. Report of 12 cases. Virchows Arch. 1999;434(5):393–400.
49. Pinkus GS, Kurtin PJ. Epithelial membrane antigen—a diagnostic discriminant in surgical pathology: immunohistochemical profile in epithelial, mesenchymal, and hematopoietic neoplasms using paraffin sections and monoclonal antibodies. Hum Pathol. 1985;16(9):929–40.
50. Bresnick AR, Weber DJ, Zimmer DB. S100 proteins in cancer. Nat Rev Cancer. 2015;15(2):96–109.
51. Hermann A, Donato R, Weiger TM, Chazin WJ. S100 calcium binding proteins and ion channels. Front Pharmacol. 2012;3:67.
52. Donato R, Cannon BR, Sorci G, Riuzzi F, Hsu K, Weber DJ, et al. Functions of S100 proteins. Curr Mol Med. 2013;13(1):24–57.
53. Truong LD, Rangdaeng S, Cagle P, Ro JY, Hawkins H, Font RL. The diagnostic utility of desmin. A study of 584 cases and review of the literature. Am J Clin Pathol. 1990;93(3):305–14.
54. Rangdaeng S, Truong LD. Comparative immunohistochemical staining for desmin and muscle-specific actin. A study of 576 cases. Am J Clin Pathol. 1991;96(1):32–45.

55. Machado I, Mayordomo-Aranda E, Giner F, Llombart-Bosch A. The role of immunohistochemistry in rhabdomyosarcoma diagnosis using tissue microarray technology and a xenograft model. Fetal Pediatr Pathol. 2015;34(5):271–81.
56. Gerald WL, Miller HK, Battifora H, Miettinen M, Silva EG, Rosai J. Intra-abdominal desmoplastic small round-cell tumor. Report of 19 cases of a distinctive type of high-grade polyphenotypic malignancy affecting young individuals. Am J Surg Pathol. 1991;15(6):499–513.
57. Ordonez NG. Desmoplastic small round cell tumor: II: an ultrastructural and immunohistochemical study with emphasis on new immunohistochemical markers. Am J Surg Pathol. 1998;22(11):1314–27.
58. Qiu X, Montgomery E, Sun B. Inflammatory myofibroblastic tumor and low-grade myofibroblastic sarcoma: a comparative study of clinicopathologic features and further observations on the immunohistochemical profile of myofibroblasts. Hum Pathol. 2008;39(6):846–56.
59. Folpe AL, Weiss SW, Fletcher CD, Gown AM. Tenosynovial giant cell tumors: evidence for a desmin-positive dendritic cell subpopulation. Mod Pathol. 1998;11(10):939–44.
60. Hornick JL. Practical soft tissue pathology: a diagnostic approach E-Book: a volume in the pattern recognition series. Amsterdam: Elsevier Health Sciences; 2017.
61. Miettinen M, Lindenmayer AE, Chaubal A. Endothelial cell markers CD31, CD34, and BNH9 antibody to H- and Y-antigens—evaluation of their specificity and sensitivity in the diagnosis of vascular tumors and comparison with von Willebrand factor. Mod Pathol. 1994;7(1):82–90.
62. Kanitakis J, Narvaez D, Claudy A. Expression of the CD34 antigen distinguishes Kaposi's sarcoma from pseudo-Kaposi's sarcoma (acroangiodermatitis). Br J Dermatol. 1996;134(1):44–6.
63. Fellinger EJ, Garin-Chesa P, Su SL, DeAngelis P, Lane JM, Rettig WJ. Biochemical and genetic characterization of the HBA71 Ewing's sarcoma cell surface antigen. Cancer Res. 1991;51(1):336–40.
64. Ambros IM, Ambros PF, Strehl S, Kovar H, Gadner H, Salzer-Kuntschik M. MIC2 is a specific marker for Ewing's sarcoma and peripheral primitive neuroectodermal tumors. Evidence for a common histogenesis of Ewing's sarcoma and peripheral primitive neuroectodermal tumors from MIC2 expression and specific chromosome aberration. Cancer. 1991;67(7):1886–93.
65. Fellinger EJ, Garin-Chesa P, Triche TJ, Huvos AG, Rettig WJ. Immunohistochemical analysis of Ewing's sarcoma cell surface antigen p30/32MIC2. Am J Pathol. 1991;139(2):317–25.
66. Folpe AL, Goldblum JR, Rubin BP, Shehata BM, Liu W, Dei Tos AP, et al. Morphologic and immunophenotypic diversity in Ewing family tumors: a study of 66 genetically confirmed cases. Am J Surg Pathol. 2005;29(8):1025–33.
67. Parham DM. Immunohistochemical markers of soft tissue tumors: pathologic diagnosis, genetic contributions, and therapeutic options. Anal Chem Insights. 2015;10(Suppl 1):1–10.
68. Folpe AL, Hill CE, Parham DM, O'Shea PA, Weiss SW. Immunohistochemical detection of FLI-1 protein expression: a study of 132 round cell tumors with emphasis on CD99-positive mimics of Ewing's sarcoma/primitive neuroectodermal tumor. Am J Surg Pathol. 2000;24(12):1657–62.
69. Turc-Carel C, Aurias A, Mugneret F, Lizard S, Sidaner I, Volk C, et al. Chromosomes in Ewing's sarcoma. I. An evaluation of 85 cases of remarkable consistency of t(11;22)(q24;q12). Cancer Genet Cytogenet. 1988;32(2):229–38.
70. Zucman J, Delattre O, Desmaze C, Plougastel B, Joubert I, Melot T, et al. Cloning and characterization of the Ewing's sarcoma and peripheral neuroepithelioma t(11;22) translocation breakpoints. Genes Chromosomes Cancer. 1992;5(4):271–7.
71. Delattre O, Zucman J, Plougastel B, Desmaze C, Melot T, Peter M, et al. Gene fusion with an ETS DNA-binding domain caused by chromosome translocation in human tumours. Nature. 1992;359(6391):162–5.
72. Nilsson G, Wang M, Wejde J, Kreicbergs A, Larsson O. Detection of EWS/FLI-1 by immunostaining. an adjunctive tool in diagnosis of Ewing's sarcoma and primitive neuroectodermal tumour on cytological samples and paraffin-embedded archival material. Sarcoma. 1999;3(1):25–32.

73. Mandahl N, Akerman M, Aman P, Dal Cin P, De Wever I, Fletcher CD, et al. Duplication of chromosome segment 12q15-24 is associated with atypical lipomatous tumors: a report of the CHAMP collaborative study group. CHromosomes And MorPhology. Int J Cancer. 1996;67(5):632–5.
74. Rosai J, Akerman M, Dal Cin P, DeWever I, Fletcher CD, Mandahl N, et al. Combined morphologic and karyotypic study of 59 atypical lipomatous tumors. Evaluation of their relationship and differential diagnosis with other adipose tissue tumors (a report of the CHAMP Study Group). Am J Surg Pathol. 1996;20(10):1182–9.
75. Binh MB, Sastre-Garau X, Guillou L, de Pinieux G, Terrier P, Lagace R, et al. MDM2 and CDK4 immunostainings are useful adjuncts in diagnosing well-differentiated and dedifferentiated liposarcoma subtypes: a comparative analysis of 559 soft tissue neoplasms with genetic data. Am J Surg Pathol. 2005;29(10):1340–7.
76. Binh MB, Garau XS, Guillou L, Aurias A, Coindre JM. Reproducibility of MDM2 and CDK4 staining in soft tissue tumors. Am J Clin Pathol. 2006;125(5):693–7.
77. Davanzo B, Emerson RE, Lisy M, Koniaris LG, Kays JK. Solitary fibrous tumor. Transl Gastroenterol Hepatol. 2018;3:94.
78. Rakheja D, Molberg KH, Roberts CA, Jaiswal VR. Immunohistochemical expression of beta-catenin in solitary fibrous tumors. Arch Pathol Lab Med. 2005;129(6):776–9.
79. Vogels RJ, Vlenterie M, Versleijen-Jonkers YM, Ruijter E, Bekers EM, Verdijk MA, et al. Solitary fibrous tumor—clinicopathologic, immunohistochemical and molecular analysis of 28 cases. Diagn Pathol. 2014;9:224.
80. Akaike K, Kurisaki-Arakawa A, Hara K, Suehara Y, Takagi T, Mitani K, et al. Distinct clinicopathological features of NAB2-STAT6 fusion gene variants in solitary fibrous tumor with emphasis on the acquisition of highly malignant potential. Hum Pathol. 2015;46(3):347–56.
81. Koelsche C, Schweizer L, Renner M, Warth A, Jones DT, Sahm F, et al. Nuclear relocation of STAT6 reliably predicts NAB2-STAT6 fusion for the diagnosis of solitary fibrous tumour. Histopathology. 2014;65(5):613–22.
82. Mohajeri A, Tayebwa J, Collin A, Nilsson J, Magnusson L, von Steyern FV, et al. Comprehensive genetic analysis identifies a pathognomonic NAB2/STAT6 fusion gene, nonrandom secondary genomic imbalances, and a characteristic gene expression profile in solitary fibrous tumor. Genes Chromosomes Cancer. 2013;52(10):873–86.
83. Yoshida A, Tsuta K, Ohno M, Yoshida M, Narita Y, Kawai A, et al. STAT6 immunohistochemistry is helpful in the diagnosis of solitary fibrous tumors. Am J Surg Pathol. 2014;38(4):552–9.
84. Rao N, Colby TV, Falconieri G, Cohen H, Moran CA, Suster S. Intrapulmonary solitary fibrous tumors: clinicopathologic and immunohistochemical study of 24 cases. Am J Surg Pathol. 2013;37(2):155–66.
85. Plaza JA, Mayerson J, Wakely PE Jr. Nodular fasciitis of the hand: a potential diagnostic pitfall in fine-needle aspiration cytopathology. Am J Clin Pathol. 2005;123(3):388–93.
86. Luna A, Molinari L, Bollea Garlatti LA, Ferrario D, Volonteri V, Roitman P, et al. Nodular fasciitis, a forgotten entity. Int J Dermatol. 2019;58(2):190–3.
87. Khanna V, Rajan M, Reddy T, Alexander N, Surendran P. Nodular fasciitis mimicking a soft tissue sarcoma—a case report. Int J Surg Case Rep. 2018;44:29–32.
88. Lu L, Lao IW, Liu X, Yu L, Wang J. Nodular fasciitis: a retrospective study of 272 cases from China with clinicopathologic and radiologic correlation. Ann Diagn Pathol. 2015;19(3):180–5.
89. Magro G. Differential diagnosis of benign spindle cell lesions. Surg Pathol Clin. 2018;11(1):91–121.
90. Wick MR, Ritter JH, Humphrey PA. Sarcomatoid carcinomas of the lung: a clinicopathologic review. Am J Clin Pathol. 1997;108(1):40–53.
91. Guarino M, Tricomi P, Giordano F, Cristofori E. Sarcomatoid carcinomas: pathological and histopathogenetic considerations. Pathology. 1996;28(4):298–305.
92. Lewis JE, Olsen KD, Sebo TJ. Spindle cell carcinoma of the larynx: review of 26 cases including DNA content and immunohistochemistry. Hum Pathol. 1997;28(6):664–73.

93. Nishihara K, Tsuneyoshi M. Undifferentiated spindle cell carcinoma of the gallbladder: a clinicopathologic, immunohistochemical, and flow cytometric study of 11 cases. Hum Pathol. 1993;24(12):1298–305.
94. Taskin OC, Akkas G, Memis B, Seven IE, Basturk O, Jang KT, et al. Sarcomatoid carcinomas of the gallbladder: clinicopathologic characteristics. Virchows Arch. 2019;475(1):59–66.
95. Wick MR, Swanson PE, Scheithauer BW, Manivel JC. Malignant peripheral nerve sheath tumor. An immunohistochemical study of 62 cases. Am J Clin Pathol. 1987;87(4):425–33.
96. Giangaspero F, Fratamico FC, Ceccarelli C, Brisigotti M. Malignant peripheral nerve sheath tumors and spindle cell sarcomas: an immunohistochemical analysis of multiple markers. Appl Pathol. 1989;7(2):134–44.
97. Romano RC, Carter JM, Folpe AL. Aberrant intermediate filament and synaptophysin expression is a frequent event in malignant melanoma: an immunohistochemical study of 73 cases. Mod Pathol. 2015;28(8):1033–42.
98. Bolander A, Agnarsdottir M, Wagenius G, Stromberg S, Ponten F, Ekman S, et al. Serological and immunohistochemical analysis of S100 and new derivatives as markers for prognosis in patients with malignant melanoma. Melanoma Res. 2008;18(6):412–9.
99. Prieto VG, Shea CR. Use of immunohistochemistry in melanocytic lesions. J Cutan Pathol. 2008;35(Suppl 2):1–10.
100. Dim DC, Cooley LD, Miranda RN. Clear cell sarcoma of tendons and aponeuroses: a review. Arch Pathol Lab Med. 2007;131(1):152–6.
101. Hisaoka M, Ishida T, Kuo TT, Matsuyama A, Imamura T, Nishida K, et al. Clear cell sarcoma of soft tissue: a clinicopathologic, immunohistochemical, and molecular analysis of 33 cases. Am J Surg Pathol. 2008;32(3):452–60.
102. Hantschke M, Mentzel T, Rutten A, Palmedo G, Calonje E, Lazar AJ, et al. Cutaneous clear cell sarcoma: a clinicopathologic, immunohistochemical, and molecular analysis of 12 cases emphasizing its distinction from dermal melanoma. Am J Surg Pathol. 2010;34(2):216–22.
103. Wang NP, Marx J, McNutt MA, Rutledge JC, Gown AM. Expression of myogenic regulatory proteins (myogenin and MyoD1) in small blue round cell tumors of childhood. Am J Pathol. 1995;147(6):1799–810.
104. Cui S, Hano H, Harada T, Takai S, Masui F, Ushigome S. Evaluation of new monoclonal anti-MyoD1 and anti-myogenin antibodies for the diagnosis of rhabdomyosarcoma. Pathol Int. 1999;49(1):62–8.
105. Kumar S, Perlman E, Harris CA, Raffeld M, Tsokos M. Myogenin is a specific marker for rhabdomyosarcoma: an immunohistochemical study in paraffin-embedded tissues. Mod Pathol. 2000;13(9):988–93.
106. Wijnaendts LC, van der Linden JC, van Unnik AJ, Delemarre JF, Voute PA, Meijer CJ. The expression pattern of contractile and intermediate filament proteins in developing skeletal muscle and rhabdomyosarcoma of childhood: diagnostic and prognostic utility. J Pathol. 1994;174(4):283–92.
107. Dias P, Chen B, Dilday B, Palmer H, Hosoi H, Singh S, et al. Strong immunostaining for myogenin in rhabdomyosarcoma is significantly associated with tumors of the alveolar subclass. Am J Pathol. 2000;156(2):399–408.
108. Heerema-McKenney A, Wijnaendts LC, Pulliam JF, Lopez-Terrada D, McKenney JK, Zhu S, et al. Diffuse myogenin expression by immunohistochemistry is an independent marker of poor survival in pediatric rhabdomyosarcoma: a tissue microarray study of 71 primary tumors including correlation with molecular phenotype. Am J Surg Pathol. 2008;32(10):1513–22.
109. Fletcher CD, Berman JJ, Corless C, Gorstein F, Lasota J, Longley BJ, et al. Diagnosis of gastrointestinal stromal tumors: a consensus approach. Int J Surg Pathol. 2002;10(2):81–9.
110. Lux ML, Rubin BP, Biase TL, Chen CJ, Maclure T, Demetri G, et al. KIT extracellular and kinase domain mutations in gastrointestinal stromal tumors. Am J Pathol. 2000;156(3):791–5.
111. Rubin BP, Singer S, Tsao C, Duensing A, Lux ML, Ruiz R, et al. KIT activation is a ubiquitous feature of gastrointestinal stromal tumors. Cancer Res. 2001;61(22):8118–21.

112. Corless CL, McGreevey L, Haley A, Town A, Heinrich MC. KIT mutations are common in incidental gastrointestinal stromal tumors one centimeter or less in size. Am J Pathol. 2002;160(5):1567–72.
113. Yarden Y, Kuang WJ, Yang-Feng T, Coussens L, Munemitsu S, Dull TJ, et al. Human proto-oncogene c-kit: a new cell surface receptor tyrosine kinase for an unidentified ligand. EMBO J. 1987;6(11):3341–51.
114. Hirota S, Isozaki K, Moriyama Y, Hashimoto K, Nishida T, Ishiguro S, et al. Gain-of-function mutations of c-kit in human gastrointestinal stromal tumors. Science. 1998;279(5350):577–80.
115. van Oosterom AT, Judson I, Verweij J, Stroobants S, Donato di Paola E, Dimitrijevic S, et al. Safety and efficacy of imatinib (STI571) in metastatic gastrointestinal stromal tumours: a phase I study. Lancet. 2001;358(9291):1421–3.
116. Demetri GD, von Mehren M, Blanke CD, Van den Abbeele AD, Eisenberg B, Roberts PJ, et al. Efficacy and safety of imatinib mesylate in advanced gastrointestinal stromal tumors. N Engl J Med. 2002;347(7):472–80.
117. Scotlandi K, Manara MC, Strammiello R, Landuzzi L, Benini S, Perdichizzi S, et al. C-kit receptor expression in Ewing's sarcoma: lack of prognostic value but therapeutic targeting opportunities in appropriate conditions. J Clin Oncol. 2003;21(10):1952–60.
118. Ahmed A, Gilbert-Barness E, Lacson A. Expression of c-kit in Ewing family of tumors: a comparison of different immunohistochemical protocols. Pediatr Dev Pathol. 2004;7(4):342–7.
119. Gonzalez I, Andreu EJ, Panizo A, Inoges S, Fontalba A, Fernandez-Luna JL, et al. Imatinib inhibits proliferation of Ewing tumor cells mediated by the stem cell factor/KIT receptor pathway, and sensitizes cells to vincristine and doxorubicin-induced apoptosis. Clin Cancer Res. 2004;10(2):751–61.
120. Miettinen M, Sarlomo-Rikala M, Lasota J. KIT expression in angiosarcomas and fetal endothelial cells: lack of mutations of exon 11 and exon 17 of C-kit. Mod Pathol. 2000;13(5):536–41.
121. Hornick JL, Fletcher CD. Immunohistochemical staining for KIT (CD117) in soft tissue sarcomas is very limited in distribution. Am J Clin Pathol. 2002;117(2):188–93.
122. Komdeur R, Hoekstra HJ, Molenaar WM, Van Den Berg E, Zwart N, Pras E, et al. Clinicopathologic assessment of postradiation sarcomas: KIT as a potential treatment target. Clin Cancer Res. 2003;9(8):2926–32.
123. Novelli M, Rossi S, Rodriguez-Justo M, Taniere P, Seddon B, Toffolatti L, et al. DOG1 and CD117 are the antibodies of choice in the diagnosis of gastrointestinal stromal tumours. Histopathology. 2010;57(2):259–70.
124. Miettinen M, Wang ZF, Lasota J. DOG1 antibody in the differential diagnosis of gastrointestinal stromal tumors: a study of 1840 cases. Am J Surg Pathol. 2009;33(9):1401–8.
125. De Young BR, Frierson HF Jr, Ly MN, Smith D, Swanson PE. CD31 immunoreactivity in carcinomas and mesotheliomas. Am J Clin Pathol. 1998;110(3):374–7.
126. Sullivan HC, Edgar MA, Cohen C, Kovach CK, HooKim K, Reid MD. The utility of ERG, CD31 and CD34 in the cytological diagnosis of angiosarcoma: an analysis of 25 cases. J Clin Pathol. 2015;68(1):44–50.
127. Suster S, Fisher C. Immunoreactivity for the human hematopoietic progenitor cell antigen (CD34) in lipomatous tumors. Am J Surg Pathol. 1997;21(2):195–200.
128. Folpe AL, Chand EM, Goldblum JR, Weiss SW. Expression of Fli-1, a nuclear transcription factor, distinguishes vascular neoplasms from potential mimics. Am J Surg Pathol. 2001;25(8):1061–6.
129. Cheuk W, Wong KO, Wong CS, Dinkel JE, Ben-Dor D, Chan JK. Immunostaining for human herpesvirus 8 latent nuclear antigen-1 helps distinguish Kaposi sarcoma from its mimickers. Am J Clin Pathol. 2004;121(3):335–42.
130. Patel RM, Goldblum JR, Hsi ED. Immunohistochemical detection of human herpes virus-8 latent nuclear antigen-1 is useful in the diagnosis of Kaposi sarcoma. Mod Pathol. 2004;17(4):456–60.

Molecular Genetics in the Multidisciplinary Management of Sarcoma

9

Vanessa Tran and John Slavin

9.1 Introduction

Sarcomas encompass a diverse, heterogeneous family of rare neoplasms arising from mesenchymal origin, accounting for only 1% of all malignant tumours [1]. This includes approximately 70 histopathological entities covering tumours of the bone, muscle, fat, vasculature and peripheral nervous system. Sarcomas are classified according to the tissue that they most closely resemble and can arise in almost any anatomical site within the body, adding to its diversity [2, 3]. Traditional classification based on these morphologic features alone is therefore insufficient in capturing the complexity of clinical behaviours encountered in practice [4]. The advent of ancillary tools such as immunohistochemistry (IHC), cytogenetics and molecular genetics has allowed stratification of sarcomas into more accurate entities that are reflective of their typical clinical characteristics [5, 6]. A better understanding of the molecular basis of bone and soft tissue tumours has widespread implications in improving patient management, including the diagnostic accuracy of sarcomas, prognostication of the disease and the development of more targeted therapies. This review will discuss the current molecular aberrations understood in sarcoma and their potential applications in sarcoma diagnosis, prognosis and treatment.

9.2 Molecular Aberrations in Sarcoma

The advent of accessible molecular testing modalities, including chromosome analysis, fluorescence in situ hybridisation (FISH) and reverse transcription polymerase

V. Tran (✉)
Department of Surgery, University of Melbourne, Melbourne, VIC, Australia

J. Slavin
Department of Anatomical Pathology, St. Vincent's Hospital Melbourne, Melbourne, VIC, Australia
e-mail: john.slavin@svha.org.au

P. F. M. Choong (ed.), *Sarcoma*, https://doi.org/10.1007/978-981-15-9414-4_9

chain reaction (RT-PCR), has enriched the characterisation of genetic abnormalities within specific sarcomas subtypes. The most common aberrations encountered are chromosomal translocations, followed by gene amplifications and activating mutations [7]. While the clinical significance of these discoveries is yet to be completely resolved, this has become a crucial aid to understanding the basis of soft tissue and bone tumours. Table 9.1 summarises the recurrent genetic abnormalities found in

Table 9.1 Common genetic alterations encountered in sarcoma

	Tumour type	Genes involved
Translocations	Alveolar rhabdomyosarcoma	PAX3-FKHR, PAX7-FKHR, PAX3-AFX, PAX3-NCOA1
	Alveolar soft-part sarcoma	ASPSCR1-TFE3
	Angiomatoid fibroid histiocytoma	EWSR1-ATF1, EWSR1-CREB1, FUS-ATF1
	Clear cell sarcoma	EWSR1-ATF1, EWSR1-CREB1
	Congenital fibrosarcoma	ETC-NTRK3
	Congenital/infantile spindle cell rhabdomyosarcoma	NCOA2-SRF, NCOA2-TEAD1
	Dermatofibrosarcoma protuberans	COL1A1-PDGFB
	Desmoplastic small round cell tumour	EWSR, WT1
	Endometrial stromal sarcoma	JAZF1-JJAZ1(SUZ12), JAZF1-PHF1, EPC-PHF1, YWHAE-FAM22
	Epithelioid haemangioendothelioma	WWTR1-CAMTA1
	Extraskeletal myxoid chondrosarcoma	EWSR1-NR4A3, TAF2N-NR4A3, TCF12-NR4A3, TFG-NR4A3
	Ewing sarcoma/PNET	EWSR1-FLI1, EWSR1-ERG, EWSR1-ETV1, EWSR1-FEV, EWSR-E1AF, FUS-ERG, FUS-FEV
	Infantile fibrosarcoma	ETC6-NTRK3
	Inflammatory myofibroblastic tumour	TPM3-ALK, TPM4-ALK, CLTC-ALK, RANBP2-ALK, CARS-ALK
	Low-grade fibromyxoid sarcoma	FUS-CREB3L2, FUS-CREB3L1
	Malignant gastrointestinal neuroectodermal tumour	EWSR1-ATF1, EWSR1-CREB1
	Mesenchymal chondrosarcoma	HEY1-NCOA2
	Myxoid/round cell liposarcoma	FUS-DDIT3, EWSR1-DDIT3
	Myxoinflammatory fibroblastic sarcoma	TGFBR3 and MGEA5
	Pulmonary myxoid sarcoma	EWSR1-CREB1
	Sclerosing epithelioid fibrosarcoma	FUS-CREB3L2
	Solitary fibrous tumour	NAB2-STAT6
	Synovial sarcoma	SSX18-SSX1, SSX2, SSX4
	Undifferentiated small round blue cell tumour	CIC-DUX4

Table 9.1 (continued)

	Tumour type	Genes involved
Amplifications	Osteosarcoma (parosteal and intramedullary)	MDM2, CDK4, HMGA2, GLI, SAS
	Leiomyosarcoma	MYOCD
	Post-radiation angiosarcoma	MYC
	Well-differentiated liposarcoma and de-differentiated liposarcoma	MDM2, CDK4
Activating mutations	Chondrosarcoma	IDH1/IDH2 COL2A1
	Desmoid-type fibromatosis	CTNNB1
	Embryonal rhabdomyosarcoma	N/K/HRAS, FGFR4
	GIST	KIT/POGFRA, SDHA/B
	Myxoid liposarcoma	PIK3CA
	Spindle cell rhabdomyosarcoma	MYOD1
Inactivating mutations or deletions	MPNST	CDKN2A
	Fibrosarcomatous DFSP	
	Advanced GIST	
	Osteosarcoma	TP53
	Leiomyosarcoma	
	Spindle cell lipoma	RB1
	Mammary-type myofibroblastoma	

sarcoma subtypes. This section of the review will present the main molecular aberrations encountered and introduce common examples of each.

9.2.1 Chromosomal Translocations

Chromosomal translocations are the most common genetic aberrations and account for 35% of all sarcomas [8]. There are two broad types of translocations: (1) non-reciprocal or unbalanced translocations, which occur when a fragment of one chromosome is transferred to another chromosome, and (2) reciprocal or balanced translocations, which describe the exchange of two chromosomal fragments between two different chromosomes (Fig. 9.1). In cancer, the chimeric gene product can produce a novel protein that is involved in the process of malignant transformation [9].

An archetypal example of a recurrent translocation-associated tumour is Ewing's sarcoma/primitive neuroectodermal tumours (PNET). Approximately 90% of Ewing sarcoma/PNET is found to harbour a translocation involving the EWSR1 gene on chromosome 22. Its fusion partners are variable and belong to collection of genes called the ETS family of transcriptional regulators. The most common of these genes is the FLI-1 gene on chromosome 11 [10–13]. Other less common fusion products include EWSR1-ERG, EWSR1-ETV and EWSR1-FEV [14–16]. The EWSR1 gene and t(11;22) translocation is also implicated in other sarcomas, such as desmoplastic round cell tumours, in which it forms a resultant EWSR1-WT1

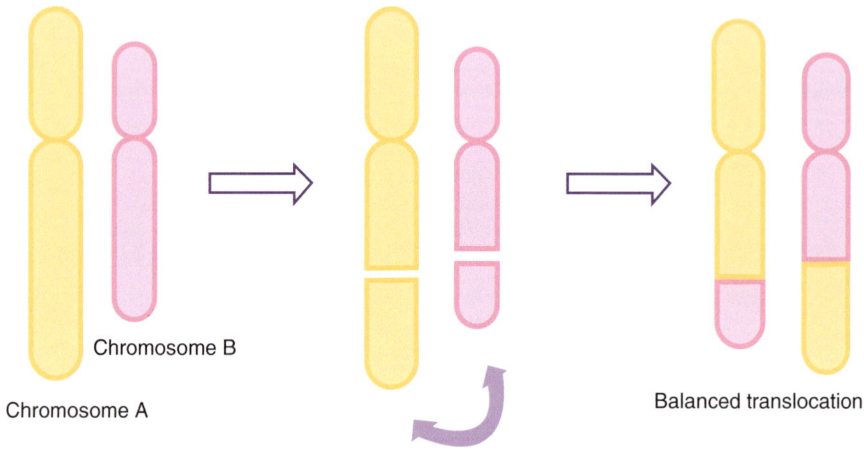

Fig. 9.1 Balanced translocation (Author's own)

fusion gene [17, 18]. In contrast, the t(X;18)(p11.2;q11.2) translocation is almost distinctively pathognomonic of synovial sarcomas, occurring uniquely within this subtype in almost 90% of cases [19–22]. This results in one of many SYT-SSX gene fusion products [23, 24]. In alveolar rhabdomyosarcoma, over three-quarters of tumours harbour either a t(2;13) or t(1;13) translocation, resulting in the chimeric PAX3-FKHR or PAX7-FKHR proteins, which are also specific to this subtype of sarcoma [25].

9.2.2 Gene Amplifications

Gene amplifications comprise around one-third of molecular abnormalities in sarcoma. Common amplifications are found in the MDM2 and CDK4 genes, and these most often occur in adipose tumours [8]. Atypical lipomatous tumours/well-differentiated liposarcoma (ALT/WDLPS) and dedifferentiated liposarcoma (DDLPS) are separate clinical entities within liposarcomas that are characterised by these molecular aberrations. These sarcomas often harbour complex genomes, characterised by an unbalanced karyotype with chromosomal instability. Karyotypes of ALT/WDLPS and DDLPS commonly reveal the presence of supernumerary ring chromosomes [26]. The genetic material within these ring chromosomes almost invariably contain amplified copies of MDM2 and CDK4 oncogenes, which can adequately be detected by FISH (gold standard) [27, 28] or IHC [29, 30]. Increased expression of MDM2 results in inactivation the p53 signalling pathway [31–33] and consequential promotion cell cycle dysregulation and cell proliferation. CDK4, on the other hand, directly promotes cell cycle progression from G1 to S phase [34]. More recently, gene amplifications have been discovered in the MYOCD gene in leiomyosarcomas [35, 36] as well as the MYC gene in radiation-associated angiosarcoma [37, 38].

9.2.3 Activating Mutations of Proto-oncogenes

An activating mutation in a proto-oncogene can lead to cell proliferation in cancer. In sarcoma, mutations may lead to deregulated kinase signalling or the production of oncometabolites, which drives tumorigenesis. A prototypical example is gain-of-function mutations in KIT and platelet-derived growth factor alpha (PDGFRA) genes in gastrointestinal stromal tumours (GIST). KIT is a member of the family of receptor tyrosine kinases [39] that is encountered in 75–80% of GISTs [40–42], while PDGFRA mutations represent 5–10% of GISTs [43–46]. Both KIT and PDGFRA are receptor tyrosine kinases that drive intracellular signalling pathways in cell differentiation, survival and proliferation [47, 48]. The responsible activating mutation in KIT is variable and includes deletions, duplications or point mutations in exons 11, 9, 13, 14, 17 and 18 [45, 48]. PDGFRA mutations may result mutations from exons 18, 12 and 14 [49].

9.2.4 Germline Mutations

An association has also been drawn between sarcoma risk and germline mutations. Li-Fraumeni syndrome is an autosomal dominant condition that is clinically characterised by its high lifetime sarcoma risk and early cancer diagnosis [50, 51]. Molecularly, it is driven by an underlying germline mutation in TP53 [52, 53]; however, diagnosis of Li-Fraumeni syndrome is in fact made clinically based on sarcoma history [51]. Additional germline mutations have been demonstrated in BRCA2, ATM, ATR, ERCC2 and DICER1 [54–56].

9.3 Molecular Techniques

In the laboratory, pathologists have access to various tools to detect genetic aberrations in tumour tissue samples. This section will highlight the main types of molecular techniques and discuss their advantages, disadvantages and clinical applications.

9.3.1 Conventional Karyotyping

Conventional karyotyping allows the visualisation under light microscope of gross structural chromosomal abnormalities, such as large deletions or duplications, chromosomal translocations or aneuploidies (Fig. 9.2). The advantage of this technique is that it does not require prior knowledge of the expected aberration. Its use, however, is limited by the availability of fresh, sterile tumour tissue and the ability to successfully culture tumour cells and subsequently capture metaphase preparations from these cultures [57]. Karyotyping of ALT/WDLPS and DDLPS, for example, can reveal giant marker or ring chromosomes, which involve the chromosomal region 12q13–15 containing amplified regions of MDM2 and CDK4 [26].

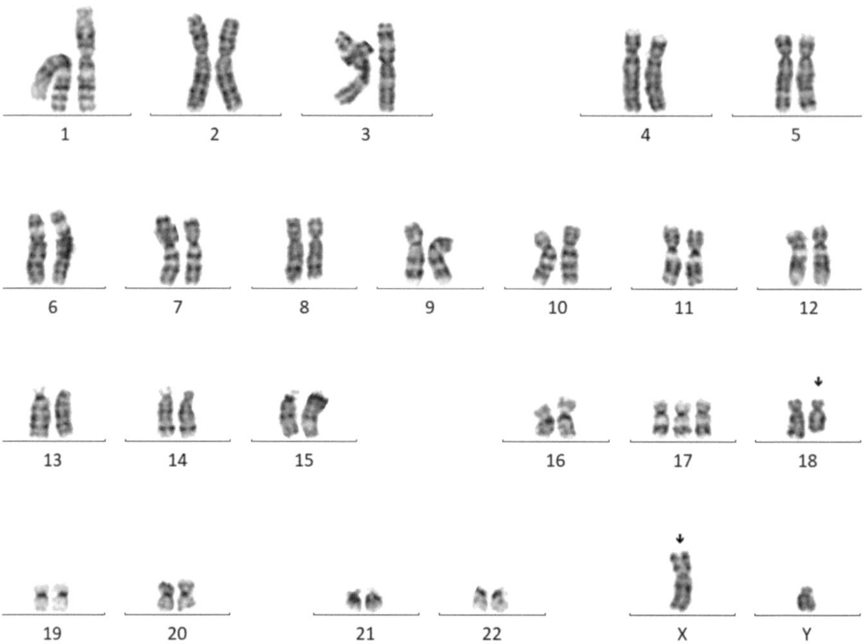

Fig. 9.2 Conventional karyotype demonstrating a t(X;18) translocation in synovial sarcoma

9.3.2 Fluorescence In Situ Hybridisation

FISH is a more recently developed molecular cytogenetic technique that detects specific DNA sequences through hybridisation with complimentary DNA probes (Fig. 9.3). Unlike conventional karyotyping, FISH can be performed on a small sample of tumour tissue of various preparations (fresh, frozen, paraffin-embedded) and can be performed relatively quickly (overnight). Its use, however, relies on knowledge of suspected molecular aberrations and is also limited by commercial availability of specific DNA probes [58]. In sarcoma, FISH has demonstrated efficacy in identifying abnormalities including chromosomal rearrangements and aneuploidies but has limited use in smaller aberrations such as point mutations due to the size of the probes [59].

9.3.3 Reverse Transcription-Polymerase Chain Reaction

RT-PCR involves the reverse transcription of known RNA transcripts into complementary DNA with subsequent amplification of these DNA targets using PCR. In sarcoma, it is useful in detecting translocation-associated chimeric RNA transcripts, such as SYT-SSX1/2 fusion transcripts in synovial sarcoma [60].

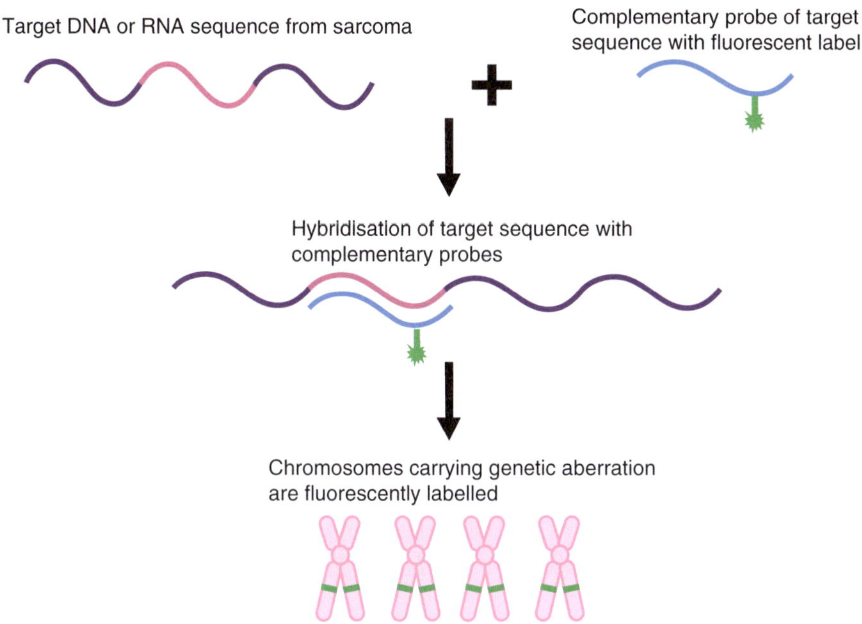

Fig. 9.3 Fluorescence in situ hybridisation (Author's own)

9.3.4 Immunohistochemistry

While immunohistochemistry is not specifically a molecular technique, genetic aberrations can be inferred from the presence of immunohistochemical surrogates in sarcoma tissue samples. Immunohistochemistry involves the detection of certain antigens in a tissue sample using antigen-specific antibodies. For example, immunohistochemical staining of MDM2 and CDK4 in well-differentiated liposarcoma is used as a surrogate marker for amplification of the respective genes [61].

9.4 Diagnosis

The challenge of sarcoma diagnosis can be attributed to both its rarity and histological heterogeneity. This difficulty is reflected in several studies, which found discrepancy rates of up to 32% for soft tissue sarcoma diagnoses between non-specialist centres and expert referral centres [62–65]. Errors in diagnosis may lead to either under- or overtreatment of tumours, both of which can adversely affect patient outcomes. Knowledge of recurrent molecular aberrations within specific sarcoma subtypes can provide supplementary information to improve diagnostic accuracy [4]. Given the vast range of treatment modalities in cancer and the frequent ambiguities in sarcoma histopathology, improvement in diagnostic precision is essential. In fact, the GENSARC study by Italiano et al. set forward the recommendation that all mesenchymal tumours, irrespective of histological certainty, undergo molecular testing as part of the diagnostic process [4]. The utility of molecular genetics can be exemplified in several contexts, particularly those in which conventional histology is insufficient as the sole investigative modality to distinguish one sarcoma variant from another.

9.4.1 Liposarcoma

ALT/WDLPS and DDLPS are both subtypes of liposarcomas that have very distinct clinical patterns of behaviour. Yet, these two separate entities both present examples of diagnostic challenges that can be assisted with adjunctive molecular testing of MDM2 amplification, as they recurrently display amplification of the MDM2 gene [28, 66]. ALT/WDLPS, on one hand, are often histologically equivocal to benign lipomatous tumours and present the challenge of distinguishing malignant from benign tumours. On the other hand, the highly heterogeneous and non-lipogenic appearance of DDLPS can be difficult to distinguish from other high-grade sarcomas [34]. MDM2 is amplified in almost 100% of all ALT/WDLPS and DDLPS and can therefore be of significant diagnostic value [29, 67]. The application of MDM2 amplification testing in identifying WDLPS among benign adipose tumours, for instance, has demonstrated sensitivity of 100% [68, 69]. MDM2 amplification, however, is not unique to liposarcomas and can be detected in numerous other sarcomas, including osteosarcoma, rhabdomyosarcoma and leiomyosarcoma [32, 70]. It is therefore insufficient alone as a diagnostic tool and its utility, rather, resides as an adjunct to traditional histopathology in distinguishing ALT/WDLPS and DDLPS from their respective histologically alike counterparts.

9.4.2 Synovial Sarcoma

Synovial sarcoma is a clinically diverse entity, with widespread anatomical localisation and histological variance. The differential list for synovial sarcomas is large and includes both mesenchymal and non-mesenchymal tumours, including cellular schwannoma, spindle cell carcinoma, spindle cell melanoma, leiomyosarcoma, malignant schwannoma and Ewing's sarcoma/PNET [71, 72]. Identification of the t(X;18)(p11.2;q11.2) translocation or a SYT-SSX fusion transcripts is a useful diagnostic marker, as this translocation exists in 90–98% of synovial sarcomas [19–22]. Moreover, characterisation of the specific fusion product may have prognostic value, which is elaborated on later in this review (see Sect. 9.5).

9.4.3 Small Round Cell Tumours

Genetic characterisation of sarcomas is also useful in the differential diagnosis of small round blue cell tumours (SRBCTs), which encompasses the Ewing's family of tumours (EWS), alveolar rhabdomyosarcoma and desmoplastic round cell tumour [59, 73, 74]. These tumours have many overlapping histological appearances and IHC features but vastly different prognoses and treatments [75, 76]. Detection of tumour-specific translocations with FISH or RT-PCR is particularly useful for the diagnosis of these SRBCTs [75–79]. Ewing's sarcoma/PNET can be diagnosed by the detection of t(11;22)(q24;q12) translocations and resultant EWS-FLI1 fusion products [11], for example, while 80% of alveolar rhabdomyosarcoma will demonstrate the PAX3-FKHR gene fusions [80, 81]. Desmoplastic round cell tumours, on the other hand, demonstrate a recurrent EWSR-WT1 fusion gene [17, 18], and more recently, a new group of Ewing-like sarcomas have been found to harbour CIC-DUX4 and BCOR-CCNB3 gene fusions [78]. Detection of these translocations or their respective fusion genes, therefore, assists in the differential diagnosis of this complex histological entity of SRBCTs.

9.4.4 Nodular Fasciitis

Molecular genetics has also demonstrated its utility in diagnosing benign soft tissue tumours, which is important in preventing overtreatment of patients and unnecessary interventions. Nodular fasciitis is a self-limiting, benign fibroblastic/myofibroblastic tumour, which displays clinical and histopathological properties that may lead to the misdiagnosis of sarcoma [62, 82, 83]. A balanced rearrangement involving a t(17;22) translocation and resultant MYH9-USP6 fusion is commonly seen in nodular fasciitis and can thus aid its diagnosis [84, 85].

9.5 Prognosis

The ability to prognosticate patients is essential in guiding both clinical and patient's decisions. Patient perspective questionnaires have revealed that patients generally wish to understand more about their prognosis; however, this information is often not received from their treating team [86–88]. Other studies have found that patients often misunderstand their prognosis [89–91] and the authors suggest that this, in part, has to do with the lack of communication from their clinicians [90]. This highlights the significance of prognosticating cancers in ensuring quality patient care. There are several molecular aberrations that have been observed to correlate with outcomes and may therefore demonstrate prognostic utility. In ESW/FLI1-associated Ewing's sarcoma/PNET, for example, there are two common fusion types (type I and type II), which can be best detected by RT-PCR [92, 93]. Detection of a type I fusion confers longer disease-free survival than other fusions in localised Ewing's sarcoma [94, 95]. In alveolar rhabdomyosarcomas, PAX7-FKHR fusion status is associated with a survival rate of 75% compared with a mere 8% in PAX3-FKHR fusion-associated tumours [25].

Some studies have also suggested prognostic value in the specific type of SYT-SSX fusion in synovial sarcomas. Retrospective analyses have demonstrated that

SYT-SSX2 fusion status supported better outcomes compared with SYT-SSX1 fusions [22, 24, 96–98], although this finding was not concluded in other studies [99, 100].

9.6 Treatment

Molecular genetics has revolutionised the approach to cancer treatment through its applications in targeted therapies. Understanding the genetic drivers of oncogenesis that distinguish cancer cells from non-cancerous cells forms the basis of developing these novel therapies [101].

9.6.1 Imatinib in GIST

At the forefront of this pursuit is the targeted inhibition of deregulated tyrosine kinase signalling in GIST. As mentioned (see Sect. 9.2.3), the majority of GIST tumours are associated with an activating mutation in KIT [40–42] and PDGFRA gene [43, 44]. Imatinib is a receptor tyrosine kinase inhibitor that has been utilised as an effective adjuvant therapy in the treatment regimen for GIST [102, 103]. Further molecular characterisation of the underlying KIT/PDGFRA mutations informs optimal treatment decisions and response outcomes [48]. For example, KIT tumours with mutations in exon 11 demonstrate the highest response rate of 67–83% compared with other KIT-mutants [104–106]. Importantly, it has been found that sunitinib, another KIT inhibitor, has greater efficacy against KIT exon 9-mutant tumours than imatinib [105]. In addition, the most common PDGFRA mutation, D842V in PDGFRA exon 18, is resistant to imatinib and sunitinib [104] but has recently been found to be sensitive to crenolanib, a novel tyrosine kinase inhibitor [107]. In summary, there is a heterogeneous response of GIST to imatinib, which can be explained by the genetic profile of the tumours. This example demonstrates the powerful utility of molecular genetics in guiding tailored therapies to patients with GIST.

9.6.2 Imatinib in the Treatment of Other Soft Tissue Tumours

The success of imatinib has established a powerful paradigm in the pursuit of more targeted therapies in sarcoma treatment. Imatinib has also shown success in the treatment of other sarcoma types, such as locally advanced or metastatic dermatofibrosarcoma protuberans (DFSP) [108–110]. These tumours harbour a characteristic t(17;22) translocation, which result in a fusion between collagen type I A1 (COL1A1) gene and PDGFB gene [111, 112]. The upregulation of the COL1A1-PDGFB fusion protein activates PDGFB receptor, a protein tyrosine kinase that forms the target of imatinib therapy [108, 113]. In addition, imatinib has shown efficacy in non-malignant tumours, such as tenosynovial giant cell tumour/

pigmented villonodular synovitis (TGCT/PVNS), a neoplasm of the synovium characterised by the overexpression of colony stimulating factor-1 (CSF1) due to a CSF1-COL6A3 fusion product [114–116]. In TGCT/PVNS, the tumour cells expressing CSF1 comprise only a minority of the tumour bulk. [114].

9.6.3 The Future of Other Targeted Therapies in Sarcoma

Beyond imatinib, there are many other targeted therapies that are showing promising results in the treatment of sarcomas. GCTB is a locally aggressive, benign tumour that causes bony destruction, a process mediated by receptor activator of nuclear factor kappa-B ligand (RANKL). Denosumab, a monoclonal antibody against RANKL that binds and prevents its interaction with RANK on osteoclast surfaces, has demonstrated success in the treatment of giant cell tumour of bone (GCTB) [117–120]. In addition, this drug has been approved for use in multiple myeloma and metastatic bone disease with further research and case studies indicating therapeutic potential in aneurysmal bone cysts [121, 122] and osteosarcoma [123–125]. In chondrosarcomas, isocitrate dehydrogenase 1 (IDH1) is found to be mutated in 56% of cases [126], resulting in the formation of an oncometabolite, 2-HG [127, 128]. A recent phase I study by Tap et al. demonstrated a disease stabilisation rate of 55% for mutant IDH1 (mIDH1) solid tumours treated with an mIDH1 inhibitor (AG-120, ivosidenib) [129]. Of note, this study presented one subject with metastatic chondrosarcoma, who demonstrated stable disease after 343 days and 4 cycles of AG-120. These promising results warrant further clinical trials of AG-120 in chondrosarcoma patients.

9.7 Conclusion

This review highlights the broad and multifaceted utility of molecular genetics in the clinical diagnosis and management of sarcomas. Its application has already shown many promising results and demonstrates great potential in for future application.

References

1. Siegel RL, Miller KD, Jemal A. Cancer statistics, 2019. CA Cancer J Clin. 2019;69(1):7–34.
2. Clark MA, Fisher C, Judson I, Thomas JM. Soft-tissue sarcomas in adults. N Engl J Med. 2005;353(7):701–11.
3. Fletcher CDM, Bridge JA, Hogendoorn PCW, Fletcher CDM, Bridge JA, Hogendoorn P. WHO classification of tumours of soft tissue and bone. Lyon: International Agency for Research on Cancer (IARC) (UN); 2013.
4. Italiano A, Di Mauro I, Rapp J, Pierron G, Auger N, Alberti L, et al. Clinical effect of molecular methods in sarcoma diagnosis (GENSARC): a prospective, multicentre, observational study. Lancet Oncol. 2016;17(4):532–8.

5. Fletcher CD. The evolving classification of soft tissue tumours—an update based on the new 2013 WHO classification. Histopathology. 2014;64(1):2–11.
6. Ladanyi M, Bridge JA. Contribution of molecular genetic data to the classification of sarcomas. Hum Pathol. 2000;31(5):532–8.
7. Hill DA, O'Sullivan MJ, Zhu X, Vollmer RT, Humphrey PA, Dehner LP, et al. Practical application of molecular genetic testing as an aid to the surgical pathologic diagnosis of sarcomas: a prospective study. Am J Surg Pathol. 2002;26(8):965–77.
8. Ducimetiere F, Lurkin A, Ranchere-Vince D, Decouvelaere AV, Peoc'h M, Istier L, et al. Incidence of sarcoma histotypes and molecular subtypes in a prospective epidemiological study with central pathology review and molecular testing. PLoS One. 2011;6(8):e20294.
9. Lazar AJ, Trent JC, Lev D. Sarcoma molecular testing: diagnosis and prognosis. Curr Oncol Rep. 2007;9(4):309–15.
10. Delattre O, Zucman J, Plougastel B, Desmaze C, Melot T, Peter M, et al. Gene fusion with an ETS DNA-binding domain caused by chromosome translocation in human tumours. Nature. 1992;359(6391):162–5.
11. Turc-Carel C, Aurias A, Mugneret F, Lizard S, Sidaner I, Volk C, et al. Chromosomes in Ewing's sarcoma. I. An evaluation of 85 cases of remarkable consistency of t(11;22)(q24;q12). Cancer Genet Cytogenet. 1988;32(2):229–38.
12. Zucman J, Delattre O, Desmaze C, Plougastel B, Joubert I, Melot T, et al. Cloning and characterization of the Ewing's sarcoma and peripheral neuroepithelioma t(11;22) translocation breakpoints. Genes Chromosomes Cancer. 1992;5(4):271–7.
13. Downing JR, Head DR, Parham DM, Douglass EC, Hulshof MG, Link MP, et al. Detection of the (11;22)(q24;q12) translocation of Ewing's sarcoma and peripheral neuroectodermal tumor by reverse transcription polymerase chain reaction. Am J Pathol. 1993;143(5):1294–300.
14. Jeon IS, Davis JN, Braun BS, Sublett JE, Roussel MF, Denny CT, et al. A variant Ewing's sarcoma translocation (7;22) fuses the EWS gene to the ETS gene ETV1. Oncogene. 1995;10(6):1229–34.
15. Peter M, Couturier J, Pacquement H, Michon J, Thomas G, Magdelenat H, et al. A new member of the ETS family fused to EWS in Ewing tumors. Oncogene. 1997;14(10):1159–64.
16. Sorensen PH, Lessnick SL, Lopez-Terrada D, Liu XF, Triche TJ, Denny CT. A second Ewing's sarcoma translocation, t(21;22), fuses the EWS gene to another ETS-family transcription factor. ERG Nat Genet. 1994;6(2):146–51.
17. Rauscher FJ 3rd, Benjamin LE, Fredericks WJ, Morris JF. Novel oncogenic mutations in the WT1 Wilms' tumor suppressor gene: a t(11;22) fuses the Ewing's sarcoma gene, EWS1, to WT1 in desmoplastic small round cell tumor. Cold Spring Harb Symp Quant Biol. 1994;59:137–46.
18. Ladanyi M, Gerald W. Fusion of the EWS and WT1 genes in the desmoplastic small round cell tumor. Cancer Res. 1994;54(11):2837–40.
19. Turc-Carel C, Dal Cin P, Limon J, Rao U, Li FP, Corson JM, et al. Involvement of chromosome X in primary cytogenetic change in human neoplasia: nonrandom translocation in synovial sarcoma. Proc Natl Acad Sci U S A. 1987;84(7):1981–5.
20. Sreekantaiah C, Ladanyi M, Rodriguez E, Chaganti RS. Chromosomal aberrations in soft tissue tumors. Relevance to diagnosis, classification, and molecular mechanisms. Am J Pathol. 1994;144(6):1121–34.
21. Wei Y, Wang J, Zhu X, Shi D, Hisaoka M, Hashimoto H. Detection of SYT-SSX fusion transcripts in paraffin-embedded tissues of synovial sarcoma by reverse transcription-polymerase chain reaction. Chin Med J. 2002;115(7):1043–7.
22. Ladanyi M, Antonescu CR, Leung DH, Woodruff JM, Kawai A, Healey JH, et al. Impact of SYT-SSX fusion type on the clinical behavior of synovial sarcoma: a multi-institutional retrospective study of 243 patients. Cancer Res. 2002;62(1):135–40.
23. Clark J, Rocques PJ, Crew AJ, Gill S, Shipley J, Chan AM, et al. Identification of novel genes, SYT and SSX, involved in the t(X;18)(p11.2;q11.2) translocation found in human synovial sarcoma. Nat Genet. 1994;7(4):502–8.

24. Kawai A, Woodruff J, Healey JH, Brennan MF, Antonescu CR, Ladanyi M. SYT-SSX gene fusion as a determinant of morphology and prognosis in synovial sarcoma. N Engl J Med. 1998;338(3):153–60.
25. Sorensen PH, Lynch JC, Qualman SJ, Tirabosco R, Lim JF, Maurer HM, et al. PAX3-FKHR and PAX7-FKHR gene fusions are prognostic indicators in alveolar rhabdomyosarcoma: a report from the children's oncology group. J Clin Oncol. 2002;20(11):2672–9.
26. Rosai J, Akerman M, Dal Cin P, DeWever I, Fletcher CD, Mandahl N, et al. Combined morphologic and karyotypic study of 59 atypical lipomatous tumors. Evaluation of their relationship and differential diagnosis with other adipose tissue tumors (a report of the CHAMP Study Group). Am J Surg Pathol. 1996;20(10):1182–9.
27. Sirvent N, Coindre JM, Maire G, Hostein I, Keslair F, Guillou L, et al. Detection of MDM2-CDK4 amplification by fluorescence in situ hybridization in 200 paraffin-embedded tumor samples: utility in diagnosing adipocytic lesions and comparison with immunohistochemistry and real-time PCR. Am J Surg Pathol. 2007;31(10):1476–89.
28. Pedeutour F, Forus A, Coindre JM, Berner JM, Nicolo G, Michiels JF, et al. Structure of the supernumerary ring and giant rod chromosomes in adipose tissue tumors. Genes Chromosomes Cancer. 1999;24(1):30–41.
29. Binh MB, Sastre-Garau X, Guillou L, de Pinieux G, Terrier P, Lagace R, et al. MDM2 and CDK4 immunostainings are useful adjuncts in diagnosing well-differentiated and dedifferentiated liposarcoma subtypes: a comparative analysis of 559 soft tissue neoplasms with genetic data. Am J Surg Pathol. 2005;29(10):1340–7.
30. Binh MB, Garau XS, Guillou L, Aurias A, Coindre JM. Reproducibility of MDM2 and CDK4 staining in soft tissue tumors. Am J Clin Pathol. 2006;125(5):693–7.
31. Leach FS, Tokino T, Meltzer P, Burrell M, Oliner JD, Smith S, et al. p53 Mutation and MDM2 amplification in human soft tissue sarcomas. Cancer Res. 1993;53(10 Suppl):2231–4.
32. Florenes VA, Maelandsmo GM, Forus A, Andreassen A, Myklebost O, Fodstad O. MDM2 gene amplification and transcript levels in human sarcomas: relationship to TP53 gene status. J Natl Cancer Inst. 1994;86(17):1297–302.
33. Miller CW, Aslo A, Won A, Tan M, Lampkin B, Koeffler HP. Alterations of the p53, Rb and MDM2 genes in osteosarcoma. J Cancer Res Clin Oncol. 1996;122(9):559–65.
34. Conyers R, Young S, Thomas DM. Liposarcoma: molecular genetics and therapeutics. Sarcoma. 2011;2011:483154.
35. Perot G, Derre J, Coindre JM, Tirode F, Lucchesi C, Mariani O, et al. Strong smooth muscle differentiation is dependent on myocardin gene amplification in most human retroperitoneal leiomyosarcomas. Cancer Res. 2009;69(6):2269–78.
36. Agaram NP, Zhang L, LeLoarer F, Silk T, Sung YS, Scott SN, et al. Targeted exome sequencing profiles genetic alterations in leiomyosarcoma. Genes Chromosomes Cancer. 2016;55(2):124–30.
37. Guo T, Zhang L, Chang NE, Singer S, Maki RG, Antonescu CR. Consistent MYC and FLT4 gene amplification in radiation-induced angiosarcoma but not in other radiation-associated atypical vascular lesions. Genes Chromosomes Cancer. 2011;50(1):25–33.
38. Mentzel T, Schildhaus HU, Palmedo G, Buttner R, Kutzner H. Postradiation cutaneous angiosarcoma after treatment of breast carcinoma is characterized by MYC amplification in contrast to atypical vascular lesions after radiotherapy and control cases: clinicopathological, immunohistochemical and molecular analysis of 66 cases. Mod Pathol. 2012;25(1):75–85.
39. Yarden Y, Kuang WJ, Yang-Feng T, Coussens L, Munemitsu S, Dull TJ, et al. Human proto-oncogene c-kit: a new cell surface receptor tyrosine kinase for an unidentified ligand. EMBO J. 1987;6(11):3341–51.
40. Hirota S, Isozaki K, Moriyama Y, Hashimoto K, Nishida T, Ishiguro S, et al. Gain-of-function mutations of c-kit in human gastrointestinal stromal tumors. Science. 1998;279(5350):577–80.
41. Singer S, Rubin BP, Lux ML, Chen CJ, Demetri GD, Fletcher CD, et al. Prognostic value of KIT mutation type, mitotic activity, and histologic subtype in gastrointestinal stromal tumors. J Clin Oncol. 2002;20(18):3898–905.

42. Rubin BP, Singer S, Tsao C, Duensing A, Lux ML, Ruiz R, et al. KIT activation is a ubiquitous feature of gastrointestinal stromal tumors. Cancer Res. 2001;61(22):8118–21.
43. Hirota S, Ohashi A, Nishida T, Isozaki K, Kinoshita K, Shinomura Y, et al. Gain-of-function mutations of platelet-derived growth factor receptor alpha gene in gastrointestinal stromal tumors. Gastroenterology. 2003;125(3):660–7.
44. Heinrich MC, Corless CL, Duensing A, McGreevey L, Chen CJ, Joseph N, et al. PDGFRA activating mutations in gastrointestinal stromal tumors. Science. 2003;299(5607):708–10.
45. Corless CL, Fletcher JA, Heinrich MC. Biology of gastrointestinal stromal tumors. J Clin Oncol. 2004;22(18):3813–25.
46. Emile JF, Brahimi S, Coindre JM, Bringuier PP, Monges G, Samb P, et al. Frequencies of KIT and PDGFRA mutations in the MolecGIST prospective population-based study differ from those of advanced GISTs. Med Oncol. 2012;29(3):1765–72.
47. Duensing A, Medeiros F, McConarty B, Joseph NE, Panigrahy D, Singer S, et al. Mechanisms of oncogenic KIT signal transduction in primary gastrointestinal stromal tumors (GISTs). Oncogene. 2004;23(22):3999–4006.
48. Bannon AE, Klug LR, Corless CL, Heinrich MC. Using molecular diagnostic testing to personalize the treatment of patients with gastrointestinal stromal tumors. Expert Rev Mol Diagn. 2017;17(5):445–57.
49. Corless CL, Schroeder A, Griffith D, Town A, McGreevey L, Harrell P, et al. PDGFRA mutations in gastrointestinal stromal tumors: frequency, spectrum and in vitro sensitivity to imatinib. J Clin Oncol. 2005;23(23):5357–64.
50. Li FP, Fraumeni JF Jr. Soft-tissue sarcomas, breast cancer, and other neoplasms. A familial syndrome? Ann Intern Med. 1969;71(4):747–52.
51. Li FP, Fraumeni JF Jr, Mulvihill JJ, Blattner WA, Dreyfus MG, Tucker MA, et al. A cancer family syndrome in twenty-four kindreds. Cancer Res. 1988;48(18):5358–62.
52. Malkin D, Li FP, Strong LC, Fraumeni JF Jr, Nelson CE, Kim DH, et al. Germ line p53 mutations in a familial syndrome of breast cancer, sarcomas, and other neoplasms. Science. 1990;250(4985):1233–8.
53. Srivastava S, Zou ZQ, Pirollo K, Blattner W, Chang EH. Germ-line transmission of a mutated p53 gene in a cancer-prone family with Li-Fraumeni syndrome. Nature. 1990;348(6303):747–9.
54. Zhang J, Walsh MF, Wu G, Edmonson MN, Gruber TA, Easton J, et al. Germline mutations in predisposition genes in pediatric cancer. N Engl J Med. 2015;373(24):2336–46.
55. Ballinger ML, Goode DL, Ray-Coquard I, James PA, Mitchell G, Niedermayr E, et al. Monogenic and polygenic determinants of sarcoma risk: an international genetic study. Lancet Oncol. 2016;17(9):1261–71.
56. Schrader KA, Cheng DT, Joseph V, Prasad M, Walsh M, Zehir A, et al. Germline variants in targeted tumor sequencing using matched normal DNA. JAMA Oncol. 2016;2(1):104–11.
57. O'Connor C. Karyotyping for chromosomal abnormalities. Nat Educ. 2008;1(1):27.
58. Antonescu CR. The role of genetic testing in soft tissue sarcoma. Histopathology. 2006;48(1):13–21.
59. Singer S. New diagnostic modalities in soft tissue sarcoma. Semin Surg Oncol. 1999;17(1):11–22.
60. Willeke F, Mechtersheimer G, Schwarzbach M, Weitz J, Zimmer D, Lehnert T, et al. Detection of SYT-SSX1/2 fusion transcripts by reverse transcriptase-polymerase chain reaction (RT-PCR) is a valuable diagnostic tool in synovial sarcoma. Eur J Cancer. 1998;34(13):2087–93.
61. Dujardin F, Binh MB, Bouvier C, Gomez-Brouchet A, Larousserie F, Muret A, et al. MDM2 and CDK4 immunohistochemistry is a valuable tool in the differential diagnosis of low-grade osteosarcomas and other primary fibro-osseous lesions of the bone. Mod Pathol. 2011;24(5):624–37.
62. Arbiser ZK, Folpe AL, Weiss SW. Consultative (expert) second opinions in soft tissue pathology. Analysis of problem-prone diagnostic situations. Am J Clin Pathol. 2001;116(4):473–6.

63. Ray-Coquard I, Montesco MC, Coindre JM, Dei Tos AP, Lurkin A, Ranchere-Vince D, et al. Sarcoma: concordance between initial diagnosis and centralized expert review in a population-based study within three European regions. Ann Oncol. 2012;23(9):2442–9.
64. Lurkin A, Ducimetiere F, Vince DR, Decouvelaere AV, Cellier D, Gilly FN, et al. Epidemiological evaluation of concordance between initial diagnosis and central pathology review in a comprehensive and prospective series of sarcoma patients in the Rhone-Alpes region. BMC Cancer. 2010;10:150.
65. Thway K, Wang J, Mubako T, Fisher C. Histopathological diagnostic discrepancies in soft tissue tumours referred to a specialist centre: reassessment in the era of ancillary molecular diagnosis. Sarcoma. 2014;2014:686902.
66. Szymanska J, Virolainen M, Tarkkanen M, Wiklund T, Asko-Seljavaara S, Tukiainen E, et al. Overrepresentation of 1q21-23 and 12q13-21 in lipoma-like liposarcomas but not in benign lipomas: a comparative genomic hybridization study. Cancer Genet Cytogenet. 1997;99(1):14–8.
67. Shimada S, Ishizawa T, Ishizawa K, Matsumura T, Hasegawa T, Hirose T. The value of MDM2 and CDK4 amplification levels using real-time polymerase chain reaction for the differential diagnosis of liposarcomas and their histologic mimickers. Hum Pathol. 2006;37(9):1123–9.
68. Aleixo PB, Hartmann AA, Menezes IC, Meurer RT, Oliveira AM. Can MDM2 and CDK4 make the diagnosis of well differentiated/dedifferentiated liposarcoma? An immunohistochemical study on 129 soft tissue tumours. J Clin Pathol. 2009;62(12):1127–35.
69. Weaver J, Downs-Kelly E, Goldblum JR, Turner S, Kulkarni S, Tubbs RR, et al. Fluorescence in situ hybridization for MDM2 gene amplification as a diagnostic tool in lipomatous neoplasms. Mod Pathol. 2008;21(8):943–9.
70. Forus A, Florenes VA, Maelandsmo GM, Meltzer PS, Fodstad O, Myklebost O. Mapping of amplification units in the q13-14 region of chromosome 12 in human sarcomas: some amplica do not include MDM2. Cell Growth Differ. 1993;4(12):1065–70.
71. Guillou L, Coindre J, Gallagher G, Terrier P, Gebhard S, de Saint Aubain Somerhausen N, et al. Detection of the synovial sarcoma translocation t(X;18) (SYT;SSX) in paraffin-embedded tissues using reverse transcriptase-polymerase chain reaction: a reliable and powerful diagnostic tool for pathologists. A molecular analysis of 221 mesenchymal tumors fixed in different fixatives. Hum Pathol. 2001;32(1):105–12.
72. Fisher C. Synovial sarcoma. Ann Diagn Pathol. 1998;2(6):401–21.
73. Wei S, Siegal GP. Round cell tumors of bone: an update on recent molecular genetic advances. Adv Anat Pathol. 2014;21(5):359–72.
74. Marino-Enriquez A, Fletcher CD. Round cell sarcomas—biologically important refinements in subclassification. Int J Biochem Cell Biol. 2014;53:493–504.
75. Lewis TB, Coffin CM, Bernard PS. Differentiating Ewing's sarcoma from other round blue cell tumors using a RT-PCR translocation panel on formalin-fixed paraffin-embedded tissues. Mod Pathol. 2007;20(3):397–404.
76. Chen QR, Vansant G, Oades K, Pickering M, Wei JS, Song YK, et al. Diagnosis of the small round blue cell tumors using multiplex polymerase chain reaction. J Mol Diagn. 2007;9(1):80–8.
77. Ptaszynski K, Szumera-Cieckiewicz A, Pekul M, Nowecki Z. Differential diagnosis of small round cell tumours (SRCT), fluorescence in situ hybridization (FISH) and immunohistochemical (IHC) study. Pol J Pathol. 2009;60(4):151–62.
78. Machado I, Navarro L, Pellin A, Navarro S, Agaimy A, Tardio JC, et al. Defining Ewing and Ewing-like small round cell tumors (SRCT): the need for molecular techniques in their categorization and differential diagnosis. A study of 200 cases. Ann Diagn Pathol. 2016;22:25–32.
79. Petrov SV, Machado I, Boulytcheva IV, Noguera R, Pellin A, Bacchini P, et al. New approaches in the diagnosis of small-cell round tumors of bone and soft tissue. Arkh Patol. 2009;71(1):34–40.
80. Barr FG, Galili N, Holick J, Biegel JA, Rovera G, Emanuel BS. Rearrangement of the PAX3 paired box gene in the paediatric solid tumour alveolar rhabdomyosarcoma. Nat Genet. 1993;3(2):113–7.

81. Shapiro DN, Sublett JE, Li B, Downing JR, Naeve CW. Fusion of PAX3 to a member of the forkhead family of transcription factors in human alveolar rhabdomyosarcoma. Cancer Res. 1993;53(21):5108–12.
82. Lu L, Lao IW, Liu X, Yu L, Wang J. Nodular fasciitis: a retrospective study of 272 cases from China with clinicopathologic and radiologic correlation. Ann Diagn Pathol. 2015;19(3):180–5.
83. Erber R, Agaimy A. Misses and near misses in diagnosing nodular fasciitis and morphologically related reactive myofibroblastic proliferations: experience of a referral center with emphasis on frequency of USP6 gene rearrangements. Virchows Arch. 2018;473(3):351–60.
84. Erickson-Johnson MR, Chou MM, Evers BR, Roth CW, Seys AR, Jin L, et al. Nodular fasciitis: a novel model of transient neoplasia induced by MYH9-USP6 gene fusion. Lab Investig. 2011;91(10):1427–33.
85. Shin C, Low I, Ng D, Oei P, Miles C, Symmans P. USP6 gene rearrangement in nodular fasciitis and histological mimics. Histopathology. 2016;69(5):784–91.
86. Butow PN, Kazemi JN, Beeney LJ, Griffin AM, Dunn SM, Tattersall MH. When the diagnosis is cancer: patient communication experiences and preferences. Cancer. 1996;77(12):2630–7.
87. Butow PN, Dowsett S, Hagerty R, Tattersall MH. Communicating prognosis to patients with metastatic disease: what do they really want to know? Support Care Cancer. 2002;10(2):161–8.
88. Hagerty RG, Butow PN, Ellis PA, Lobb EA, Pendlebury S, Leighl N, et al. Cancer patient preferences for communication of prognosis in the metastatic setting. J Clin Oncol. 2004;22(9):1721–30.
89. Mackillop WJ, Stewart WE, Ginsburg AD, Stewart SS. Cancer patients' perceptions of their disease and its treatment. Br J Cancer. 1988;58(3):355–8.
90. Siminoff LA, Ravdin P, Colabianchi N, Sturm CM. Doctor-patient communication patterns in breast cancer adjuvant therapy discussions. Health Expect. 2000;3(1):26–36.
91. Soylu C, Babacan T, Sever AR, Altundag K. Patients' understanding of treatment goals and disease course and their relationship with optimism, hope, and quality of life: a preliminary study among advanced breast cancer outpatients before receiving palliative treatment. Support Care Cancer. 2016;24(8):3481–8.
92. Jain S, Xu R, Prieto VG, Lee P. Molecular classification of soft tissue sarcomas and its clinical applications. Int J Clin Exp Pathol. 2010;3(4):416–28.
93. Hameed M. Molecular diagnosis of soft tissue neoplasia: clinical applications and recent advances. Expert Rev Mol Diagn. 2014;14(8):961–77.
94. de Alava E, Kawai A, Healey JH, Fligman I, Meyers PA, Huvos AG, et al. EWS-FLI1 fusion transcript structure is an independent determinant of prognosis in Ewing's sarcoma. J Clin Oncol. 1998;16(4):1248–55.
95. Riley RD, Burchill SA, Abrams KR, Heney D, Sutton AJ, Jones DR, et al. A systematic review of molecular and biological markers in tumours of the Ewing's sarcoma family. Eur J Cancer. 2003;39(1):19–30.
96. Sun Y, Sun B, Wang J, Cai W, Zhao X, Zhang S, et al. Prognostic implication of SYT-SSX fusion type and clinicopathological parameters for tumor-related death, recurrence, and metastasis in synovial sarcoma. Cancer Sci. 2009;100(6):1018–25.
97. Nilsson G, Skytting B, Xie Y, Brodin B, Perfekt R, Mandahl N, et al. The SYT-SSX1 variant of synovial sarcoma is associated with a high rate of tumor cell proliferation and poor clinical outcome. Cancer Res. 1999;59(13):3180–4.
98. Inagaki H, Murase T, Otsuka T, Eimoto T. Detection of SYT-SSX fusion transcript in synovial sarcoma using archival cytologic specimens. Am J Clin Pathol. 1999;111(4):528–33.
99. Takenaka S, Ueda T, Naka N, Araki N, Hashimoto N, Myoui A, et al. Prognostic implication of SYT-SSX fusion type in synovial sarcoma: a multi-institutional retrospective analysis in Japan. Oncol Rep. 2008;19(2):467–76.
100. Stegmaier S, Leuschner I, Poremba C, Ladenstein R, Kazanowska B, Ljungman G, et al. The prognostic impact of SYT-SSX fusion type and histological grade in pediatric patients with synovial sarcoma treated according to the CWS (Cooperative Weichteilsarkom Studie) trials. Pediatr Blood Cancer. 2017;64(1):89–95.

101. Lee YT, Tan YJ, Oon CE. Molecular targeted therapy: treating cancer with specificity. Eur J Pharmacol. 2018;834:188–96.
102. Demetri GD, von Mehren M, Blanke CD, Van den Abbeele AD, Eisenberg B, Roberts PJ, et al. Efficacy and safety of imatinib mesylate in advanced gastrointestinal stromal tumors. N Engl J Med. 2002;347(7):472–80.
103. van Oosterom AT, Judson I, Verweij J, Stroobants S, Donato di Paola E, Dimitrijevic S, et al. Safety and efficacy of imatinib (STI571) in metastatic gastrointestinal stromal tumours: a phase I study. Lancet. 2001;358(9291):1421–3.
104. Heinrich MC, Corless CL, Demetri GD, Blanke CD, von Mehren M, Joensuu H, et al. Kinase mutations and imatinib response in patients with metastatic gastrointestinal stromal tumor. J Clin Oncol. 2003;21(23):4342–9.
105. Heinrich MC, Maki RG, Corless CL, Antonescu CR, Harlow A, Griffith D, et al. Primary and secondary kinase genotypes correlate with the biological and clinical activity of sunitinib in imatinib-resistant gastrointestinal stromal tumor. J Clin Oncol. 2008;26(33):5352–9.
106. Heinrich MC, Owzar K, Corless CL, Hollis D, Borden EC, Fletcher CD, et al. Correlation of kinase genotype and clinical outcome in the North American Intergroup Phase III Trial of imatinib mesylate for treatment of advanced gastrointestinal stromal tumor: CALGB 150105 Study by Cancer and Leukemia Group B and Southwest Oncology Group. J Clin Oncol. 2008;26(33):5360–7.
107. Heinrich MC, Griffith D, McKinley A, Patterson J, Presnell A, Ramachandran A, et al. Crenolanib inhibits the drug-resistant PDGFRA D842V mutation associated with imatinib-resistant gastrointestinal stromal tumors. Clin Cancer Res. 2012;18(16):4375–84.
108. Rutkowski P, Van Glabbeke M, Rankin CJ, Ruka W, Rubin BP, Debiec-Rychter M, et al. Imatinib mesylate in advanced dermatofibrosarcoma protuberans: pooled analysis of two phase II clinical trials. J Clin Oncol. 2010;28(10):1772–9.
109. Rutkowski P, Debiec-Rychter M, Nowecki Z, Michej W, Symonides M, Ptaszynski K, et al. Treatment of advanced dermatofibrosarcoma protuberans with imatinib mesylate with or without surgical resection. J Eur Acad Dermatol Venereol. 2011;25(3):264–70.
110. Rutkowski P, Klimczak A, Lugowska I, Jagielska B, Wagrodzki M, Debiec-Rychter M, et al. Long-term results of treatment of advanced dermatofibrosarcoma protuberans (DFSP) with imatinib mesylate—the impact of fibrosarcomatous transformation. Eur J Surg Oncol. 2017;43(6):1134–41.
111. Pedeutour F, Coindre JM, Sozzi G, Nicolo G, Leroux A, Toma S, et al. Supernumerary ring chromosomes containing chromosome 17 sequences. A specific feature of dermatofibrosarcoma protuberans? Cancer Genet Cytogenet. 1994;76(1):1–9.
112. Pedeutour F, Simon MP, Minoletti F, Sozzi G, Pierotti MA, Hecht F, et al. Ring 22 chromosomes in dermatofibrosarcoma protuberans are low-level amplifiers of chromosome 17 and 22 sequences. Cancer Res. 1995;55(11):2400–3.
113. Shimizu A, O'Brien KP, Sjoblom T, Pietras K, Buchdunger E, Collins VP, et al. The dermatofibrosarcoma protuberans-associated collagen type Ialpha1/platelet-derived growth factor (PDGF) B-chain fusion gene generates a transforming protein that is processed to functional PDGF-BB. Cancer Res. 1999;59(15):3719–23.
114. West RB, Rubin BP, Miller MA, Subramanian S, Kaygusuz G, Montgomery K, et al. A landscape effect in tenosynovial giant-cell tumor from activation of CSF1 expression by a translocation in a minority of tumor cells. Proc Natl Acad Sci U S A. 2006;103(3):690–5.
115. Ravi V, Wang WL, Lewis VO. Treatment of tenosynovial giant cell tumor and pigmented villonodular synovitis. Curr Opin Oncol. 2011;23(4):361–6.
116. Cassier PA, Gelderblom H, Stacchiotti S, Thomas D, Maki RG, Kroep JR, et al. Efficacy of imatinib mesylate for the treatment of locally advanced and/or metastatic tenosynovial giant cell tumor/pigmented villonodular synovitis. Cancer. 2012;118(6):1649–55.
117. Thomas D, Henshaw R, Skubitz K, Chawla S, Staddon A, Blay JY, et al. Denosumab in patients with giant-cell tumour of bone: an open-label, phase 2 study. Lancet Oncol. 2010;11(3):275–80.

118. Muller DA, Beltrami G, Scoccianti G, Campanacci DA, Franchi A, Capanna R. Risks and benefits of combining denosumab and surgery in giant cell tumor of bone-a case series. World J Surg Oncol. 2016;14(1):281.
119. Rekhi B, Verma V, Gulia A, Jambhekar NA, Desai S, Juvekar SL, et al. Clinicopathological features of a series of 27 cases of post-denosumab treated giant cell tumors of bones: a single institutional experience at a Tertiary Cancer Referral Centre. India Pathol Oncol Res. 2017;23(1):157–64.
120. Branstetter DG, Nelson SD, Manivel JC, Blay JY, Chawla S, Thomas DM, et al. Denosumab induces tumor reduction and bone formation in patients with giant-cell tumor of bone. Clin Cancer Res. 2012;18(16):4415–24.
121. Lange T, Stehling C, Frohlich B, Klingenhofer M, Kunkel P, Schneppenheim R, et al. Denosumab: a potential new and innovative treatment option for aneurysmal bone cysts. Eur Spine J. 2013;22(6):1417–22.
122. Pauli C, Fuchs B, Pfirrmann C, Bridge JA, Hofer S, Bode B. Response of an aggressive periosteal aneurysmal bone cyst (ABC) of the radius to denosumab therapy. World J Surg Oncol. 2014;12:17.
123. Branstetter D, Rohrbach K, Huang LY, Soriano R, Tometsko M, Blake M, et al. RANK and RANK ligand expression in primary human osteosarcoma. J Bone Oncol. 2015;4(3):59–68.
124. Chen Y, Di Grappa MA, Molyneux SD, McKee TD, Waterhouse P, Penninger JM, et al. RANKL blockade prevents and treats aggressive osteosarcomas. Sci Transl Med. 2015;7(317):317ra197.
125. Cathomas R, Rothermundt C, Bode B, Fuchs B, von Moos R, Schwitter M. RANK ligand blockade with denosumab in combination with sorafenib in chemorefractory osteosarcoma: a possible step forward? Oncology. 2015;88(4):257–60.
126. Amary MF, Bacsi K, Maggiani F, Damato S, Halai D, Berisha F, et al. IDH1 and IDH2 mutations are frequent events in central chondrosarcoma and central and periosteal chondromas but not in other mesenchymal tumours. J Pathol. 2011;224(3):334–43.
127. Dang L, White DW, Gross S, Bennett BD, Bittinger MA, Driggers EM, et al. Cancer-associated IDH1 mutations produce 2-hydroxyglutarate. Nature. 2009;462(7274):739–44.
128. Xu W, Yang H, Liu Y, Yang Y, Wang P, Kim SH, et al. Oncometabolite 2-hydroxyglutarate is a competitive inhibitor of alpha-ketoglutarate-dependent dioxygenases. Cancer Cell. 2011;19(1):17–30.
129. Tap WD, Villalobos V, Cote GM, Burris H, Janku F, Mir O, et al. A phase 1 study of AG-120, an IDH1 mutant enzyme inhibitor: results from the chondrosarcoma dose escalation and expansion cohorts. In: Connective Tissue Oncology Society Annual Meeting, 2016.

The Role of Radiotherapy for Sarcoma 10

Samuel Y. Ngan, Julie Chu, and Sarat Chander

10.1 Introduction

Sarcomas are rare cancers and occur in 1% of the Australian population. Sarcomas consist of soft tissue and bone tumours. Soft tissue sarcomas (STS) are a heterogeneous group of mesenchymal tumours that can arise anywhere in the body and can affect all age groups. Majority of soft tissue sarcoma arise in the extremity (60%). Other sites include truncal wall, retroperitoneum, head and neck and mediastinum. Gastrointestinal stromal tumour (GIST), which accounts for majority of sarcomas arising from the gastrointestinal tract, is included in the fourth edition of WHO classification (2013).

The management of such a diverse group of tumours has evolved over the last few decades. In addition to tumour control, retaining limb function is equally important. The goal is to achieve tumour control, retain limb function and free from treatment-related long-term morbidity such as chronic pain or severe oedema. Radical ablative surgery has been replaced with limb-sparing surgery combined with radiotherapy to achieve these goals.

10.2 The Role of External Beam Radiotherapy in Soft Tissue Sarcoma of Extremity

Prior to the early 1980s, amputation for extremity soft tissue sarcoma was frequently performed. Local control was excellent with this approach, but the rate of metastatic relapse remained [1]. Retaining limb function became an issue that needed to be

S. Y. Ngan (✉) · J. Chu · S. Chander
Bone & Soft Tissue Sarcoma Unit, Peter MacCallum Cancer Centre,
Melbourne, VIC, Australia

Division of Radiation Oncology, Peter MacCallum Cancer Centre, Melbourne, VIC, Australia
e-mail: sam.ngan@petermac.org; julie.chu@petermac.org; sarat.chander@petermac.org

P. F. M. Choong (ed.), *Sarcoma*, https://doi.org/10.1007/978-981-15-9414-4_10

addressed. Studies to explore the role of radiation therapy started in the 1970s. These studies provided evidence that radiotherapy could result in adequate local control without increasing the risk of distant relapse. There was increasing interest in determining how best to integrate radiation therapy with surgical management. In 1982, Rosenberg et al. published the landmark prospective randomised trial which proved to be practice changing [2]. In the National Cancer Institute (NCI) study, a total of 43 patients with high-grade soft tissue sarcomas of the extremity were randomised to amputation or limb-sparing surgery followed by adjuvant radiotherapy. Both groups received post-operative chemotherapy (doxorubicin, cyclophosphamide and high-dose methotrexate). There were four local recurrences in the limb-sparing group and none in the amputation group; the difference was not statistically significant. There was no significant difference in disease-free and overall survival between the study arms.

A subsequent NCI prospective randomised trial reported by Yang et al. further confirmed the role of adjuvant external beam radiotherapy (EBRT) in the setting of limb-sparing resection [3]. A total of 141 patients with both high- and low-grade sarcomas were randomised to receive adjuvant radiotherapy or without. Those with high-grade tumours also received post-operative chemotherapy (doxorubicin and cyclophosphamide). There was no local recurrence in the group received radiotherapy. The local recurrence rate was 22% in the group who did not have radiotherapy. Improved local control was seen in both low-grade and high-grade sarcomas treated with adjuvant radiotherapy.

An update on long-term overall survival, local control and limb function was published in 2014 [4]. The median follow-up was 17.9 years. The 10- and 20-year overall survival (OS) was 77% and 64%, respectively, for patients who had surgery alone and 82% and 71%, respectively, for those who received adjuvant radiotherapy. There was no difference in OS when stratified against tumour grade. The rate of local recurrence was 25% following limb-sparing surgery (LSS). Almost all 18 recurrences were early recurrences. In contrast, only one recurrence was reported following LSS and adjuvant radiotherapy. In terms of functional limb deficits, there were no deficits observed in patients with upper limb STS. Of those with lower limb STS, 15% of the surgery-alone group required an assist device to ambulate compared to 8% of those treated with adjuvant radiotherapy. Two patients developed complications related to radiotherapy.

10.3 Tumour Grade and Radiotherapy

Long-term data from the NCI study by Yang et al. confirmed improved local control in patients who received external beam radiotherapy. This improvement was evident for both high-grade and low-grade sarcomas. Choong et al. reported on their study of 132 patients who received radiotherapy and surgery for low-grade sarcoma. They observed that tumours greater than 5 cm which were not also treated with radiotherapy were associated with a higher incidence of local recurrence. Radiotherapy was particularly effective in reducing local recurrence when applied to patients treated with marginal surgical margins. Adjuvant radiotherapy did not seem to confer a local recurrence benefit when applied to tumours that were treated with wide surgical margins or which were ≤5 cm [5]. In cases where brachytherapy is being contemplated, improved local control was only evident for high-grade tumours [6]. A prospective trial by the French Sarcoma Group randomising patients to adjuvant radiotherapy versus no radiotherapy after complete excision of extremity soft tissue sarcoma is ongoing.

Factors to be considered in determining combining radiotherapy with surgery include proximity to a major nerve or blood supply and proximity to the joint. In general, if amputation is necessary to salvage a local recurrence, radiotherapy is usually indicated. Tumour grade is not a major factor in most situations.

10.4 The Timing of External Beam Radiotherapy

National Cancer Institute of Canada Clinical Trials Group SR-2 trial randomised patients with extremity sarcoma to preoperative vs. post-operative radiotherapy and found no difference in local control, progression-free survival or overall survival between the two groups [7]. Preoperative radiotherapy is associated with lower rates of late toxicities, namely, oedema, fibrosis and joint stiffness. This translates to better limb function. However, wound complication rate was higher in the preoperative group.

There are many advantages for delivering external beam radiotherapy in the preoperative setting. In majority of cases, the gross tumour is intact and readily visualised on MRI. In some cases, peri-tumoural oedema may be present. Given peri-tumoural oedema can harbour tumour cells, it is essential to include this in the clinical target volume (CTV). Accurate target delineation and no tumour bed, drain sites and surgical wound to include lead to smaller treatment volume. Not only is the treatment volume smaller; the prescribed dose is also lower in the preoperative setting to achieve equivalent tumour control. Delivering radiotherapy preoperatively also avoid unforeseeable delay and irradiating healthy tissue that has been brought in to repair surgical defect.

10.5 Target Delineation and Definition of Margins

The development of multi-detector CT in the mid-1990s has revolutionised radiotherapy planning. 3D conformal radiotherapy (3DCRT) has become the new standard. Fusion of MRI and functional images are possible due to improvement in planning software and tools.

In 2010, a consensus meeting on gross tumour volume (GTV) and clinical target volume (CTV) on computed tomographic images for preoperative radiotherapy for extremity high-grade soft tissue sarcoma was held during the Radiation Therapy Oncology Group (RTOG) meeting. The RTOG consensus atlas was published in the red journal the following year [8]. Based on this consensus, the GTV is gross tumour defined by T1 contrast-enhanced magnetic resonance images. CTV includes gross tumour and clinical microscopic margins, typically 3 cm in the cranio-caudal directions. The radial margin from gross tumour should be 1.5 cm including any portion of the tumour not confined by intact fascial barrier, bone or skin surface. In cases where the field extends beyond the compartment, the field can be shortened to include the end of a compartment. In other case where peri-tumoural oedema as defined by T2 magnetic resonance images extends beyond the field, clinical judgement is needed to determine if the risk of oedema harbouring sarcoma is high or low. If the risk is low, there is no need to modify the field. Alternatively, if the risk is high, the decision to extend the field must be balanced against potential excessive toxicity. A 1–1.5-cm margin for planning target volume (PTV) is generally acceptable.

In terms of radial margin, our preference is to include a minimum of 2 cm or the intact fascial boundary or the muscle bundle radially. This is to ensure that the CTV is no less than the surgical margin. In some cases, individualising margin is required.

Individualised margin that should be applied in preoperative radiotherapy is particularly relevant in superficial myxofibrosarcoma (MFS) and undifferentiated pleomorphic sarcoma (UPS) as these histological subtypes are frequently associated with an infiltrative growth or tail sign and local recurrence [9]. In this series by Imanishi et al., local recurrence occurred in three out of the eight pathologically viable tail cases following preoperative radiotherapy but in none of the cases without tail or with non-viable tail. It is imperative to adequately cover these tails by the preoperative radiotherapy field and to employ wider surgical margins to maximise local control.

Radiation dose of 50–50.4 Gy is recommended for preoperative radiotherapy. Intensity modulated radiotherapy (IMRT) or volumetric modulated arc radiotherapy (VMAT) is superior to 3DCRT in terms of dose homogeneity for a long tumour. In post-operative radiotherapy, the CTV includes operative bed, drain site and incision scar. A total dose of 60–64 Gy is recommended, and shrinking field technique is usually applied for the tumour bed.

10.6 Chemoradiotherapy

In pursuit of improving survival for high-grade sarcoma, chemotherapy is combined with radiotherapy in order to address local disease and potential micro-metastatic disease at the same time. The chemotherapeutic agent or targeted agent will need to have an intrinsic effect on the tumour by itself as well as radiosensitising effect. Ideally the agent can improve the therapeutic ratio, that is, improving the tumour control with the same level of toxicity or maintaining the same level of tumour control with lower toxicity. The ultimate goal is to improve survival without compromising local control. In order to achieve this goal, dose intensity of chemotherapy and radiotherapy is critical.

Preoperative radiotherapy is generally preferred for a high-grade sarcoma. As surgery remains the cornerstone of success, it is important that preoperative chemoradiotherapy does not lead to severe toxicity, which may delay surgery, leading to increased surgical morbidity or worsened functional outcomes. A number of different strategies have been studied.

One approach is to administer doxorubicin, an active agent for sarcoma and a potent radiosensitiser, immediately before commencing reduced dose of preoperative radiotherapy. Temple et al. reported a series with a protocol of 60–90 mg of doxorubicin infused intra-arterially or intravenously over 3 days into a vessel feeding the involved area, 30 Gy of radiotherapy given over 10 days [10].

Another approach is concomitant chemotherapy and radiotherapy. In a report of a phase I study at MD Anderson Cancer Center (MDACC) with 50 Gy radiotherapy with escalating dose of doxorubicin, the maximum tolerance dose of doxorubicin was found to be 17.5 mg/m^2/week. Half of the patients had 90% or greater tumour necrosis [11]. In another study from MDACC local and systemic toxicities after the administration of therapeutic doses of ifosfamide with concomitant radiotherapy were comparable to those observed with either treatment alone [12].

Combination chemotherapy has been studied. At Mayo Clinic, two cycles of neoadjuvant ifosfamide, mitomycin, doxorubicin and cisplatin (IMAP) were followed by chemoradiotherapy 45 Gy and reduced doses of MAP and then surgery. Radiation to total doses of 55–65 Gy was accomplished by delivery of an additional 10–20 Gy to the tumour bed via intraoperative electron beam, brachytherapy or external beam irradiation at the completion of surgery. Chemotherapy toxicity grade three or higher consisted primarily of vomiting (23%), leukopaenia (54%) and thrombocytopaenia (77%). The estimated 5-year survival was 80% approximately [13].

An innovative approach which combined radiotherapy with neoadjuvant mesna, doxorubicin, ifosfamide and dacarbazine (MAID) followed by resection and adjuvant chemotherapy was studied at Massachusetts General Hospital (MGH). Chemoradiotherapy 44 Gy, split into two equal halves, were administered in between three courses of MAID. This regiment of therapies led to a significant decrease in systemic metastases and an increase in disease-free and overall survival when compared with a historical control group. These results led to a multi-institutional trial by RTOG [14].

The RTOG 9514 study included high-grade soft tissue sarcoma, ≥8 cm in diameter of the extremities and body wall. Three patients (5%) experienced fatal grade 5 toxicities (myelodysplasias, two patients; infection, one patient). Another 53 patients (83%) experienced grade 4 toxicities, 78% experienced grade 4 haematologic toxicity, and 19% experienced grade 4 nonhaematologic toxicity. Estimated 3-year rates for disease-free, distant disease-free and overall survival are 56.6%, 64.5% and 75.1%, respectively [15].

After a median follow-up period of 9.3 years in patients treated with a similar protocol at MGH, 7-year disease-specific and overall survival rates were 81% and 79%, respectively [16]. With a median follow-up of 7.7 years in patients treated in RTOG 9514, estimated 5-year rates of disease-free survival, distant disease-free survival and overall survival were 56.1%, 64.1% and 71.2%, respectively [17].

Biological agents including bevacizumab, sorafenib, pazopanib and sunitinib were also studied with radiotherapy.

In a critical review of current evidence of preoperative radiotherapy by sarcoma experts, it was concluded that outside the setting of well-designed prospective clinical trials, the conventional 50 Gy in 5–6-week schedule should be considered as standard [18].

10.7 Brachytherapy

Brachytherapy is a form of radiation therapy delivery in which a radiation source is placed in close proximity or inside the target tissue (Brachy = close). There is a rapid fall off in dose with relatively short distance and hence has the advantage of delivering high doses of radiation to the tumour while reducing the dose to the surrounding normal tissues.

Brachytherapy can be delivered with either a low-dose rate (LDR) or high-dose rate (HDR) system. The International Commission on Radiation Units (ICRU) defines LDR brachytherapy as 0.4–2 Gy per hour, whereas HDR brachytherapy is delivered at >12 Gy per hour.

For soft tissue sarcoma brachytherapy, afterloading catheters are placed in the operative tumour bed which is defined by the surgeon and spaced at 1 cm intervals to cover the entire area of risk. Usually a single-plane implant is used. Traditionally, LDR brachytherapy with an iridium-192 source was used to deliver radiotherapy completely in this manner. The treatment was delivered over 48–72 h or more in a shielded room as an inpatient. Technological advances have made HDR brachytherapy feasible. This method of delivery uses a higher-strength radioactive source and delivers the source for a brief period of time to catheters (minutes versus days) but unlike LDR requires treatment over multiple days.

Typically the afterloading catheters are loaded with the radioactive source usually around the 5th to 8th post-operative day, and treatment is given over a few fractions and can be delivered as an outpatient. Currently most centres around the world have abandoned the iridium wire-based LDR brachytherapy for the convenience and safety of the HDR.

Indications for brachytherapy are similar to those for external beam radiotherapy (EBRT) and include surgery with close or intralesional margins, local recurrences, high-grade tumours, size greater than 5 cm, and deep lesions.

Adjuvant brachytherapy alone may be applicable in patients with high-grade trunk wall or extremity sarcomas that have undergone complete surgical excision with negative margin [19]. It remains unclear whether brachytherapy in combination with EBRT or as a single modality is preferable with positive surgical margins. Factors that may influence the use of EBRT and brachytherapy in scenarios with positive margins include the tumour grade, prior surgeries and tumour size.

Adjuvant brachytherapy has been shown to enhance local control of disease over surgery alone for high-grade soft tissue sarcomas of the extremity and superficial trunk [20]. However, it is controversial if the same can be concluded from studies of low-grade tumours [6, 21]. Like preoperative EBRT, the addition of brachytherapy is associated with a higher early wound complication rate [22, 23].

An improvement in local control of disease in retroperitoneal sarcomas has been observed in several case series where brachytherapy has been combined with preoperative [24] or post-operative external beam [25] radiotherapy. A small randomised study showed benefit with the use of HDR-IORT [26]. However, superiority over preoperative radiotherapy for local control or overall survival could not be established at 10 years [27].

There have been no randomised comparisons of the relative efficacy or morbidity of post-operative EBRT compared with brachytherapy. In a retrospective comparison of patients treated by IMRT or brachytherapy, the IMRT group appeared to have somewhat worse prognostic features, but the 5-year local control rate was significantly higher with IMRT (92% vs. 82%) [28].

At our centre, we reserve brachytherapy as an adjuvant therapy (either as boost or definitive treatment) for patients who have had a recurrence of sarcoma in a previously irradiated field.

10.8 The Role of Radiotherapy in Primary Bone Sarcoma

Primary bone tumours are rare. The three most common types of malignant primary bone tumours are osteosarcoma, chondrosarcoma and Ewing sarcoma. Osteosarcomas commonly arise in extremities and rarely in axial sites such as the jaw. Osteosarcoma of the jaw affects either mandible or maxilla. It is characterised by high propensity for local invasion but rarely metastasise. In contrast, high-grade osteosarcoma of extremities often metastasises, and the most frequent metastatic site is the lung. Chondrosarcoma frequently arises in the axial skeleton and the metaphyseal region of long bones. Majority are low-grade locally aggressive tumours and do not metastasise. Ewing sarcoma affects mainly children and adolescents. They are all high-grade tumours, arising commonly in extremities, pelvis, vertebrae and ribs. Almost all Ewing sarcoma share EWSR1 gene rearrangement making molecular testing mandatory.

10.9 Osteosarcoma

Unlike soft issue sarcomas, the role of radiotherapy is limited in primary bone tumours. Current standard therapy for high-grade osteosarcoma is neoadjuvant chemotherapy and surgical resection of the primary tumour. In cases of resectable osteosarcoma, there is no role for radiotherapy. However, for tumours where complete resection is not possible, adjuvant radiotherapy or definitive radiotherapy may be used to improve local control and extend progression-free survival.

Retrospective series from MGH by DeLaney et al. reported patients with either gross or subtotal resection had a greater rate of local control, survival and disease-free survival with radiotherapy. Although no radiation dose-response relationship for local control was shown, the effectiveness of radiation appears to correlate with the extent of resection [29].

Experience from Cooperative Osteosarkomstudiengruppe (COSS) Registry by Schwarz et al. also helped to define the role of radiotherapy in osteosarcoma [30]. Of the patients who were analysed, majority received external beam radiotherapy, and the rest received proton therapy, neutron therapy, intraoperative radiotherapy or radionuclide therapy by samarium-153. The median dose for external beam radiotherapy was 55.8 Gy. Local control for the entire group was 30%. However, local control rates for the group received surgery and radiotherapy were significantly superior than the group received radiotherapy alone (48% vs. 22%, $p = 0.002$).

Osteosarcoma is traditionally considered a radio-resistant tumour. The high radiation dose required to eradicate it is challenging with conventional external beam radiotherapy approach. New radiotherapy techniques such as proton and carbon ion aim to bridge the gap. Single institutional experience of unresectable osteosarcoma treated with proton therapy reported local control rate of 72% and overall survival of 67% at 5 years [31]. In a report from Chiba, Japan, using carbon ion for unresectable OS of the trunk and spine, local control rate of 62% and 79% at 5 years were achieved in those with unresectable truncal and spinal osteosarcoma, respectively [32]. Despite these early encouraging results, a systematic review of the clinical effectiveness of proton therapy in children by Leroy concluded that there was insufficient evidence to either support or refute the role of proton [33].

Stereotactic body radiotherapy (SBRT) is another radiotherapy technique that enables highly focus and precise delivery of large doses of radiation per fraction and thereby increases biologically effective doses beyond what is achievable with conventional fractionated radiotherapy. Single institutional series by Brown et al. reported their experience using SBRT for recurrent and metastatic osteosarcoma and Ewing sarcoma [34]. Of patients treated with curative intent, the estimated local control at 2 years was 85%. For those treated with palliative intent, majority progressed. However, many did experience symptomatic improvement. Significant late toxicities such as sacral plexopathy and femoral head necrosis/fracture occurred in the setting of re-irradiation and when established dose constraints were knowingly exceeded. SBRT is a promising technique, but more data is needed to establish its role in primary bone tumours.

10.10 Ewing Sarcoma

Contrary to osteosarcoma, Ewing sarcoma is a radiosensitive tumour. Complete surgical resection remains the gold standard for resectable tumour. Post-operative radiotherapy is indicated in cases of inadequate surgical margins or those with poor histological response. In cases where complete surgical resection of all tissues originally involved with tumour prior to chemotherapy is not possible, conventionally fractionated radiotherapy in the dose range of 45–60 Gy should be used to achieve local control. A randomised controlled trial INT-0091 assigned patients with Ewing sarcoma, peripheral neuroectodermal tumour (PNET) of the bone or primitive sarcoma of the bone to VACA-IE chemotherapy versus VACA chemotherapy alone [35]. An analysis of a subgroup of patients with non-metastatic pelvic Ewing sarcoma treated on this study was undertaken to investigate the relationship between the type of local control modality and the risk of local failure. It did not demonstrate a statistically significant difference in local control between different treatment modalities. Local failure rates at 5 years were 25% each for surgery and radiotherapy but only 11% for a combination of surgery and radiotherapy [36]. A more contemporary series from Mayo Clinic of patients with pelvic Ewing sarcoma reported a 5-year local recurrence rate of 26%, 13% and 0% for those treated with radiation alone, surgery alone and a combination of surgery and radiotherapy, respectively [37]. This is, however, not statistically significant. It also reported a lower local recurrence rate in those treated with radiation doses of no less than 56 Gy. This is again not statistically significant, but suggesting dose intensification may improve local control.

MRI and PET scans, both pre- and post-chemotherapy, are used for planning the treatment. The GTV usually consists of the initial extent of the tumour at diagnosis, but allowances are often made for responses to neoadjuvant chemotherapy in the chest and pelvic cavities. The CTV includes an additional 1.5–2 cm margin to the GTV to ensure inclusion of the inflammatory zone around a tumour which is known to contain satellite disease, and this zone is clipped at normal anatomical structures such as vessels and normal bone. The PTV routinely includes a 1-cm margin to the CTV for variability in set-up. The timing of when RT is delivered (preoperative, post-operative), the treatment protocol, the reason why (definitive, multimodality) or patient/tumour characteristics and location will determine the dose of delivery. In general, definitive RT or where there is gross residual disease after surgery, 55–59 Gy is used. For narrow margins or positive margins and/or poor response to chemotherapy, 45–50.4 Gy is used. Should preoperative RT be decided, then 45–50.4 Gy is delivered preoperatively. Most patients these days are treated with an IMRT or VMAT.

10.11 Chondrosarcoma

The most common histologic subtype of chondrosarcoma is conventional chondrosarcoma, and majority are low-grade but locally aggressive and do not generally metastasise. The other subtypes are rare and consist of dedifferentiated chondrosarcoma, clear cell and mesenchymal chondrosarcoma. These subtypes are usually high-grade and have a greater propensity to metastasise. Chondrosarcomas commonly arise from metaphysis of the long bone and the axial skeleton such as skull base and sacrum. As an entity, chondrosarcoma is considered relatively radio-resistant. Hence, high doses of radiation are required. In attempts to enhance biological effective dose, therefore, efficacy was made using charged particles such as protons and carbon ions. Institutional series of skull base chondrosarcoma treated by proton or carbon ions reported excellent local control rates of 75–95% [38, 39]. Single institutional experience of fractionated stereotactic radiotherapy (FSRT) concluded its use is associated with high rates of overall survival and local control [36]. Nearly half the patients experienced acute toxicity, but majority resolved spontaneously within 6 months of FSRT. Late toxicity was uncommon and mainly occurred in patients who received prior radiation therapy. More data is needed to establish the role of FSRT in chondrosarcoma.

10.12 Whole-Lung Irradiation

Whole-lung irradiation (WLI) is considered standard treatment for children with metastatic Ewing Sarcoma. However, its role in the adult population remains controversial. Retrospective studies comparing patients treated with multi-agent chemotherapy and local therapy of the primary tumour with or without WLI reported improvement in event-free survival and reduction in pulmonary relapse which were not statistically significant [40, 41]. A randomised trial by Razek et al. randomly assigned 193 patients with primary Ewing sarcoma to vincristine, actinomycin and cyclophosphamide (VAC) and Adriamycin (arm 1), VAC alone (arm 2) and VAC plus WLI (arm 3) [42]. The incidence of pulmonary metastases was the lowest at 10% in arm 1 while the incidence in arm 2 was 38% ($p = 0.001$). WLI reduced the incidence of pulmonary metastases to 20%. The difference in EFS and OS between different arms was not statistically significant. A single institutional series from MSKCC reported outcomes and patterns of failure in adult patients with Ewing sarcoma treated with WLI for pulmonary metastases. The overall 3-year EFS, OS and pulmonary relapse rate (PRR) were 38%, 45% and 55%, respectively. All 26 patients received VAC-IE chemotherapy. Those who received 15 Gy in 1.5 Gy per fraction WLI had a superior OS of 51%. Those without extra-pulmonary metastases also had a much better prognosis with a 3-year EFS and OS of 61% and 49%, respectively. Many of these studies reported no severe acute lung toxicity. In general, the incidence of severe pulmonary complications appeared relatively low. The dose and fractionation of WLI following completion of chemotherapy and metastasectomy as per NCCN guideline is 18 Gy in 1.5 Gy fraction for patients >14 years [43]. Given the lack of clear evidence to support the use of WLI in adult patients with metastatic Ewing sarcoma, its use should be individualised balancing the risk of lung metastases and the risk of pulmonary complications. WLI should only be carried out in specialised sarcoma centres with multidisciplinary expertise.

10.13 Chordoma

Chordoma arise from remnants of the notochord. It can occur in mobile and sacral spine. Its management is particularly difficult due to close proximity to the spinal cord and adjacent vital structures. En bloc excision with clear margins is the cornerstone of treatment success. However, morbidity is high. In a study at MSKCC, three-quarter of patients after radical sacral surgery reported sexual dysfunction, bowel dysfunction (including colostomies) or the need to self-catheterise.

Radiotherapy is often combined with surgery. In a retrospective study, adjuvant radiotherapy reduced the risk of local recurrence after en bloc resection of sacrococcygeal chordoma when compared with no adjuvant radiotherapy [44]. When resection is not possible without severe morbidity, high-dose radiotherapy is used as a definitive treatment.

Treating chordoma with radiotherapy alone is equally challenging. It is generally agreed that radiation dose in the region of at least 70 Gy will be necessary to eradicate the tumour. It is well beyond the tolerance of surrounding structures. Highly conformal techniques with IMRT, VMAT or SBRT are some of the tools to achieve high tumour dose while sparing surrounding tissue. When it is given after resection, artefacts from surgical implant hamper accurate target volume delineation and negatively impact dosimetry.

High-dose spine stereotactic radiotherapy can offer patients with chordoma the chance of durable control. A recent series from MSKCC of 35 patients treated with single-fraction stereotactic radiotherapy to a median PTV dose 24 Gy reported 3- and 5-year LRFS of 96.3% and 90.0%, respectively [45].

Hadron therapy (protons or charged particles such as carbon ions) is used taking advantage of the Bragg peak to achieve a steep dose gradient between the target and the surrounding tissues.

Long-term results of a phase II study at MGH using high-dose photon/proton radiotherapy given before and after surgery showed promising results. Eight-year actuarial local control rate was 85% for primary tumours. The 8-year actuarial risk of grades 3–4 late RT morbidity was 13% [46].

Carbon ions are heavier than protons. Their greater relative biologic effectiveness (RBE) leads to a greater probability of achieving tumour control. The National Institute of Radiological Sciences in Chiba, Japan, has offered carbon ion since 1994. In a retrospective study of patients with unresectable sacral chordoma, 188 patients treated with carbon ion radiation therapy between 1996 and 2013 were analysed. The highest proximal invasion reached past S2 level in 137 patients. The median clinical target volume was 345 cm^3. One hundred six patients received 67.2 grey equivalents (GyE)/16 fractions (fr), 74 patients received 70.4 GyE/16 fr, 7 patients received 73.6 GyE/16 fr, and 1 patient received 64.0 GyE/16 fr. The 5-year local control, overall survival and disease-free survival rates were 77.2%, 81.1% and 50.3%, respectively. Forty-one patients had a local recurrence [48].

10.14 Retroperitoneal Sarcoma

Retroperitoneal sarcomas (RPS) are rare soft tissue tumours, representing 10–15% of all soft tissue sarcomas [47]. They are a heterogeneous group of tumours. It is often large in size. Together with its location and proximity to abdominal organs, it poses technical surgical challenges. Local recurrence is common (at least 40–50%) and remains a major cause of morbidity and mortality, with up to 75% of RPS-related deaths attributable to locally recurrent disease.

High tumour grade and macroscopically incomplete resection are predictors of local relapse.

Salvage procedure for residual disease after resection or recurrent disease is often not successful. In a retrospective review of 33 patients with recurrent RPS and 12 with residual disease after resection, 15 patients were deemed inappropriate for further resection, with a subsequent median overall survival period of 15 months. Among the 30 resected patients, the median and 5-year overall survival was 53 months (50%). Overall survival was better in the recurrent group than in the residual group [49].

Radiotherapy for RPS includes preoperative external beam radiotherapy, post-operative EBRT, intraoperative radiotherapy (IORT) or combination. In a case-control propensity score-matched analysis of 9068 patients with localised retroperitoneal sarcoma identified from a nationwide clinical oncology database treated with preoperative or post-operative radiotherapy versus surgery alone from 2003 to 2011, both preoperative radiotherapy and post-operative radiotherapy were significantly associated with improved overall survival compared with surgery alone [50]. In another study in patients who underwent resection with curative intent for retroperitoneal liposarcoma and who received preoperative radiotherapy or surgery alone identified in the US National Cancer Data Base (2004–2013), in the propensity score-matched cohort, preoperative radiotherapy was associated with an improvement in survival (median overall survival 129.2 versus 84.3 months; $P = 0.046$). This effect appeared most pronounced for tumours with adjacent organ invasion (median overall survival not reached versus 63.8 months; $P = 0.044$) [51].

Preoperative radiotherapy is the preferred method for retroperitoneal sarcoma. Radiation enteritis is significantly lower than post-operative radiotherapy as the tumour mass displaces small intestine away from the radiation volume. The radiation target is much better defined before resection [27]. Histologic diagnosis is usually obtained by CT-guided core biopsy with posterior approach. PET CT increases the diagnostic yield of the core biopsy by identifying the most metabolically active part of the tumour. In order to ensure that the biopsy track is within the radiation target, the biopsy tract can be documented by CT at the time of biopsy. A renal DMSA scan for split renal function is recommended when nephrectomy is expected.

A radiation dose of 45 Gy to 50 Gy is recommended for preoperative radiotherapy. VMAT or IMRT is vastly superior to 3DCRT in terms of radiation dose homogeneity, dose to organs at risk and ability to dose paint.

In a study conducted by NRG Oncology, CT scans for 2 cases of RPS were distributed among 12 sarcoma radiation oncologists with instructions for contouring GTV, CTV, areas judged to be at high risk of resulting in positive margins after resection and organs at risk (OARs). There was high level of agreement in GTV, CTV and most OARs. Contours of areas of potential positive margins were more variable [52]. Surgical input in clarification of high-risk area is recommended.

Well-differentiated liposarcoma is the commonest type of retroperitoneal sarcoma. They are often large and present several challenges. Defining GTV accurately of a large well-differentiated lipoma-like liposarcoma can be difficult as it is not too dissimilar to normal abdominal fat. In the course of radiotherapy, inter-fraction displacement of the tumour is more pronounced for superior positioned tumour.

Volumetric changes of the tumour are common. In a clinical study, it was observed GTV volumetric increase during the first 2 weeks of treatment was followed by GTV volumetric decrease by completion of radiotherapy [53].

References

1. Hoekstra HJ, Thijssens K, van Ginkel RJ. Role of surgery as primary treatment and as intervention in the multidisciplinary treatment of soft tissue sarcoma. Ann Oncol. 2004;15(Suppl 4):iv181–6.
2. Rosenberg SA, Tepper J, Glatstein E, Costa J, Baker A, Brennan M, et al. The treatment of soft-tissue sarcomas of the extremities: prospective randomized evaluations of (1) limb-sparing surgery plus radiation therapy compared with amputation and (2) the role of adjuvant chemotherapy. Ann Surg. 1982;196(3):305–15.
3. Yang JC, Chang AE, Baker AR, Sindelar WF, Danforth DN, Topalian SL, et al. Randomized prospective study of the benefit of adjuvant radiation therapy in the treatment of soft tissue sarcomas of the extremity. J Clin Oncol. 1998;16(1):197–203.
4. Beane JD, Yang JC, White D, Steinberg SM, Rosenberg SA, Rudloff U. Efficacy of adjuvant radiation therapy in the treatment of soft tissue sarcoma of the extremity: 20-year follow-up of a randomized prospective trial. Ann Surg Oncol. 2014;21(8):2484–9.
5. Choong PF, Petersen IA, Nascimento AG, Sim FH. Is radiotherapy important for low-grade soft tissue sarcoma of the extremity? Clin Orthop Relat Res. 2001;387:191–9.
6. Pisters PW, Harrison LB, Leung DH, Woodruff JM, Casper ES, Brennan MF. Long-term results of a prospective randomized trial of adjuvant brachytherapy in soft tissue sarcoma. J Clin Oncol. 1996;14(3):859–68.
7. O'Sullivan B, Davis AM, Turcotte R, Bell R, Catton C, Chabot P, et al. Preoperative versus postoperative radiotherapy in soft-tissue sarcoma of the limbs: a randomised trial. Lancet. 2002;359(9325):2235–41.
8. Wang D, Bosch W, Roberge D, Finkelstein SE, Petersen I, Haddock M, et al. RTOG sarcoma radiation oncologists reach consensus on gross tumor volume and clinical target volume on computed tomographic images for preoperative radiotherapy of primary soft tissue sarcoma of extremity in Radiation Therapy Oncology Group studies. Int J Radiat Oncol Biol Phys. 2011;81(4):e525–8.
9. Imanishi J, Slavin J, Pianta M, Jackett L, Ngan SY, Tanaka T, et al. Tail of superficial myxofibrosarcoma and undifferentiated pleomorphic sarcoma after preoperative radiotherapy. Anticancer Res. 2016;36(5):2339–44.
10. Temple WJ, Temple CL, Arthur K, Schachar NS, Paterson AH, Crabtree TS. Prospective cohort study of neoadjuvant treatment in conservative surgery of soft tissue sarcomas. Ann Surg Oncol. 1997;4(7):586–90.
11. Pisters PW, Patel SR, Prieto VG, Thall PF, Lewis VO, Feig BW, et al. Phase I trial of preoperative doxorubicin-based concurrent chemoradiation and surgical resection for localized extremity and body wall soft tissue sarcomas. J Clin Oncol. 2004;22(16):3375–80.
12. Cormier JN, Patel SR, Herzog CE, Ballo MT, Burgess MA, Feig BW, et al. Concurrent ifosfamide-based chemotherapy and irradiation. Analysis of treatment-related toxicity in 43 patients with sarcoma. Cancer. 2001;92(6):1550–5.
13. Edmonson JH, Petersen IA, Shives TC, Mahoney MR, Rock MG, Haddock MG, et al. Chemotherapy, irradiation, and surgery for function-preserving therapy of primary extremity soft tissue sarcomas: initial treatment with ifosfamide, mitomycin, doxorubicin, and cisplatin plus granulocyte macrophage-colony-stimulating factor. Cancer. 2002;94(3):786–92.
14. DeLaney TF, Spiro IJ, Suit HD, Gebhardt MC, Hornicek FJ, Mankin HJ, et al. Neoadjuvant chemotherapy and radiotherapy for large extremity soft-tissue sarcomas. Int J Radiat Oncol Biol Phys. 2003;56(4):1117–27.

15. Kraybill WG, Harris J, Spiro IJ, Ettinger DS, DeLaney TF, Blum RH, et al. Phase II study of neoadjuvant chemotherapy and radiation therapy in the management of high-risk, high-grade, soft tissue sarcomas of the extremities and body wall: Radiation Therapy Oncology Group Trial 9514. J Clin Oncol. 2006;24(4):619–25.
16. Mullen JT, Kobayashi W, Wang JJ, Harmon DC, Choy E, Hornicek FJ, et al. Long-term follow-up of patients treated with neoadjuvant chemotherapy and radiotherapy for large, extremity soft tissue sarcomas. Cancer. 2012;118(15):3758–65.
17. Kraybill WG, Harris J, Spiro IJ, Ettinger DS, DeLaney TF, Blum RH, et al. Long-term results of a phase 2 study of neoadjuvant chemotherapy and radiotherapy in the management of high-risk, high-grade, soft tissue sarcomas of the extremities and body wall: Radiation Therapy Oncology Group Trial 9514. Cancer. 2010;116(19):4613–21.
18. Haas RL, Miah AB, LePechoux C, DeLaney TF, Baldini EH, Alektiar K, et al. Preoperative radiotherapy for extremity soft tissue sarcoma; past, present and future perspectives on dose fractionation regimens and combined modality strategies. Radiother Oncol. 2016;119(1):14–21.
19. Andrews SF, Anderson PR, Eisenberg BL, Hanlon AL, Pollack A. Soft tissue sarcomas treated with postoperative external beam radiotherapy with and without low-dose-rate brachytherapy. Int J Radiat Oncol Biol Phys. 2004;59(2):475–80.
20. Harrison LB, Franzese F, Gaynor JJ, Brennan MF. Long-term results of a prospective randomized trial of adjuvant brachytherapy in the management of completely resected soft tissue sarcomas of the extremity and superficial trunk. Int J Radiat Oncol Biol Phys. 1993;27(2):259–65.
21. Pisters PW, Harrison LB, Woodruff JM, Gaynor JJ, Brennan MF. A prospective randomized trial of adjuvant brachytherapy in the management of low-grade soft tissue sarcomas of the extremity and superficial trunk. J Clin Oncol. 1994;12(6):1150–5.
22. Alektiar KM, Zelefsky MJ, Brennan MF. Morbidity of adjuvant brachytherapy in soft tissue sarcoma of the extremity and superficial trunk. Int J Radiat Oncol Biol Phys. 2000;47(5):1273–9.
23. Emory CL, Montgomery CO, Potter BK, Keisch ME, Conway SA. Early complications of high-dose-rate brachytherapy in soft tissue sarcoma: a comparison with traditional external-beam radiotherapy. Clin Orthop Relat Res. 2012;470(3):751–8.
24. Petera J, Soumarova R, Ruzickova J, Neumanova R, Dusek L, Sirak I, et al. Perioperative hyperfractionated high-dose rate brachytherapy for the treatment of soft tissue sarcomas: multicentric experience. Ann Surg Oncol. 2010;17(1):206–10.
25. Alektiar KM, Hu K, Anderson L, Brennan MF, Harrison LB. High-dose-rate intraoperative radiation therapy (HDR-IORT) for retroperitoneal sarcomas. Int J Radiat Oncol Biol Phys. 2000;47(1):157–63.
26. Sindelar WF, Kinsella TJ, Chen PW, DeLaney TF, Tepper JE, Rosenberg SA, et al. Intraoperative radiotherapy in retroperitoneal sarcomas. Final results of a prospective, randomized, clinical trial. Arch Surg. 1993;128(4):402–10.
27. Smith MJ, Ridgway PF, Catton CN, Cannell AJ, O'Sullivan B, Mikula LA, et al. Combined management of retroperitoneal sarcoma with dose intensification radiotherapy and resection: long-term results of a prospective trial. Radiother Oncol. 2014;110(1):165–71.
28. Alektiar KM, Brennan MF, Singer S. Local control comparison of adjuvant brachytherapy to intensity-modulated radiotherapy in primary high-grade sarcoma of the extremity. Cancer. 2011;117(14):3229–34.
29. DeLaney TF, Park L, Goldberg SI, Hug EB, Liebsch NJ, Munzenrider JE, et al. Radiotherapy for local control of osteosarcoma. Int J Radiat Oncol Biol Phys. 2005;61(2):492–8.
30. Schwarz R, Bruland O, Cassoni A, Schomberg P, Bielack S. The role of radiotherapy in oseosarcoma. Cancer Treat Res. 2009;152:147–64.
31. Ciernik IF, Niemierko A, Harmon DC, Kobayashi W, Chen YL, Yock TI, et al. Proton-based radiotherapy for unresectable or incompletely resected osteosarcoma. Cancer. 2011;117(19):4522–30.
32. Matsunobu A, Imai R, Kamada T, Imaizumi T, Tsuji H, Tsujii H, et al. Impact of carbon ion radiotherapy for unresectable osteosarcoma of the trunk. Cancer. 2012;118(18):4555–63.
33. Leroy R, Benahmed N, Hulstaert F, Van Damme N, De Ruysscher D. Proton therapy in children: a systematic review of clinical effectiveness in 15 pediatric cancers. Int J Radiat Oncol Biol Phys. 2016;95(1):267–78.

34. Brown LC, Lester RA, Grams MP, Haddock MG, Olivier KR, Arndt CA, et al. Stereotactic body radiotherapy for metastatic and recurrent Ewing sarcoma and osteosarcoma. Sarcoma. 2014;2014:418270.
35. Yock TI, Krailo M, Fryer CJ, Donaldson SS, Miser JS, Chen Z, et al. Local control in pelvic Ewing sarcoma: analysis from INT-0091—a report from the Children's Oncology Group. J Clin Oncol. 2006;24(24):3838–43.
36. Vasudevan HN, Raleigh DR, Johnson J, Garsa AA, Theodosopoulos PV, Aghi MK, et al. Management of chordoma and chondrosarcoma with fractionated stereotactic radiotherapy. Front Surg. 2017;4:35.
37. Ahmed SK, Robinson SI, Arndt CAS, Petersen IA, Haddock MG, Rose PS, et al. Pelvis Ewing sarcoma: local control and survival in the modern era. Pediatr Blood Cancer. 2017;64(9)
38. Ares C, Hug EB, Lomax AJ, Bolsi A, Timmermann B, Rutz HP, et al. Effectiveness and safety of spot scanning proton radiation therapy for chordomas and chondrosarcomas of the skull base: first long-term report. Int J Radiat Oncol Biol Phys. 2009;75(4):1111–8.
39. Weber DC, Malyapa R, Albertini F, Bolsi A, Kliebsch U, Walser M, et al. Long term outcomes of patients with skull-base low-grade chondrosarcoma and chordoma patients treated with pencil beam scanning proton therapy. Radiother Oncol. 2016;120(1):169–74.
40. Bolling T, Schuck A, Paulussen M, Dirksen U, Ranft A, Konemann S, et al. Whole lung irradiation in patients with exclusively pulmonary metastases of Ewing tumors. Toxicity analysis and treatment results of the EICESS-92 trial. Strahlenther Onkol. 2008;184(4):193–7.
41. Paulussen M, Ahrens S, Burdach S, Craft A, Dockhorn-Dworniczak B, Dunst J, et al. Primary metastatic (stage IV) Ewing tumor: survival analysis of 171 patients from the EICESS studies. European Intergroup Cooperative Ewing Sarcoma Studies. Ann Oncol. 1998;9(3):275–81.
42. Razek A, Perez CA, Tefft M, Nesbit M, Vietti T, Burgert EO Jr, et al. Intergroup Ewing's Sarcoma Study: local control related to radiation dose, volume, and site of primary lesion in Ewing's sarcoma. Cancer. 1980;46(3):516–21.
43. Biermann JS, Chow W, Reed DR, Lucas D, Adkins DR, Agulnik M, et al. NCCN guidelines insights: bone cancer, version 2.2017. J Natl Compr Cancer Netw. 2017;15(2):155–67.
44. Moojen WA, Vleggeert-Lankamp CL, Krol AD, Dijkstra SP. Long-term results: adjuvant radiotherapy in en bloc resection of sacrococcygeal chordoma is advisable. Spine (Phila Pa 1976). 2011;36(10):E656–61.
45. Jin CJ, Berry-Candelario J, Reiner AS, Laufer I, Higginson DS, Schmitt AM, Lis E, Barzilai O, Boland P, Yamada Y, Bilsky MH. Long-term outcomes of high-dose single-fraction radiosurgery for chordomas of the spine and sacrum. J Neurosurg Spine. 2019:1–10. https://doi.org/10.3171/2019.7.SPINE19515. Epub ahead of print. PMID: 31628294.
46. DeLaney TF, Liebsch NJ, Pedlow FX, Adams J, Weyman EA, Yeap BY, et al. Long-term results of Phase II study of high dose photon/proton radiotherapy in the management of spine chordomas, chondrosarcomas, and other sarcomas. J Surg Oncol. 2014;110(2):115–22.
47. Porter GA, Baxter NN, Pisters PW. Retroperitoneal sarcoma: a population-based analysis of epidemiology, surgery, and radiotherapy. Cancer. 2006;106(7):1610–6. https://doi.org/10.1002/cncr.21761. PMID: 16518798.
48. Imai R, Kamada T, Araki N, Working Group for Bone, Soft Tissue Sarcoma. Carbon ion radiation therapy for unresectable sacral chordoma: an analysis of 188 cases. Int J Radiat Oncol Biol Phys. 2016;95(1):322–7.
49. Hamilton TD, Cannell AJ, Kim M, Catton CN, Blackstein ME, Dickson BC, et al. Results of resection for recurrent or residual retroperitoneal sarcoma after failed primary treatment. Ann Surg Oncol. 2017;24(1):211–8.
50. Nussbaum DP, Rushing CN, Lane WO, Cardona DM, Kirsch DG, Peterson BL, et al. Preoperative or postoperative radiotherapy versus surgery alone for retroperitoneal sarcoma: a case-control, propensity score-matched analysis of a nationwide clinical oncology database. Lancet Oncol. 2016;17(7):966–75.
51. Ecker BL, Peters MG, McMillan MT, Sinnamon AJ, Zhang PJ, Fraker DL, et al. Preoperative radiotherapy in the management of retroperitoneal liposarcoma. Br J Surg. 2016;103(13):1839–46.

52. Baldini EH, Abrams RA, Bosch W, Roberge D, Haas RLM, Catton CN, et al. Retroperitoneal sarcoma target volume and organ at risk contour delineation agreement among NRG sarcoma radiation oncologists. Int J Radiat Oncol Biol Phys. 2015;92(5):1053–9.
53. Wong P, Dickie C, Lee D, Chung P, O'Sullivan B, Letourneau D, et al. Spatial and volumetric changes of retroperitoneal sarcomas during pre-operative radiotherapy. Radiother Oncol. 2014;112(2):308–13.

The Role of Systemic Therapies in the Management of Soft Tissue Sarcoma

11

Nikki Burdett, Susie Bae, Anne Hamilton, and Jayesh Desai

11.1 Introduction

Soft tissue sarcomas (STS) are solid tumours that originate from mesenchymal cells and can be subclassified into over 50 subtypes. Representing 1% of adult tumours and 15% of paediatric malignancies, their rarity and diversity has traditionally made clinical trial design and thereby the provision of a strong evidence base to guide individual patient management challenging. As therapeutic options as a whole have increased for solid cancers in the context of an increased understanding of molecular drivers that predict response to those therapies, the challenges faced by the STS community have meant that the overall pace of drug development has been slower, with some notable exceptions in selected sarcoma subtypes in which clear molecular drivers have been identified (e.g. gastrointestinal stromal tumours). However, the recognition that "splitting" these requisite subtypes even if based on classical histopathological features into their respective individual entities over the last two decades, rather than "lumping" all STS together, has helped advance the field considerably. In addition, international collaborative efforts have advanced in parallel, facilitating the successful conduct of trials in specific subtypes to be conducted, including randomized phase III trials.

11.2 Systemic Therapy in Localized STS

For most limb and truncal STS without distant metastases, surgery with or without pre-/post-operative radiotherapy is standard treatment and achieves high rates of

N. Burdett · S. Bae · A. Hamilton · J. Desai (✉)
Bone and Soft Tissue Sarcoma Service, Peter MacCallum Cancer Centre, Melbourne, VIC, Australia

Division of Medical Oncology, Peter MacCallum Cancer Centre, Melbourne, VIC, Australia
e-mail: Nikki.Burdett@petermac.org.au; susie.bae@petermac.org; anne.hamilton@petermac.org.au; jayesh.desai@petermac.org.au

P. F. M. Choong (ed.), *Sarcoma*, https://doi.org/10.1007/978-981-15-9414-4_11

local control while maintaining optimal function. The role of systemic therapy for localized STS remains controversial although frequently debated in multidisciplinary meetings. Although currently not regarded as standard treatment in Australia, it should be considered for individual patients with high-risk disease and potentially chemosensitive subtypes on the basis that benefit cannot be excluded, with conflicting evidence in the literature. An earlier meta-analysis published in 1997 reported a benefit in improving local control and distant recurrence-free survival; however, the overall survival benefit was not statistically significant [1]. Two subsequent meta-analyses supported these data. Interestingly, one of these studies reported a significant survival benefit for adjuvant chemotherapy; however this was not maintained with long-term follow-up [2, 3]. The most recent EORTC 62931 study, published in 2012, failed to demonstrate any clear improvement in local control, relapse-free survival or overall survival in patients treated with adjuvant chemotherapy [4].

The role of neoadjuvant chemotherapy is increasingly debated in multidisciplinary meetings, particularly for patients with large high-grade STS that is considered borderline resectable. However, the data supporting the use of neoadjuvant chemotherapy for STS is more notably limited and mainly derived from retrospective series and phase I trials [5, 6]. Patient factors including age and comorbidity, together with the tumour factors including histology subtype, stage and surgical resectability, all need to be considered in discussing the appropriateness of this approach. A multidisciplinary team discussion remains essential in selecting patients on a case-by-case basis.

11.3 Systemic Therapy in Advanced/Metastatic STS

Most STS are treated empirically with traditional cytotoxic chemotherapy. However, it is critically important to be aware of some of the specific subtypes that need to be approached differently (including diagnostically) as outcomes can be vastly different in some of these cases. Improving the outcome of patients with advanced/metastatic STS will therefore need to continue to focus on refining existing treatments and combinations in parallel with efforts to better predict specific molecular drivers of STS subtypes that are potentially targetable.

At present, the selection of systemic therapies is individualized based on disease tempo, histology, patient preference and comorbidities. The biological tempo can be especially important as the natural history of advanced/metastatic STS can be variable, with significant differences seen between low- and high-grade histology. Additionally, it is recognized that certain histological subtypes may have higher rates of chemosensitivity, which may factor into the decision process for timing and type of treatment, for example, ifosfamide with synovial sarcoma, doxorubicin with myxoid/round cell liposarcoma, eribulin with liposarcoma, taxanes with angiosarcoma and trabectedin in myxoid/round cell liposarcomas.

Until we develop molecular biomarkers capable of predicting response for individual subsets of STS, clinicians need to rely on existing data in the optimal use of systemic therapies in the aim of assisting palliation and potentially improving survival. This review will focus on traditional and evolving options available for management of advanced STS for both cytotoxic and targeted agents but will not encompass the role of adjuvant or neoadjuvant use of these agents.

11.4 Traditional Cytotoxic Agents

11.4.1 Doxorubicin and/or Ifosfamide

Historically, the single agents in STS with the highest recorded levels of activity have been doxorubicin (or epirubicin) and ifosfamide. Additionally, the range of responses is highly variable reflecting the biologic heterogeneity and chemosensitivity of tumoural subclass in each individual trial. Median survival after metastatic disease is 12–18 months but may extend out to 2 years in approximately one quarter of patients with unresectable disease [7, 8].

Since the first studies in the 1970s, doxorubicin has been and remains the single most active agent for the treatment of STS. There is much variation in its reported response rate given the underlying tumour heterogeneity of early trials, which customarily included multiple STS subtypes. Modern-day studies in unselected STS reported response rates of 10–25% [9–11].

It is important to recognize that there is a dose-response relationship with doxorubicin, seen at doses between 60 and 75 mg/m^2 per cycle [12]. Other agents have been investigated to try and avoid dose-limiting cumulative cardiotoxicity. Epirubicin has equimolar dosing with less cardiotoxicity and a similar toxicity profile and response rate, but with most data generated with the use of doxorubicin rather than epirubicin, doxorubicin remains the better established therapy in most regions of the world [13–15]. Alternatively, liposomal doxorubicin, in phase II studies, has similar activity to doxorubicin with response rates between 10 and 50% and an improved toxicity profile [11]. Although widely used, phase III studies have yet to be conducted to show non-inferiority to doxorubicin, and its higher cost has also limited its global use.

Single-agent ifosfamide has comparable activity to doxorubicin and has response rates between 7 and 41% for patients who have failed front-line doxorubicin. Its differing safety profile is related to its metabolites (haemorrhagic cystitis, renal tubular acidosis and encephalopathy), and although a dose-response relationship exists supporting doses as high as 12 g/m^2, it can be associated with excess toxicity [16, 17]. Although difficult to clearly define, the "low threshold" for ifosfamide is considered to be at least 6 g/m^2, but additional responses are noted even with doses with $\geq$10 g/m^2 [16, 18].

The combination of doxorubicin and ifosfamide has been explored since the 1970s, with multiple randomized trials failing to provide definitive, practice-changing evidence for the advantage of a combination approach versus single-agent doxorubicin. Several randomized studies have compared varying (in dose and schedule) doxorubicin-based combinations to single-agent doxorubicin. While these are associated with higher response rates (range of 15–46%) when compared with single-agent doxorubicin (10–18%), these have not improved overall survival. Moreover, toxicity was significantly greater for the combination group [8, 19–21].

Most earlier trials were criticized for various reasons, the inclusion or lumping together of "outliers" such as GIST that were less responsive or unresponsive to chemotherapy, being underpowered or utilizing an inadequate dose intensity of either doxorubicin or especially ifosfamide. The issue has perhaps finally been put to rest however, with the completion of a well-conducted randomized trial, the EORTC 62012 trial. A total of 455 patients were enrolled from 38 centres in 10 countries to doxorubicin (at 75 mg/m^2) vs doxorubicin plus ifosfamide (75 mg/m^2 and 10 g/m^2, respectively) [22]. Results from this trial showed no survival advantage with the combination approach and with a considerably higher rate of serious toxicities (febrile neutropenia of 46% vs. 13%). The authors concluded that these results do not support the routine use of this combination in the palliation of patients with advanced STS. Of note, the response rate was significantly higher in the combination group (RECIST-defined objective responses of 26% vs. 14%), suggesting that the combination may have a role to play in selected patients where tumour shrinkage is an important goal of treatment, e.g. neoadjuvant chemotherapy, or in patients with highly symptomatic lesions but minimal other comorbidities allowing them to tolerate a more aggressive approach.

11.4.2 Other Traditional Cytotoxic Agents

Gemcitabine as a single agent has inconsistent data supporting its utility. One trial showed that fixed dose rate infusions were associated with a partial response with non-GI leiomyosarcoma, yet other reports including data from the control arms of randomized phase II trials with gemcitabine have consistently shown little single-agent activity [23]. This is in contrast to combination therapy with gemcitabine and other agents (e.g. docetaxel or vinorelbine), which has considerably more activity [24]. The combination with most noted activity, and the one most studied, is with gemcitabine and docetaxel. This was initially compared to gemcitabine alone in a multicentre randomized phase II study with a response rate (16% vs. 8%) and survival (17.9 vs. 11.5 months) favouring combination treatment, with the most benefit seen in those with leiomyosarcoma and undifferentiated STS [25]. Given its clear activity in STS, gemcitabine plus docetaxel has since been compared to doxorubicin alone in a first-line setting. The GeDDis trial compared the combination of gemcitabine plus docetaxel with single-agent doxorubicin in chemo-naive patients with a variety of histologies of advanced and metastatic STS in a randomized phase III trial [26]. The results of the GeDDis trial revealed almost identical outcomes (46% progression-free) in both study arms at 24 weeks (the primary endpoint) and median overall survival slightly favouring doxorubicin (76 versus 67 weeks, HR for death 1.14, 95% CI 0.83–1.57), though this was not statistically significant. Of note, gemcitabine plus docetaxel was more toxic and harder to administer than single-agent doxorubicin. In addition, the lack of histological stratification (pleomorphic sarcoma/malignant fibrous histiocytoma) which is of importance when translating this into practice was underrepresented in this trial. This is important because pleomorphic sarcoma and malignant fibrous histiocytoma are known to be responsive to gemcitabine and docetaxel. Additionally, the dose of gemcitabine and docetaxel used in this UK-led trial was lower than that used in the earlier phase II (and American-led) trials, which may have impacted on the efficacy of the combination in more responsive subtypes such as leiomyosarcoma. These results have again confirmed the place of doxorubicin as the standard of care in the first-line setting.

Other combinations with gemcitabine including dacarbazine (DTIC) or vinorelbine have been tested in the phase II setting with modest activity and would therefore not be considered a standard of care option in most centres.

Dacarbazine has been used for many years and is the control arm on several phase III studies, and although it has less activity than doxorubicin and ifosfamide, it still has activity in the second-line setting and beyond [27].

11.4.3 Histotype-Specific Cytotoxic Agents

A number of "new" cytotoxic therapies for soft tissue sarcoma have been developed over the last decade, with notable activity in STS, and unique mechanisms of action when compared to traditional cytotoxic therapies such as alkylating agents.

11.4.3.1 Trabectedin

The most compelling of these "histocyte-specific cytotoxics" in sarcoma is trabectedin (ET-743; ecteinascidin), with activity thought to be related to its binding to the minor groove of DNA, leading to cytotoxicity via damaging the DNA nucleotide excision repair machinery [28, 29]. Trabectedin's development, and proven efficacy leading to its regulatory approval (particularly in the USA), was a long and complex process, perhaps mostly due to its histotype specificity in an era of generic STS trials, relatively low response rates but prolonged disease control, as well as additional efforts required to determine optimal scheduling (24-h vs. 3-h infusions). A series of trials eventually led to a phase II trial, with promising activity noted in pretreated leiomyosarcoma and myxoid/round cell liposarcoma [30]. The definitive randomized phase III multicentre trial of trabectedin was conducted in the USA, and compared trabectedin (given as a 24-h infusion, on a three weekly basis) to dacarbazine, in a large cohort of 518 patients with advanced LMS or liposarcoma previously exposed to conventional chemotherapy [31]. Although the primary endpoint of median overall survival was not significantly different with trabectedin (12.4 vs. 12.9 months), PFS was significantly improved with trabectedin (4.2 vs. 1.5 months). In addition, while the objective response rate was not significantly better with trabectedin, the clinical benefit rate was significantly better with trabectedin (34% versus 19%). Benefit was seen in both uterine and non-uterine LMS and in all liposarcoma subtypes. The benefit of trabectedin over dacarbazine was almost three times (median PFS 5.6 versus 1.5 months) in myxoid/round cell liposarcomas while only marginal (median PFS 2.2 versus 1.9 months) in dedifferentiated liposarcoma. Other studies have also noted particularly striking responses in patients with advanced myxoid/round cell liposarcoma, with a 51% response rate in 1 study of 51 patients. Importantly, these responses were sustained, with 88% progression-free at 6 months [32]. Other key points noted in this trial were the types of response, with clear early radiologic changes (decreased tumour density on CT or contrast enhancement on MRI) followed by delayed tumour shrinkage, which are markedly different to what has been seen with traditional cytotoxic agents and perhaps more akin to changes seen with kinase inhibitors in GIST [33].

11.4.3.2 Eribulin

Eribulin, an analog of halichrondrin B, inhibits microtubule function but in a manner that is distinct from taxanes. Following a signal-seeking multi-arm EORTC-led phase II trial in different STS subtypes, a randomized phase III trial was conducted in the two subtypes with highest activity, leiomyosarcoma and adipocytic (lipo) sarcomas [34]. When compared to the control group of dacarbazine in the phase III trial, the overall results suggested only modest improvements in the eribulin group. However, a preplanned subgroup analysis demonstrated a significant difference in the liposarcoma arm, with an overall survival of 15.5 vs. 8.4 months. Interestingly, both response rates and progression-free survival were not appreciably different between the two arms, a result that was also noted in a previous trial of eribulin in breast cancer, observations that may perhaps relate to its unique mechanism of action [35].

11.4.4 Molecularly Targeted Agents

Many subtypes of STS have demonstrated minimal chemosensitivity, but interestingly the rare "chemoresistant" subtypes such as clear cell sarcoma and alveolar soft part sarcoma are increasingly identified as being driven through specific molecular pathways. Conversely, many of the other more common sarcoma subtypes such as liposarcoma, leiomyosarcoma, synovial sarcoma and angiosarcoma have a moderate response to chemotherapy but less clearly defined molecular drivers. Sarcomas can, to some extent, be distinguished by specific genotypes, including those with simple or complex karyotypes [36–39]. Multiple efforts using genomic analyses have identified point mutations or deletions, which may inform future strategies of molecularly targeted agents for preclinical or clinical studies. While the link between the molecular biology and response to targeted therapies are few, certain tumours (e.g. alveolar soft part sarcoma and well-differentiated/dedifferentiated liposarcoma) may be candidates for novel therapies.

11.4.5 Tyrosine Kinase Inhibitors (TKIs) or Multi-targeted Kinase Inhibitors

TKIs as they are called here, and usually in reference to agents used in diseases such as sarcomas, are small multifunctional molecules that induce downstream effects such as inhibition of angiogenesis, cell growth and proliferation.

11.4.5.1 Pazopanib

Pazopanib was the first targeted substance to be approved in non-GIST STS and was indicated in patients who had demonstrated poor response to earlier chemotherapy. It is a multi-kinase inhibitor (VEGF, PDGF, c-KIT). Pazopanib was compared to placebo in the international multicentre randomized phase III PALETTE (Pazopanib for Metastatic Soft Tissue Sarcoma) trial of 369 patients with systemic disease (excluding GIST and adipocytic sarcomas), who had received at least 1 anthracycline-containing regimen [40]. The pazopanib group achieved a statistically significant improvement in PFS of 4.6 months compared to 1.6 months in the placebo group ($p < 0.0001$). However, there was no overall survival benefit. A number of reasons have been proposed to explain this, including a higher than expected rate of post-progression therapy with other potentially active agents.

11.5 Treatment Considerations for Certain STS Histology Subtypes

As our understanding about the complex genetic landscape of STS expands, the management of STS is increasingly becoming subtype-dependent. As described above, STS subtypes such as undifferentiated pleomorphic sarcoma, dedifferentiated/myxoid liposarcoma and synovial sarcoma are mostly sensitive to conventional cytotoxic therapies. There are other STS subtypes, which inherently have unique characteristics, which are worth noting.

11.5.1 Angiosarcoma

Angiosarcoma often arises as primary cutaneous or soft tissue tumour. It can also develop secondary to radiotherapy. Weekly paclitaxel is the preferred first-line therapy for advanced angiosarcoma, with its activity demonstrated from a phase II study and a retrospective series [41, 42]. Disappointingly the addition of an anti-angiogenetic drug, bevacizumab, to paclitaxel did not improve progression-free survival in advanced angiosarcomas [43]. Further studies are ongoing exploring potential escape pathways other than VEGF (NCT02979899).

11.5.2 Solitary Fibrous Tumour (SFT)

Most SFTs treated surgically do not recur; however, approximately 10–20% will have more aggressive features. A NAB2-STAT6 gene fusion is the diagnostic marker of SFTs and is responsible for the genetic alteration [44]. Anti-angiogenetic agents such as pazopanib, sunitinib and sorafenib are shown to be active in this entity [45–47]. It tends to be refractory to doxorubicin, but there has been variable response seen with other cytotoxic agents, including dacarbazine and trabectedin [48, 49].

11.5.3 Perivascular Epithelioid Cell tumour (PEComa)

PEComa is a family of rare mesenchymal tumours consisting of perivascular epithelioid cells. TSC1 and TSC2 mutations disrupting the mTOR signaling pathway led to exploration of mTOR inhibitors in PEComas. Activity of sirolimus and temsirolimus have been reported in small case series [50–52], and newer more potent agents targeting the mTOR pathway are also in development. PEComas are considered less responsive to chemotherapy—reinforcing the importance of an accurate diagnosis both in opening up potentially promising targeted approaches and in avoiding traditional cytotoxics [53].

11.5.4 Alveolar Soft Part Sarcoma (ASPS)

ASPS is a rare, translocation-driven t(X;17)(p11;q25) STS that is characterized by indolent behaviour but its propensity to metastasize to the lung and brain. It is regarded as inherently resistant to chemotherapy. Tyrosine kinase inhibitors such as sunitinib, cediranib and pazopanib have shown activity with tumour responses or disease stabilization in more than half of the cases [54–56]. Immune checkpoint inhibitors have also shown promising activity in ASPS based on early-phase immunotherapy trials [57].

11.6 Treatment Considerations for Certain Benign/ Intermediate-Grade Soft Tissue Tumours

Although most soft tissue tumours of various histological subtypes are classified as either benign or malignant, many are of an intermediate nature, which typically implies aggressive local behaviour with a low-to-moderate propensity for metastasis. There have been remarkable advances in the field of cancer biology in the past two decades, which have improved our understanding of specific molecular pathways responsible for pathogenesis of soft tissue tumours. Targeted therapy options are now often discussed at multidisciplinary meetings for patients affected by unresectable soft tissue tumours such as dermatofibrosarcoma protuberans, pigmented villonodular synovitis and desmoid-type fibromatosis.

11.6.1 Dermatofibrosarcoma Protuberans (DFSP)

Dermatofibrosarcoma protuberans is a rare type of cutaneous soft tissue sarcoma. They rarely metastasize but have propensity to recur locally and can lead to significant morbidity. The majority of DFSPs are characterized by a unique translocation t(17;22)(q22;q13), resulting in the *COL1A1/PDGFB* fusion gene, responsible for platelet-derived growth factor-beta receptor activation [58, 59]. This explains its sensitivity to imatinib, an inhibitor of PDGF, with consistent and notable activity demonstrated in multiple small studies [60–66]. The mainstay of optimal treatment for localized DFSP is complete resection with negative margins. Radiotherapy may be delivered as an adjunctive treatment to improve local control. For patients with locally advanced unresectable and/or metastatic DFSP, imatinib can often provide meaningful tumour shrinkage and disease control [66]. Imatinib's use for this indication has been approved in multiple regions globally.

11.6.2 Pigmented Villonodular Synovitis (PVNS)

PVNS, otherwise known as tenosynovial giant cell tumour, is a rare but well-recognized proliferative disorder of synovial tissue. It is considered as a benign neoplasm, lacking malignant and metastatic potential. There are two histopathological forms: a localized form, which involves a discrete section of the synovium, amenable to surgical resection, and a diffuse form, which involves the entire synovium, often associated with multiple recurrences and bulky disease, resulting in significant bone destruction. In PVNS, a translocation in *CSF1-COL6A3*, t(1;2)(p13;q35), leads to overexpression of colony-stimulating factor 1 receptor (CSF1R). In a recent international randomized, placebo-controlled, double-blinded phase III trial (ENLIVEN), a potent CSF1R inhibitor, pexidartinib, showed an impressive overall response rates in patients with unresectable PVNS, coupled with corresponding improvement in functional outcomes [67]. Based on these results, pexidartinib recently received FDA approval for its use in the USA, with applications for approval in other regions also underway at the time of this writing. Other less potent CSF1R inhibitors, such as imatinib and nilotinib, have also been tried, showing less pronounced activity [68, 69].

11.6.3 Desmoid-Type Fibromatosis

Desmoid-type fibromatosis (DTF) is a rare mesenchymal tumour that has a variable and unpredictable clinical course. Although lacking metastatic potential, it can behave aggressively, leading to significant morbidity from locoregional complications. Two different clinico-pathological entities have been described: sporadic DTF associated with *CTNNB1* mutation and DTF associated with germline mutation of *APC*. Wnt/APC/β-catenin pathway alterations are considered to be the driver of tumour proliferation; however, drugs targeting this pathway are not yet available in the clinic [70–72] for routine use. A multidisciplinary approach is the key to the appropriate management of DTF and requires careful assessment of the expected benefit and risks associated with any proposed treatment. Currently, an initial period of observation is universally considered the preferred and acceptable strategy for well-selected patients with asymptomatic or minimally symptomatic tumours, and recent revisions to national and regional guidelines reflect this. Large en bloc surgery is no longer regarded as the cornerstone treatment for DTF, because of the high relapse rate after surgery [73]. For those who fail the "wait and see" management, either surgery or radiotherapy can be considered for those in whom local control is the primary treatment goal. As a general principle, the approach to systemic therapy is based on the urgency of the clinical situation, which takes into account tumour location, symptom burden, growth rate and patient preference. For those who require rapid response, cytotoxic chemotherapy such as pegylated liposomal doxorubicin or combinations of methotrexate and vinblastine are reasonable options, with responses noted in small published case series studies [74–77]. Tyrosine kinase inhibitors such as sorafenib or pazopanib are also reasonable first-line alternatives although drug access may be more difficult [78–80]. Other patients who qualify for systemic therapy should be managed with less toxic approaches such as NSAIDs and/or tamoxifen based on limited data [81–83]. It should be noted that DTFs are typically slow growing, and due to its unpredictable natural history, up to 20% of patients on the placebo arm of interventional studies have shown tumour regression. There are ongoing global efforts in exploring other novel agents such as small molecular inhibitors inhibiting the Notch signaling pathway [84, 85].

11.7 Gynaecological Sarcomas

Gynaecological sarcomas are universally rare cancers. The incidence in developed countries lies between 8 and 9.6 per million [86–88]. Gynaecological carcinosarcomas are regarded as poorly differentiated epithelial malignancies after WHO reclassification in 2003, and are not addressed here [89].

11.7.1 Uterine Sarcoma

Uterine sarcomas are the most common gynaecological sarcomas. As with other STS and osteosarcomas, Li-Fraumeni syndrome should be considered in young patients and those with significant family histories [90]. Histologically, these are categorized into tumours of myometrial (leiomyosarcoma, LMS) and endometrial (endometrial stromal sarcoma, ESS) origin. Clinically, the grade of the tumour, the presence or absence of hormone receptors and the clinical pace of disease are the most important prognostic factors. Unlike soft tissue sarcomas arising in non-gynaecological organ systems, uterine sarcomas are rarely diagnosed prior to definitive surgery, due to their radiological resemblance to common atypical fibroids and endometrial carcinomas. Accordingly, pre-operative treatment is rarely considered. Surgical procedures such as morcellation may inadvertently compromise outcomes for patients diagnosed with an occult sarcoma after a hysterectomy for a benign uterine condition [91, 92]. Adjuvant pelvic radiotherapy is frequently offered for local control of high-risk tumours, but no survival benefit from this has been demonstrated [93].

Likewise, the role of adjuvant systemic therapy is not established. A trial of 156 patients with stage I or II uterine sarcoma (all histotypes) randomized to doxorubicin for 6 months or no further treatment did not demonstrate a recurrence-free or overall survival benefit. Though this trial included carcinosarcoma, which is now not considered a true uterine sarcoma, there were no differences between histological subtypes to suggest this may have affected the outcome [94]. SARC005 was a single-arm phase II trial of four cycles of gemcitabine plus docetaxel, followed by four cycles of doxorubicin for those who remained disease-free. At 2 years, the progression-free survival rate was 78%; at 3 years it was 57% [95]. A randomized phase III trial of this combination versus observation was commenced, but closed prematurely due to poor accrual, despite opening at 701 sites internationally [96]. A phase III trial of adjuvant ifosfamide, cisplatin plus doxorubicin in addition to sequential radiotherapy demonstrated an improvement in disease-free survival, accompanied by significant toxicity. With only nine patients with a high-grade undifferentiated sarcoma included, and the confounder of the inclusion of carcinosarcomas, the benefit for this subtype is somewhat inconclusive [97]. Based on the limited evidence available, there are insufficient data to support the use of adjuvant therapy.

11.7.2 Uterine Undifferentiated Pleomorphic Sarcoma (UUPS)

Uterine UPS are high-grade tumours, with immunohistochemical profiling inconclusive as to tissue of origin. They frequently carry a p53 mutation [98]. They are managed clinically according to guidelines for other non-gynaecological UPS. There are no data to support the routine use of adjuvant systemic therapy. Chemotherapeutic agents including doxorubicin, ifosfamide, dacarbazine and docetaxel and gemcitabine are all used in the metastatic setting [99]. Pazopanib is registered in some countries for improvement of progression-free survival [100]. As with non-uterine UPS, the role of immunotherapy is currently under active investigation but is regarded as experimental [101].

11.7.3 Uterine Leiomyosarcoma (ULMS)

ULMS exhibit a range of clinical behaviours. Histological grading does not always correlate with clinical behaviour, but extremes of Ki67 can be predictive. The Cancer Genome Atlas Network described a low tumour mutational burden in both uterine and soft tissue LMS, as well as PI3K/AKT signaling alterations, and mutations in *p53*, *RB1* and *PTEN* [102]. It may be that the PI3K-AKT-MTOR pathway will be an actionable target in the future, though this remains speculative at present. Pathogenic *BRCA2* variants have been identified in a small subset (<10%), and a small number of those patients have been demonstrated to have a durable response to poly (ADP-ribose) polymerase inhibitor therapy [103].

ULMS are usually included in clinical trials of therapies in metastatic LMS, but outcomes are rarely reported for them as a distinct subgroup. They respond to the standard agents used in other soft tissue sarcomas, including doxorubicin, ifosfamide, dacarbazine, trabectedin and gemcitabine in combination with docetaxel

[22, 29, 31, 40, 104–108]. There are more specific data, either from dedicated trials or large predefined subsets using doxorubicin with or without ifosfamide and gemcitabine with or without docetaxel [104–106, 109]. The highest response rates were seen with gemcitabine and docetaxel combination [106, 110]. Uterine LMS were included in the trials of the PDGFR-alpha monoclonal antibody olaratumab, which looked promising in phase II trials, but failed to meet its primary endpoint in the phase III trial of its use in combination with gemcitabine and docetaxel [111]. Uterine leiomyosarcoma was included in two trials of PD-1 inhibitor therapy in LMS, with discouraging results. Tawbi et al. identified no responses in 10 patients with ULMS who received pembrolizumab, and Ben-Ami et al. reported no responses in 12 patients who received nivolumab [112, 113]. Alternative immunotherapeutic approaches will therefore be needed if this modality is to find a role for patients with this histology.

High-grade ULMS are aggressive soft tissue malignancies. They are more likely to carry *p53* mutations than their lower-grade counterparts and express high Ki67, with low or no hormone receptor expression. Lower-grade ULMS follow a more indolent disease course and frequently express oestrogen and progesterone receptors. Hormonal therapies have been used historically for indolent disease, without a strong evidence base. A single-arm phase II trial of letrozole for the treatment of ULMS demonstrated a 12-week progression-free survival rate of 50%, with a best objective response of stable disease [114]. Friedlander et al. have formally studied anastrozole in patients with hormone receptor-positive gynaecological sarcoma but are yet to publish results [115]. Tumours progressing through hormonal therapy are offered standard chemotherapeutic options.

Benign metastasizing leiomyomata are an extremely indolent, low-grade myometrial variant, most commonly identified in the lung. They strongly express hormonal receptors. The primary tumour may not be identified if the patient has undergone a previous hysterectomy, as features of malignancy may not have been identified. Primary tumours may have been reported as atypical fibroids, or smooth muscle tumours of uncertain malignant potential. Observation or hormonal therapy is the most common initial management [116, 117].

11.7.4 Endometrial Stromal Sarcoma (ESS)

Low-grade ESS are the most common subtype of ESS. They are indolent tumours, characterized by strong expression of hormone receptors, CD10 and Bcl2. At a molecular level, *JAZF1* rearrangements are common and are regarded as diagnostic [118]. They are highly sensitive to progestins, such as medroxyprogesterone (Provera), and hormonal therapy is favoured over cytotoxic agents in the first line. Chemotherapeutic agents are generally reserved for patients with hormone-resistant disease [118–120].

High-grade ESS have an aggressive natural history, are characterized by a lack of hormone receptor and CD10 expression and may have a translocation which results in the in-frame fusion gene, *YWHAE-FAM22* [121, 122]. They are managed with the same chemotherapeutic agents as other high-grade soft tissue sarcomas.

11.7.5 Ovarian Sarcoma

Pure ovarian sarcomas are extremely rare tumours, and there are no prospective trials to guide management. Their prognosis is worse than epithelial tumours of the same stage [123]. In the absence of robust tumour-specific data, management is often extrapolated from uterine leiomyosarcoma.

References

1. Tierney JF, Sylvester RJ. Adjuvant chemotherapy for localised resectable soft-tissue sarcoma of adults: meta-analysis of individual data. Lancet. 1997;350(9092):1647.
2. Pervaiz N, Colterjohn N, Farrokhyar F, Tozer R, Figueredo A, Ghert M. A systematic meta-analysis of randomized controlled trials of adjuvant chemotherapy for localized resectable soft-tissue sarcoma. Cancer. 2008;113(3):573–81.
3. Sarcoma Meta-analysis Collaboration—see acknowledgement section for list of a. Adjuvant chemotherapy for localised resectable soft tissue sarcoma in adults. Cochrane Database of Systematic Reviews. 2000;(4).
4. Woll PJ, Reichardt P, Le Cesne A, Bonvalot S, Azzarelli A, Hoekstra HJ, et al. Adjuvant chemotherapy with doxorubicin, ifosfamide, and lenograstim for resected soft-tissue sarcoma (EORTC 62931): a multicentre randomised controlled trial. Lancet Oncol. 2012;13(10):1045–54.
5. Gortzak E, Azzarelli A, Buesa J, Bramwell V, Van Coevorden F, Van Geel A, et al. A randomised phase II study on neo-adjuvant chemotherapy for 'high-risk' adult soft-tissue sarcoma. Eur J Cancer. 2001;37(9):1096–103.
6. Palassini E, Ferrari S, Verderio P, De Paoli A, Martin Broto J, Quagliuolo V, et al. Feasibility of preoperative chemotherapy with or without radiation therapy in localized soft tissue sarcomas of limbs and superficial trunk in the Italian sarcoma Group/Grupo Espanol de Investigacion en Sarcomas Randomized Clinical Trial: three versus five cycles of full-dose epirubicin plus ifosfamide. J Clin Oncol. 2015;33(31):3628–34.
7. Van Glabbeke M, Van Oosterom A, Oosterhuis J, Mouridsen H, Crowther D, Somers R, et al. Prognostic factors for the outcome of chemotherapy in advanced soft tissue sarcoma: an analysis of 2185 patients treated with anthracycline-containing first-line regimens-a European Organization for Research and Treatment of Cancer Soft Tissue and Bone Sarcoma Group Study. J Clin Oncol. 1999;17:150–7.
8. Ryan CW, Merimsky O, Agulnik M, Blay J-Y, Schuetze SM, Van Tine BA, et al. PICASSO III: a phase III, placebo-controlled study of doxorubicin with or without palifosfamide in patients with metastatic soft tissue sarcoma. J Clin Oncol. 2016;34(32):3898–905.
9. Lorigan P, Verweij J, Papai Z, Rodenhuis S, Le Cesne A, Leahy MG, et al. Phase III trial of two investigational schedules of ifosfamide compared with standard-dose doxorubicin in advanced or metastatic soft tissue sarcoma: a European Organisation for Research and Treatment of Cancer Soft Tissue and Bone Sarcoma Group Study. J Clin Oncol. 2007;25(21):3144–50.
10. Borden EC, Amato DA, Rosenbaum C, Enterline HT, Shiraki MJ, Creech RH, et al. Randomized comparison of three adriamycin regimens for metastatic soft tissue sarcomas. J Clin Oncol. 1987;5(6):840–50.

11. Judson I, Radford JA, Harris M, Blay J-Y, van Hoesel Q, Le Cesne A, et al. Randomised phase II trial of pegylated liposomal doxorubicin (DOXIL®/CAELYX®) versus doxorubicin in the treatment of advanced or metastatic soft tissue sarcoma: a study by the EORTC Soft Tissue and Bone Sarcoma Group. Eur J Cancer. 2001;37(7):870–7.
12. O'Bryan R, Baker L, Gottlieb J, Rivkin S, Balcerzak S, Grumet G, et al. Dose response evaluation of adriamycin in human neoplasia. Cancer. 1977;39(5):1940–8.
13. Mouridsen H, Bastholt L, Somers R, Santoro A, Bramwell V, Mulder J, et al. Adriamycin versus epirubicin in advanced soft tissue sarcomas. A randomized phase II/phase III study of the EORTC Soft Tissue and Bone Sarcoma Group. Eur J Cancer Clin Oncol. 1987;23(10):1477–83.
14. Nielsen OS, Dombernowsky P, Mouridsen H, Crowther D, Verweij J, Buesa J, et al. High-dose epirubicin is not an alternative to standard-dose doxorubicin in the treatment of advanced soft tissue sarcomas. A study of the EORTC soft tissue and bone sarcoma group. Br J Cancer. 1998;78(12):1634.
15. Nielsen OS, Dombernowsky P, Mouridsen H, Daugaard S, Van Glabbeke M, Kirkpatrick A, et al. Epirubicin is not superior to doxorubicin in the treatment of advanced soft tissue sarcomas. The experience of the EORTC soft tissue and bone sarcoma group. Sarcoma. 2000;4(1–2):31–5.
16. Patel SR, Vadhan-Raj S, Papadopolous N, Plager C, Burgess MA, Hays C, et al. High-dose ifosfamide in bone and soft tissue sarcomas: results of phase II and pilot studies--dose-response and schedule dependence. J Clin Oncol. 1997;15(6):2378–84.
17. Nielsen OS, Judson I, van Hoesel Q, le Cesne A, Keizer HJ, Blay JY, et al. Effect of high-dose ifosfamide in advanced soft tissue sarcomas. A multicentre phase II study of the EORTC Soft Tissue and Bone Sarcoma Group. Eur J Cancer. 2000;36(1):61–7.
18. Le Cesne A, Antoine E, Spielmann M, Le Chevalier T, Brain E, Toussaint C, et al. High-dose ifosfamide: circumvention of resistance to standard-dose ifosfamide in advanced soft tissue sarcomas. J Clin Oncol. 1995;13(7):1600–8.
19. Edmonson J, Ryan L, Blum R, Brooks J, Shiraki M, Frytak S, et al. Randomized comparison of doxorubicin alone versus ifosfamide plus doxorubicin or mitomycin, doxorubicin, and cisplatin against advanced soft tissue sarcomas. J Clin Oncol. 1993;11(7):1269–75.
20. Santoro A, Tursz T, Mouridsen H, Verweij J, Steward W, Somers R, et al. Doxorubicin versus CYVADIC versus doxorubicin plus ifosfamide in first-line treatment of advanced soft tissue sarcomas: a randomized study of the European Organization for Research and Treatment of Cancer Soft Tissue and Bone Sarcoma Group. J Clin Oncol. 1995;13(7):1537–45.
21. Maurel J, López-Pousa A, de Las PR, Fra J, Martín J, Cruz J, et al. Efficacy of sequential high-dose doxorubicin and ifosfamide compared with standard-dose doxorubicin in patients with advanced soft tissue sarcoma: an open-label randomized phase II study of the Spanish group for research on sarcomas. J Clin Oncol. 2009;27(11):1893–8.
22. Judson I, Verweij J, Gelderblom H, Hartmann JT, Schöffski P, Blay J-Y, et al. Doxorubicin alone versus intensified doxorubicin plus ifosfamide for first-line treatment of advanced or metastatic soft-tissue sarcoma: a randomised controlled phase 3 trial. Lancet Oncol. 2014;15(4):415–23.
23. Patel SR, Gandhi V, Jenkins J, Papadopolous N, Burgess MA, Plager C, et al. Phase II clinical investigation of gemcitabine in advanced soft tissue sarcomas and window evaluation of dose rate on gemcitabine triphosphate accumulation. J Clin Oncol. 2001;19(15):3483–9.
24. Dileo P, Morgan JA, Zahrieh D, Desai J, Salesi JM, Harmon DC, et al. Gemcitabine and vinorelbine combination chemotherapy for patients with advanced soft tissue sarcomas: results of a phase II trial. Cancer. 2007;109(9):1863–9.
25. Maki RG, Wathen JK, Patel SR, Priebat DA, Okuno SH, Samuels B, et al. Randomized phase II study of gemcitabine and docetaxel compared with gemcitabine alone in patients with metastatic soft tissue sarcomas: results of sarcoma alliance for research through collaboration study 002 [corrected]. J Clin Oncol. 2007;25(19):2755–63.
26. Seddon B, Strauss SJ, Whelan J, Leahy M, Woll PJ, Cowie F, et al. Gemcitabine and docetaxel versus doxorubicin as first-line treatment in previously untreated advanced unresectable or

metastatic soft-tissue sarcomas (GeDDiS): a randomised controlled phase 3 trial. Lancet Oncol. 2017;18(10):1397–410.
27. Zucali PA, Bertuzzi A, Parra HJS, Campagnoli E, Quagliuolo V, Santoro A. The "old drug" dacarbazine as a second/third line chemotherapy in advanced soft tissue sarcomas. Invest New Drugs. 2008;26(2):175–81.
28. Pommier Y, Kohlhagen G, Bailly C, Waring M, Mazumder A, Kohn KW. DNA sequence- and structure-selective alkylation of guanine N2 in the DNA minor groove by ecteinascidin 743, a potent antitumor compound from the Caribbean tunicate Ecteinascidia turbinata. Biochemistry. 1996;35(41):13303–9.
29. Demetri GD, Chawla SP, von Mehren M, Ritch P, Baker LH, Blay JY, et al. Efficacy and safety of trabectedin in patients with advanced or metastatic liposarcoma or leiomyosarcoma after failure of prior anthracyclines and ifosfamide: results of a randomized phase II study of two different schedules. J Clin Oncol. 2009;27(25):4188–96.
30. Kawai A, Araki N, Sugiura H, Ueda T, Yonemoto T, Takahashi M, et al. Trabectedin monotherapy after standard chemotherapy versus best supportive care in patients with advanced, translocation-related sarcoma: a randomised, open-label, phase 2 study. Lancet Oncol. 2015;16(4):406–16.
31. Demetri GD, Von Mehren M, Jones RL, Hensley ML, Schuetze SM, Staddon A, et al. Efficacy and safety of trabectedin or dacarbazine for metastatic liposarcoma or leiomyosarcoma after failure of conventional chemotherapy: results of a phase III randomized multicenter clinical trial. J Clin Oncol. 2016;34(8):786.
32. Grosso F, Jones RL, Demetri GD, Judson IR, Blay J-Y, Le Cesne A, et al. Efficacy of trabectedin (ecteinascidin-743) in advanced pretreated myxoid liposarcomas: a retrospective study. Lancet Oncol. 2007;8(7):595–602.
33. Choi H, Charnsangavej C, Faria SC, Macapinlac HA, Burgess MA, Patel SR, et al. Correlation of computed tomography and positron emission tomography in patients with metastatic gastrointestinal stromal tumor treated at a single institution with imatinib mesylate: proposal of new computed tomography response criteria. J Clin Oncol. 2007;25(13):1753–9.
34. Schöffski P, Ray-Coquard IL, Cioffi A, Bui NB, Bauer S, Hartmann JT, et al. Activity of eribulin mesylate in patients with soft-tissue sarcoma: a phase 2 study in four independent histological subtypes. Lancet Oncol. 2011;12(11):1045–52.
35. Demetri GD, Schöffski P, Grignani G, Blay J-Y, Maki RG, Van Tine BA, et al. Activity of eribulin in patients with advanced liposarcoma demonstrated in a subgroup analysis from a randomized phase III study of eribulin versus dacarbazine. J Clin Oncol. 2017;35(30):3433–9.
36. Quesada J, Amato R. The molecular biology of soft-tissue sarcomas and current trends in therapy. Sarcoma. 2012;2012:849456.
37. Ryan C, Desai J, editors. The past, present, and future of cytotoxic chemotherapy and pathway-directed targeted agents for soft tissue sarcoma. American Society of Clinical Oncology educational book. In: American Society of Clinical Oncology Annual Meeting; 2013.
38. Riedel RF. Targeted agents for sarcoma: is individualized therapy possible in such a diverse tumor type? Semin Oncol. 2011;38(Suppl 3):S30–42.
39. Taylor BS, Barretina J, Maki RG, Antonescu CR, Singer S, Ladanyi M. Advances in sarcoma genomics and new therapeutic targets. Nat Rev Cancer. 2011;11(8):541.
40. Van Der Graaf WT, Blay J-Y, Chawla SP, Kim D-W, Bui-Nguyen B, Casali PG, et al. Pazopanib for metastatic soft-tissue sarcoma (PALETTE): a randomised, double-blind, placebo-controlled phase 3 trial. The Lancet. 2012;379(9829):1879–86.
41. Schlemmer M, Reichardt P, Verweij J, Hartmann J, Judson I, Thyss A, et al. Paclitaxel in patients with advanced angiosarcomas of soft tissue: a retrospective study of the EORTC soft tissue and bone sarcoma group. Eur J Cancer. 2008;44(16):2433–6.
42. Penel N, Bui BN, Bay J-O, Cupissol D, Ray-Coquard I, Piperno-Neumann S, et al. Phase II trial of weekly paclitaxel for unresectable angiosarcoma: the ANGIOTAX Study. J Clin Oncol. 2008;26(32):5269–74.

43. Ray-Coquard IL, Domont J, Tresch-Bruneel E, Bompas E, Cassier PA, Mir O, et al. Paclitaxel given once per week with or without bevacizumab in patients with advanced angiosarcoma: a randomized phase II trial. J Clin Oncol. 2015;33(25):2797–802.
44. Robinson DR, Wu Y-M, Kalyana-Sundaram S, Cao X, Lonigro RJ, Sung Y-S, et al. Identification of recurrent NAB2-STAT6 gene fusions in solitary fibrous tumor by integrative sequencing. Nat Genet. 2013;45(2):180.
45. Maruzzo M, Martin-Liberal J, Messiou C, Miah A, Thway K, Alvarado R, et al. Pazopanib as first line treatment for solitary fibrous tumours: the Royal Marsden Hospital experience. Clin Sarcoma Res. 2015;5(1):5.
46. Stacchiotti S, Negri T, Libertini M, Palassini E, Marrari A, De Troia B, et al. Sunitinib malate in solitary fibrous tumor (SFT). Ann Oncol. 2012;23(12):3171–9.
47. Valentin T, Fournier C, Penel N, Bompas E, Chaigneau L, Isambert N, et al. Sorafenib in patients with progressive malignant solitary fibrous tumors: a subgroup analysis from a phase II study of the French Sarcoma Group (GSF/GETO). Invest New Drugs. 2013;31(6):1626–7.
48. Stacchiotti S, Tortoreto M, Bozzi F, Tamborini E, Morosi C, Messina A, et al. Dacarbazine in solitary fibrous tumor: a case series analysis and preclinical evidence vis-a-vis temozolomide and antiangiogenics. Clin Cancer Res. 2013;19(18):5192–201.
49. Khalifa J, Ouali M, Chaltiel L, Le Guellec S, Le Cesne A, Blay J, et al. Efficacy of trabectedin in malignant solitary fibrous tumors: a retrospective analysis from the French Sarcoma Group. BMC Cancer. 2015;15(1):700.
50. Wagner AJ, Malinowska-Kolodziej I, Morgan JA, Qin W, Fletcher CD, Vena N, et al. Clinical activity of mTOR inhibition with sirolimus in malignant perivascular epithelioid cell tumors: targeting the pathogenic activation of mTORC1 in tumors. J Clin Oncol. 2010;28(5):835.
51. Batereau C, Knösel T, Angele M, Dürr HR, D'Anastasi M, Kampmann E, et al. Neoadjuvant or adjuvant sirolimus for malignant metastatic or locally advanced perivascular epithelioid cell tumors: two case reports. Anticancer Drugs. 2016;27(3):254–8.
52. Benson C, Vitfell-Rasmussen J, Maruzzo M, Fisher C, Tunariu N, Mitchell S, et al. A retrospective study of patients with malignant PEComa receiving treatment with sirolimus or temsirolimus: the Royal Marsden Hospital experience. Anticancer Res. 2014;34(7):3663–8.
53. Hindi N, Sanfilippo R, Stacchiotti S, Fumagalli E, Libertini M, Provenzano S, et al. 1450P Systemic therapy in perivascular epithelioid cell tumors (PECOMA). Ann Oncol. 2014;25(Suppl_4):iv506-iv.
54. Stacchiotti S, Mir O, Le Cesne A, Vincenzi B, Fedenko A, Maki RG, et al. Activity of pazopanib and trabectedin in advanced alveolar soft part sarcoma. Oncologist. 2018;23(1):62–70.
55. Stacchiotti S, Tamborini E, Marrari A, Brich S, Rota SA, Orsenigo M, et al. Response to sunitinib malate in advanced alveolar soft part sarcoma. Clin Cancer Res. 2009;15(3):1096–104.
56. Judson I, Morden JP, Kilburn L, Leahy M, Benson C, Bhadri V, et al. Cediranib in patients with alveolar soft-part sarcoma (CASPS): a double-blind, placebo-controlled, randomised, phase 2 trial. Lancet Oncol. 2019;20(7):1023–34.
57. Folpe A, Deyrup A. Alveolar soft-part sarcoma: a review and update. J Clin Pathol. 2006;59(11):1127–32.
58. Simon M-P, Pedeutour F, Sirvent N, Grosgeorge J, Minoletti F, Coindre J-M, et al. Deregulation of the platelet-derived growth factor β-chain gene via fusion with collagen gene COL1A1 in dermatof ibrosarcoma protuberans and giant-cell fibroblastoma. Nat Genet. 1997;15(1):95.
59. Sirvent N, Maire G, Pedeutour F. Genetics of dermatofibrosarcoma protuberans family of tumors: from ring chromosomes to tyrosine kinase inhibitor treatment. Genes Chromosomes Cancer. 2003;37(1):1–19.
60. McArthur GA, Demetri GD, Van Oosterom A, Heinrich MC, Debiec-Rychter M, Corless CL, et al. Molecular and clinical analysis of locally advanced dermatofibrosarcoma protuberans treated with imatinib: Imatinib Target Exploration Consortium Study B2225. J Clin Oncol. 2005;23(4):866–73.
61. Mizutani K, Tamada Y, Hara K, Tsuzuki T, Saeki H, Tamaki K, et al. Imatinib mesylate inhibits the growth of metastatic lung lesions in a patient with dermatofibrosarcoma protuberans. British Journal of Dermatology. 2004;151(1):235–7.

62. Rubin BP, Schuetze SM, Eary JF, Norwood TH, Mirza S, Conrad EU, et al. Molecular targeting of platelet-derived growth factor B by imatinib mesylate in a patient with metastatic dermatofibrosarcoma protuberans. J Clin Oncol. 2002;20(17):3586–91.
63. Rutkowski P, Van Glabbeke M, Rankin CJ, Ruka W, Rubin BP, Debiec-Rychter M, et al. Imatinib mesylate in advanced dermatofibrosarcoma protuberans: pooled analysis of two phase II clinical trials. J Clin Oncol. 2010;28(10):1772.
64. Stacchiotti S, Pantaleo MA, Negri T, Astolfi A, Tazzari M, Dagrada GP, et al. Efficacy and biological activity of imatinib in metastatic dermatofibrosarcoma protuberans (DFSP). Clin Cancer Res. 2016;22(4):837–46.
65. Ugurel S, Mentzel T, Utikal J, Helmbold P, Mohr P, Pföhler C, et al. Neoadjuvant imatinib in advanced primary or locally recurrent dermatofibrosarcoma protuberans: a multicenter phase II DeCOG trial with long-term follow-up. Clin Cancer Res. 2014;20(2):499–510.
66. Navarrete-Dechent C, Mori S, Barker CA, Dickson MA, Nehal KS. Imatinib treatment for locally advanced or metastatic dermatofibrosarcoma protuberans: a systematic review. JAMA Dermatol. 2019;155(3):361–9.
67. Tap WD, Gelderblom H, Palmerini E, Desai J, Bauer S, Blay J-Y, et al. Pexidartinib versus placebo for advanced tenosynovial giant cell tumour (ENLIVEN): a randomised phase 3 trial. Lancet. 2019;394(10197):478–87.
68. Blay J-Y, El Sayadi H, Thiesse P, Garret J, Ray-Coquard I. Complete response to imatinib in relapsing pigmented villonodular synovitis/tenosynovial giant cell tumor (PVNS/TGCT). Ann Oncol. 2008;19(4):821–2.
69. Cassier PA, Gelderblom H, Stacchiotti S, Thomas D, Maki RG, Kroep JR, et al. Efficacy of imatinib mesylate for the treatment of locally advanced and/or metastatic tenosynovial giant cell tumor/pigmented villonodular synovitis. Cancer. 2012;118(6):1649–55.
70. Tejpar S, Nollet F, Li C, Wunder JS, Michils G, Dal Cin P, et al. Predominance of beta-catenin mutations and beta-catenin dysregulation in sporadic aggressive fibromatosis (desmoid tumor). Oncogene. 1999;18(47):6615.
71. Le Guellec S, Soubeyran I, Rochaix P, Filleron T, Neuville A, Hostein I, et al. CTNNB1 mutation analysis is a useful tool for the diagnosis of desmoid tumors: a study of 260 desmoid tumors and 191 potential morphologic mimics. Mod Pathol. 2012;25(12):1551.
72. Dômont J, Salas S, Lacroix L, Brouste V, Saulnier P, Terrier P, et al. High frequency of β-catenin heterozygous mutations in extra-abdominal fibromatosis: a potential molecular tool for disease management. Br J Cancer. 2010;102(6):1032.
73. Crago AM, Denton B, Salas S, Dufresne A, Mezhir JJ, Hameed M, et al. A prognostic nomogram for prediction of recurrence in desmoid fibromatosis. Ann Surg. 2013;258(2):347.
74. de Camargo VP, Keohan ML, D'Adamo DR, Antonescu CR, Brennan MF, Singer S, et al. Clinical outcomes of systemic therapy for patients with deep fibromatosis (desmoid tumor). Cancer. 2010;116(9):2258–65.
75. Wehl G, Rossler J, Otten J, Boehm N, Uhl M, Kontny U, et al. Response of progressive fibromatosis to therapy with liposomal doxorubicin. Oncol Res Treat. 2004;27(6):552–6.
76. Constantinidou A, Jones RL, Scurr M, Al-Muderis O, Judson I. Pegylated liposomal doxorubicin, an effective, well-tolerated treatment for refractory aggressive fibromatosis. Eur J Cancer. 2009;45(17):2930–4.
77. Reich S, Overberg-Schmidt US, Bührer C, Henze GN. Low-dose chemotherapy with vinblastine and methotrexate in childhood desmoid tumors. J Clin Oncol. 1999;17(3):1086.
78. Gounder MM, Lefkowitz RA, Keohan ML, D'Adamo DR, Hameed M, Antonescu CR, et al. Activity of sorafenib against desmoid tumor/deep fibromatosis. Clin Cancer Res. 2011;17(12):4082–90.
79. Bulut G, Ozluk A, Erdogan AP, Uslu R, Elmas N, Karaca B. Pazopanib: a novel treatment option for aggressive fibromatosis. Clin Sarcoma Res. 2016;6(1):22.
80. Szucs Z, Messiou C, Wong HH, Hatcher H, Miah A, Zaidi S, et al. Pazopanib, a promising option for the treatment of aggressive fibromatosis. Anticancer Drugs. 2017;28(4):421.
81. Wilcken N, Tattersall MH. Endocrine therapy for desmoid tumors. Cancer. 1991;68(6):1384–8.
82. Sportiello DJ, Hoogerland DL. A recurrent pelvic desmoid tumor successfully treated with tamoxifen. Cancer. 1991;67(5):1443–6.

83. Hansmann A, Adolph C, Vogel T, Unger A, Moeslein G. High-dose tamoxifen and sulindac as first-line treatment for desmoid tumors. Cancer. 2004;100(3):612–20.
84. Villalobos VM, Hall F, Jimeno A, Gore L, Kern K, Cesari R, et al. Long-term follow-up of desmoid fibromatosis treated with PF-03084014, an oral gamma secretase inhibitor. Ann Surg Oncol. 2018;25(3):768–75.
85. Kummar S, Coyne GOS, Do KT, Turkbey B, Meltzer PS, Polley E, et al. Clinical activity of the γ-secretase inhibitor PF-03084014 in adults with desmoid tumors (aggressive fibromatosis). J Clin Oncol. 2017;35(14):1561.
86. Francis M, Dennis NL, Hirschowitz L, Grimer R, Poole J, Lawrence G, et al. Incidence and survival of gynecologic sarcomas in England. Int J Gynecol Cancer. 2015;25(5):850–7.
87. Pietzner K, Buttmann-Schweiger N, Sehouli J, Kraywinkel K. Incidence patterns and survival of gynecological sarcoma in Germany: analysis of population-based cancer registry data on 1066 women. Int J Gynecol Cancer. 2018;28(1):134–8.
88. Jiang X, Tang H, Chen T. Epidemiology of gynecologic cancers in China. J Gynecol Oncol. 2017;29(1):e7.
89. Eble JN, Tavassoli FA, Devilee P. Pathology and genetics of tumours of the breast and female genital organs. Lyon: IARC; 2003.
90. Bougeard G, Renaux-Petel M, Flaman J-M, Charbonnier C, Fermey P, Belotti M, et al. Revisiting Li-Fraumeni syndrome from TP53 mutation carriers. J Clin Oncol. 2015;33(21):2345–52.
91. Ricci S, Stone RL, Fader AN. Uterine leiomyosarcoma: epidemiology, contemporary treatment strategies and the impact of uterine morcellation. Gynecol Oncol. 2017;145(1):208–16.
92. Park J-Y, Park S-K, Kim D-Y, Kim J-H, Kim Y-M, Kim Y-T, et al. The impact of tumor morcellation during surgery on the prognosis of patients with apparently early uterine leiomyosarcoma. Gynecol Oncol. 2011;122(2):255–9.
93. Reed N, Mangioni C, Malmström H, Scarfone G, Poveda A, Pecorelli S, et al. Phase III randomised study to evaluate the role of adjuvant pelvic radiotherapy in the treatment of uterine sarcomas stages I and II: an European Organisation for Research and Treatment of Cancer Gynaecological Cancer Group Study (protocol 55,874). Eur J Cancer. 2008;44(6):808–18.
94. Omura GA, Blessing JA, Major F, Lifshitz S, Ehrlich CE, Mangan C, et al. A randomized clinical trial of adjuvant adriamycin in uterine sarcomas: a Gynecologic Oncology Group Study. J Clin Oncol. 1985;3(9):1240–5.
95. Hensley ML, Wathen JK, Maki RG, Araujo DM, Sutton G, Priebat DA, et al. Adjuvant therapy for high-grade, uterus-limited leiomyosarcoma: results of a phase 2 trial (SARC 005). Cancer. 2013;119(8):1555–61.
96. Hensley ML, Enserro D, Hatcher H, Ottevanger PB, Krarup-Hansen A, Blay J-Y, et al. Adjuvant gemcitabine plus docetaxel followed by doxorubicin versus observation for uterus-limited, high-grade leiomyosarcoma: a phase III GOG study. J Clin Oncol. 2018;36(15_Suppl):5505.
97. Pautier P, Floquet A, Gladieff L, Bompas E, Ray-Coquard I, Piperno-Neumann S, et al. A randomized clinical trial of adjuvant chemotherapy with doxorubicin, ifosfamide, and cisplatin followed by radiotherapy versus radiotherapy alone in patients with localized uterine sarcomas (SARCGYN study). A study of the French Sarcoma Group. Ann Oncol. 2012;24(4):1099–104.
98. Kurihara S, Oda Y, Ohishi Y, Iwasa A, Takahira T, Kaneki E, et al. Endometrial stromal sarcomas and related high-grade sarcomas: immunohistochemical and molecular genetic study of 31 cases. Am J Surg Pathol. 2008;32(8):1228–38.
99. Tanner EJ, Garg K, Leitao MM Jr, Soslow RA, Hensley ML. High grade undifferentiated uterine sarcoma: surgery, treatment, and survival outcomes. Gynecol Oncol. 2012;127(1):27–31.
100. Kim H-J, Kim Y, Lee SJ, Lee J, Park SH. Pazopanib monotherapy in the treatment of pretreated, metastatic uterine sarcoma: a single-center retrospective study. J Gynecol Oncol. 2017;29(1):e3.
101. Burgess MA, Bolejack V, Schuetze S, Tine BAV, Attia S, Riedel RF, et al. Clinical activity of pembrolizumab (P) in undifferentiated pleomorphic sarcoma (UPS) and dedifferentiated/

pleomorphic liposarcoma (LPS): final results of SARC028 expansion cohorts. J Clin Oncol. 2019;37(15_Suppl):11015.
102. CGAR Network. Comprehensive and integrated genomic characterization of adult soft tissue sarcomas. Cell. 2017;171(4):950.
103. Seligson ND, Kautto EA, Passen EN, Stets C, Toland AE, Millis SZ, et al. BRCA1/2 functional loss defines a targetable subset in leiomyosarcoma. Oncologist. 2019;24(7):973–9.
104. Muss HB, Bundy B, Disaia PJ, Homesley HD, Fowler WC Jr, Creasman W, et al. Treatment of recurrent or advanced uterine sarcoma. A randomized trial of doxorubicin versus doxorubicin and cyclophosphamide (a phase III trial of the Gynecologic Oncology Group). Cancer. 1985;55(8):1648–53.
105. Look KY, Sandler A, Blessing JA, Lucci JA III, Rose PG. Phase II trial of gemcitabine as second-line chemotherapy of uterine leiomyosarcoma: a Gynecologic Oncology Group (GOG) Study. Gynecol Oncol. 2004;92(2):644–7.
106. Hensley ML, Blessing JA, Mannel R, Rose PG. Fixed-dose rate gemcitabine plus docetaxel as first-line therapy for metastatic uterine leiomyosarcoma: a Gynecologic Oncology Group phase II trial. Gynecol Oncol. 2008;109(3):329–34.
107. Pautier P, Floquet A, Penel N, Piperno-Neumann S, Isambert N, Rey A, et al. Randomized multicenter and stratified phase II study of gemcitabine alone versus gemcitabine and docetaxel in patients with metastatic or relapsed leiomyosarcomas: a Federation Nationale des Centres de Lutte Contre le Cancer (FNCLCC) French Sarcoma Group Study (TAXOGEM study). Oncologist. 2012;17(9):1213–20.
108. García-del-Muro X, López-Pousa A, Maurel J, Martín J, Martínez-Trufero J, Casado A, et al. Randomized phase II study comparing gemcitabine plus dacarbazine versus dacarbazine alone in patients with previously treated soft tissue sarcoma: a Spanish Group for Research on Sarcomas study. J Clin Oncol. 2011;29(18):2528–33.
109. Sutton G, Blessing JA, Malfetano JH. Ifosfamide and doxorubicin in the treatment of advanced leiomyosarcomas of the uterus: a Gynecologic Oncology Group study. Gynecol Oncol. 1996;62(2):226–9.
110. Hensley ML, Blessing JA, DeGeest K, Abulafia O, Rose PG, Homesley HD. Fixed-dose rate gemcitabine plus docetaxel as second-line therapy for metastatic uterine leiomyosarcoma: a Gynecologic Oncology Group phase II study. Gynecol Oncol. 2008;109(3):323–8.
111. Tap WD, Wagner AJ, Papai Z, Ganjoo KN, Yen C-C, Schoffski P, et al. ANNOUNCE: a randomized, placebo (PBO)-controlled, double-blind, phase (Ph) III trial of doxorubicin (dox) + olaratumab versus dox + PBO in patients (pts) with advanced soft tissue sarcomas (STS). Alexandria: American Society of Clinical Oncology; 2019.
112. Tawbi HA, Burgess M, Bolejack V, Van Tine BA, Schuetze SM, Hu J, et al. Pembrolizumab in advanced soft-tissue sarcoma and bone sarcoma (SARC028): a multicentre, two-cohort, single-arm, open-label, phase 2 trial. Lancet Oncol. 2017;18(11):1493–501.
113. Ben-Ami E, Barysauskas CM, Solomon S, Tahlil K, Malley R, Hohos M, et al. Immunotherapy with single agent nivolumab for advanced leiomyosarcoma of the uterus: results of a phase 2 study. Cancer. 2017;123(17):3285–90.
114. George S, Feng Y, Manola J, Nucci MR, Butrynski JE, Morgan JA, et al. Phase 2 trial of aromatase inhibition with letrozole in patients with uterine leiomyosarcomas expressing estrogen and/or progesterone receptors. Cancer. 2014;120(5):738–43.
115. Friedlander M, Sjoquist KM, Sommeijer DW, Bailey L, Martyn J, Gillies K, et al. PARAGON: Phase II study of aromatase inhibitors in women with potentially hormone responsive recurrent/metastatic gynecologic neoplasms: ANZGOG 0903. J Clin Oncol. 2013;31(15_Suppl):TPS5614-TPS.
116. Miller J, Shoni M, Siegert C, Lebenthal A, Godleski J, McNamee C. Benign metastasizing leiomyomas to the lungs: an institutional case series and a review of the recent literature. Ann Thorac Surg. 2016;101(1):253–8.
117. Rivera J, Christopoulos S, Small D, Trifiro M. Hormonal manipulation of benign metastasizing leiomyomas: report of two cases and review of the literature. J Clin Endocrinol Metabol. 2004;89(7):3183–8.

118. Jakate K, Azimi F, Ali RH, Lee C-H, Clarke BA, Rasty G, et al. Endometrial sarcomas: an immunohistochemical and JAZF1 re-arrangement study in low-grade and undifferentiated tumors. Mod Pathol. 2013;26(1):95.
119. Seagle B-LL, Shilpi A, Buchanan S, Goodman C, Shahabi S. Low-grade and high-grade endometrial stromal sarcoma: A National Cancer Database study. Gynecol Oncol. 2017;146(2):254–62.
120. Yamaguchi M, Erdenebaatar C, Saito F, Motohara T, Miyahara Y, Tashiro H, et al. Long-term outcome of aromatase inhibitor therapy with letrozole in patients with advanced low-grade endometrial stromal sarcoma. Int J Gynecol Cancer. 2015;25(9):1645–51.
121. Pautier P, Nam EJ, Provencher DM, Hamilton AL, Mangili G, Siddiqui NA, et al. Gynecologic Cancer InterGroup (GCIG) consensus review for high-grade undifferentiated sarcomas of the uterus. Int J Gynecol Cancer. 2014;24(Suppl 3):S73–7.
122. Kurman RJ, Carcangiu ML, Herrington S, Young RH. WHO classification of tumours of female reproductive organs. Lyon: IARC; 2014.
123. Bacalbasa N, Balescu I, Dima S, Popescu I. Ovarian sarcoma carries a poorer prognosis than ovarian epithelial cancer throughout all FIGO stages: a single-center case–control matched study. Anticancer Res. 2014;34(12):7303–8.

12 The Role of Systemic Therapies in the Management of Bone Sarcoma

Yat Hang To, Lisa Orme, and Jeremy Lewin

12.1 Introduction

Primary malignant bone tumours are rare, accounting for an estimated 0.2% of all newly diagnosed cancer case with approximately 255 new cases diagnosed in Australia per year [1, 2]. Although relatively rare on a population level, the majority of bone sarcomas occur within adolescent and young adults (AYA), representing the third most frequent cancer within this group. They encompass an array of histological and genetic subtypes of mesenchymal origin with the 2013 World Health Organisation classification defining more than 30 different types of primary bone cancers [3]. Of these, the most common types are osteosarcoma (35%) and Ewing sarcoma (16%) in children and AYA patients, and chondrosarcoma (30%) in older individuals (16%) [1].

The dramatic improvement in outcomes for patients with Ewing sarcoma and osteosarcoma is predicated on a multidisciplinary approach with routine administration of multi-agent chemotherapy regimens. Although 80–85% of individuals will present with localised lesions, control with surgical resection alone is

Y. H. To · J. Lewin (✉)
Bone & Soft Tissue Sarcoma Service, Peter MacCallum Cancer Centre,
Melbourne, VIC, Australia

Division of Medical Oncology, Peter MacCallum Cancer Centre, Melbourne, VIC, Australia
e-mail: jeremy.lewin@petermac.org

L. Orme
Bone & Soft Tissue Sarcoma Service, Peter MacCallum Cancer Centre,
Melbourne, VIC, Australia

Division of Medical Oncology, Peter MacCallum Cancer Centre, Melbourne, VIC, Australia

Department of Paediatric Oncology, Royal Children's Hospital, Melbourne, VIC, Australia
e-mail: lisa.orme@petermac.org

P. F. M. Choong (ed.), *Sarcoma*, https://doi.org/10.1007/978-981-15-9414-4_12

inadequate to optimise cure on the basis that the majority of patients with high-grade bone sarcoma will have subclinical micrometastatic disease [4–7]. With current approaches, contemporary series have demonstrated that approximately 70–80% of patients with localised osteosarcoma or Ewing sarcoma are cured of disease [8, 9]. Even in metastatic disease, cure is often achievable in selected individuals, particularly for those with metastasis limited to the lungs [10–12].

Beyond osteosarcoma and Ewing sarcoma, there are a heterogenous group of additional bone tumours that require nuanced consideration in the utility of systemic therapies. For example, chondrosarcoma is the most frequent sarcoma in adulthood with the majority being low-grade lesions where chemotherapy is typically ineffective [13]. However, systemic therapy may be appropriate in certain situations: for example, in those with dedifferentiated or mesenchymal subtypes, or those with targetable driver mutations [14, 15]. Similarly, the treatment of giant cell tumour of bone (GCTB), which is a benign but locally aggressive neoplasm, has been revolutionised with the use of denosumab, a fully humanised monoclonal antibody to receptor activator of nuclear factor kinase ligand (RANKL), for those with unresectable disease [16].

12.2 Special Considerations

Given the rarity of sarcoma, experience and caseload are associated with improved outcomes. The importance of having patients managed in high volume multidisciplinary expert sarcoma centres embedded with clinical trials cannot be understated. In addition, both the disease and its treatment carry the risk of significant morbidity and premature mortality that leads to long-term physical and psychological sequelae that requires particular consideration.

12.2.1 Genetic

The diagnosis of bone sarcoma, particularly in children, should heighten clinicians to the potential for germline genetic abnormalities and referral to a familial cancer clinic. For example, mutations in *TP53,* or Li-Fraumeni syndrome are associated with osteosarcoma, Ewing sarcoma and rhabdomyosarcoma [17]. Similarly, individuals who survive childhood retinoblastoma with a germline RB1 mutation are at particular risk of developing subsequent osteosarcoma [18].

12.2.2 Adolescent and Young Adults

AYA (aged 15–25 years in the Australian setting) experience poorer outcomes compared to paediatric and older patients [19, 20]. Although specific causes are unclear, there is likely to be multiple contributing factors such as delayed diagnosis, decreased rates of participation in clinical trials, altered biology and differences in chemotherapy metabolism [21–25]. In addition, AYA require specific consideration given their unique developmental and psychosocial concerns thus referral to dedicated services that focus on positive adolescent development and provision of youth relevant health interventions is strongly encouraged.

12.2.3 Fertility Preservation

Given the younger age demographics of this cohort, patients of reproductive age planned to receive gonadotoxic chemotherapy or pelvic irradiation should have discussion regarding fertility preservation prior to commencing treatment. Sperm storage is recommended for male patients. For female patients, a fertility specialist should be consulted about potential oocyte cryopreservation or ovarian tissue sampling and cryopreservation if time permits [26, 27].

12.2.4 Disease and Late Effects Surveillance

With improving survival, follow-up approaches for patients with bone sarcoma are increasingly important. Post-treatment assessment includes radiological surveillance, managing chronic toxicities and addressing the survivorship concerns of individuals [28]. Increasing literature stemming from paediatric late effects surveillance continues to define the cumulative post-treatment burden experienced by survivors of bone sarcoma. These include cardiac complications [29], impaired physical performance [30], obesity [31], infertility and neuro-cognitive impairment [32]. Of additional concern, survivors face an increased risk of secondary malignancies and premature mortality from non-cancer causes [33, 34]. The Children Oncology Group has published guidelines for long-term survivorship follow-up to guide management [35].

12.3 Osteosarcoma

Multi-modality therapy including neoadjuvant chemotherapy followed by wide resection of the primary tumour and further adjuvant chemotherapy is the current standard of care for localised osteosarcoma. Induction chemotherapy in particular offers several distinct advantages:

- Increase time for patient and surgeon to discuss and plan resection and reconstruction.
- Lead time for multidisciplinary planning of surgery, method of limb reconstruction (if appropriate) to allow optimal outcome for both disease control and function.

- Down-staging of primary tumours to facilitate limb-sparing surgery [36].
- Better demarcation of the tumour against surrounding tissue and improving surgical outcomes [36].
- Providing prognostic information; the degree of tumour response to neoadjuvant treatment is one of the most reliable prognostic factors in osteosarcoma [37, 38].

The four key cytotoxic drugs that have shown activity in osteosarcoma are doxorubicin, cisplatin, high-dose methotrexate (HDMTX) with leucovorin rescue and ifosfamide [11, 39]. Of these, doxorubicin has the greatest single agent activity but is limited by cardiotoxicity [40]. Preferred chemotherapy regimens are therefore based on various combinations of these drugs. A meta-analysis of 19 studies, most of which were based on paediatric patients, demonstrated that a combination of three drugs is superior to two but there are no further benefits in using a four-drug regimen [40].

In our centre, the most commonly accepted approach we use in younger patients (those aged below 30 years and in selected cases below 40 years) is high-dose methotrexate, doxorubicin and cisplatin (MAP regimen). There are various permutations of this treatment with varying doses and schedules [41–43]. Given its general acceptance, MAP is used as the control arm in a number of prospective studies, demonstrating 5-year survival rates of 70 to 80% [41–43]. Generally, two cycles of MAP are given prior to local therapy with a further four cycles given post-operatively. An example (Fig. 12.1) is the regimen used in the control arm of the international multicentre collaborative EURAMOS-1 trial, as shown below [43]:

Careful monitoring of organ function is required. Baseline assessment of renal function and audiology is performed and cisplatin is omitted in the final two cycles at a cumulative dose of 480 mg/m^2 to avoid significant accumulative nephro- and ototoxicity. Assessment of baseline cardiac function is mandated with either a gated blood pool scan or transthoracic echocardiogram and is repeated during therapy for early detection of cardiotoxicity that may require omission of doxorubicin as the dose approaches its final cumulative total of 450 mg/m^2 [44]. Furthermore, doxorubicin and cisplatin can be given as split-dosing over days 1 and 2 of each cycle.

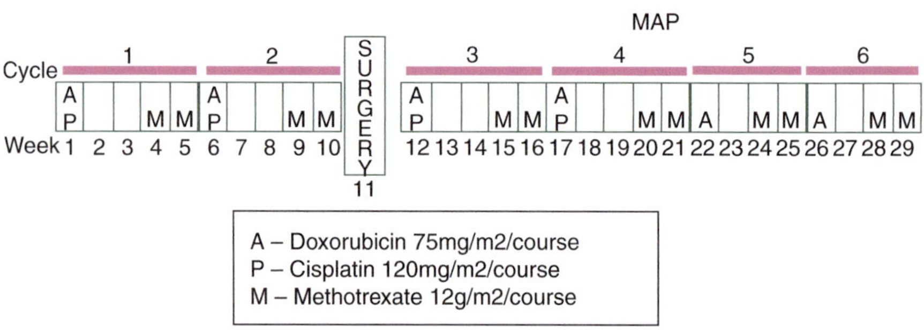

Fig. 12.1 Multi-agent chemotherapy regimen for osteosarcoma

The role of HDMTX in adults is unclear as nearly all trials exploring HDMTX have been conducted in children or patients aged up to 40 years [43, 45]. Increasing age is associated with important differences such as the increased incidence of histologic variants of osteosarcoma (including secondary osteosarcomas), medical co-morbidities that may limit tolerance to dose-intensive chemotherapies and less efficient clearance of MTx [46]. Given these factors, we recommend that HDMTX be given only to children and adults aged below 30 years or in selected cases for those aged below 40 years. For older patients, it is our practice that a combination of cisplatin and doxorubicin alone be given for a total of six cycles, two delivered pre-operatively and four post-operatively,

Response to induction chemotherapy is a major prognostic factor. "Good responders" have tumour necrosis greater than 90% on histological examination of the primary tumour. This is associated with a more favourable survival compared to poor responders with histological tumour necrosis <90% [11, 45]. In one series of 1058 patients with osteosarcoma, a good histological response was achieved in 59% treated with pre-operative chemotherapy. The 5-year survival rate was significantly higher in good responders (68% compared to 52%) [45]. The Children's Oncology Group also published a report that demonstrated 8 year survival rates of 87% for good responders, compared to 52% for poor responders [47].

Aiming to improve the inferior outcomes seen in poor responders, there has been interest in modifying post-operative chemotherapy based on histopathological response. In the international EURAMOS-1 trial, 618 patients with a poor histopathological response after induction chemotherapy were randomly assigned to MAP with or without ifosfamide and etoposide (IE) after surgery [43]. The addition of IE did not appear to improve event-free survival and was associated with increased toxicities. As such, MAP remains the standard adjuvant chemotherapy regardless of the degree of histological response and should be resumed promptly as a delay of greater than 21 days after definitive surgery is associated with poorer outcomes [48].

Investigational agents have included liposomal muramyl tripeptide phosphatidyl ethanolamine, commonly known as mifamurtide, an immunomodulatory agent that binds to macrophages and monocytes, inducing interleukin and cytokine production [49]. The addition of mifamurtide to three or four drug combination chemotherapy (MAP with or without ifosfamide) appeared to improve six-year overall survival in a large phase III study (78% versus 70%) of newly diagnosed, resectable, localised osteosarcoma [50]. However, in subsequent analyses, there appeared to be a significant interaction between mifamurtide and ifosfamide, ultimately obscuring its potential benefit [51]. This uncertainty has led to the approval of mifamurtide by European regulatory bodies but not the US Food and Drug administration (FDA).

12.3.1 Metastatic Disease

Approximately 20% of patients will present with macro-metastatic disease at diagnosis, with estimated 5-year survival rates of only 20%, compared to 80% seen in non-metastatic presentations [52–54]. Any chance of cure is predicated upon achieving complete surgical resection of all disease. As such, an aggressive multi-modality approach aiming for complete surgical resection of disease is usually adopted.

Lung is the most common site of metastasis, with bone and soft tissue being less common [55]. The number of metastases at diagnosis is considered prognostic [56, 57]. Complete resection of all clinically detectable lung metastases has been shown to improve outcomes, with 5-year event-free survival rates of 20 to 30% [58, 59]. Therefore, metastasectomy is usually pursued where feasible.

The same active chemotherapy agents are considered to treat metastatic osteosarcoma and the MAP backbone is utilised if a curative approach to therapy is undertaken. In our centre, we would suggest MAP for patients aged below 30 to 40 years of age and combination of cisplatin and doxorubicin alone for older patients. Other regimens can be considered. Of note, the combination of etoposide and high-dose ifosfamide was explored in a study of forty-three patients with primary metastatic osteosarcoma. This study demonstrated a projected 2-year progression-free survival rate of 39% for those with lung metastases and 58% of those with bone metastases albeit with significant haematological and renal toxicities [60]. However other studies using other cytotoxic combinations demonstrate only modest disease-free survival rates [61]. More intensive approaches incorporating high-dose chemotherapy with stem cell rescue have failed to significantly improve long-term survival beyond 20% [62].

In general, complete resection of all sites of metastatic disease should be undertaken. Failing this, outcomes are poor and enrolment into clinical trials should be considered.

12.3.2 Post-Treatment Surveillance

Surveillance is based on consensus-based guidelines rather than prospective data and survival benefits are unclear. The National Comprehensive Cancer Network (NCCN) and Children's Oncology Group (COG) have recommended physical examination, chest imaging, and local imaging of the primary site every three months for two years, every four months for year 3, then every 6 months of years 4 and 5, and annually thereafter [63, 64]. CT rather than chest x-ray is utilised to maximise early detection of oligometastatic lung recurrence that may be offered curative resection. A head-to-toe PET/CT or bone scan may also be considered.

Other consensus guidelines, including those published by the European Society of Medical Oncology (ESMO), vary in regard to recommended timing of disease surveillance resulting in uncertainty over the optimal scheduling [26]. Consideration also needs to be given for patients transitioning from paediatric to adult centres. There is significant variation between the practice of paediatric and non-paediatric oncologists in regard to long-term follow-up and this places AYA at risk of disengagement [28]. Further work is needed to ensure greater uniformity in follow-up practices and guidelines.

As stated, survivors of primary bone cancers have overall worse morbidity and premature mortality. Therefore, long-term follow-up for treatment-related toxicity should continue indefinitely. The COG has published survivorship guidelines to guide management in this area [35].

12.3.3 Recurrent and Relapsed Disease

About 30% of patients with disease remission after primary treatment for localised disease and 80% of patients with primary metastatic disease will relapse [63]. In a series of 564 patients, the median time to recurrence was 13 months and overall medial survival was poor at 14 months, with those recurring within 2 years having the worst prognosis [65]. Salvage is still possible, particularly in those with limited pulmonary disease and in whom a second surgical remission is possible [66]. Therefore, resection of recurrences should be undertaken where possible, especially in those with isolated pulmonary disease. The role of post-surgery chemotherapy in these cases is still unclear but can be considered.

Osteosarcoma is less chemo-responsive than Ewing sarcoma and disease control periods are generally short without a defined optimal salvage chemotherapy regimen [66]. Studied combinations include ifosfamide plus etoposide, cyclophosphamide plus etoposide and gemcitabine plus docetaxel, with varying response rates of around 13% to 48% [67–69]. Our practice is to offer combination of ifosfamide and etoposide to patients if there is a possibility of cytoreductive surgery following a significant chemotherapy response. However, long-term survival is poor and treatment of recurrent osteosarcomas is still an area of unmet need. Enrolment in clinical trials where available is suggested.

Investigational agents have included radiopharmaceutical approaches such as samarium-153 ethylenediamine tetramethylene phosphate (Sm153-EDTMP) and radium-223 dichloride (Ra-223), particularly in bone metastases but is limited by myelotoxicity [70, 71]. Sorafenib, a vascular endothelial growth factor receptor (VEGFR) inhibitor, has also been demonstrated to have activity in patients with relapsed and unresectable osteosarcoma after failure of standard multi-modality therapy [72]. A phase II study of regorafenib, an oral multi-kinase inhibitor, has demonstrated an 8-week clinical benefit rate of 65% in 43 patients with progressive osteosarcoma after one to two lines of chemotherapy [73]. In the SARC024 study, regorafenib was demonstrated to have improved median PFS compared to placebo (3.6 versus 1.7 months) in patients with progressive metastatic osteosarcoma who had received an average of 2.3 lines of prior chemotherapy [74].

12.4 Ewing Sarcoma Family of Tumours

The Ewing sarcoma family of tumours (ESFTs) are a group of cancers that includes Ewing sarcoma of bone, extraosseous Ewing tumours, primitive neuroectodermal tumours (pNET) and Askin's tumour of the chest wall. These are all thought to arise from a common mesenchymal progenitor cell origin and are histologically characterised by sheets of small, round, blue cells [75]. ESFT share and are distinguished from other small round cell tumours by a distinct reciprocal chromosomal translocation, all involving the *EWS* gene on chromosome 22 [76]. The most common is a reciprocal translocation between chromosome 11 and 22, resulting in the formation of the *EWS-FLI1* fusion gene, an aberrant transcription factor found in 90% of all ESFT [77, 78]. In a minority of Ewing sarcoma, the *EWS* has a different fusion partner including *ERG*, *ETV1* and *EAIF* genes [78].

Ewing-like tumour is a term used to describe a subset of round cell sarcomas occurring in children or young adults that share similar microscopic features of ESFT but lacking the reciprocal translocation in the *EWS* gene. In one case series of 22 patients, 68% were found to harbour *CIC* rearrangements [79]. *CIC* is a transcriptional repressor and mutations in this gene are associated with other cancers such as glioblastomas [80]. Alternative fusions involving the *BCOR* gene, another transcription repressor, have also been described [81]. Ewing-like tumours can have atypical features such as angulated nuclei or spindle cell morphology and are thought to be more aggressive than classical ESFT [82, 83]. Whilst they are thought to be less responsive to standard ESFT chemotherapy, the same management principles and chemotherapy regimens are applied to these tumours [84].

Multi-agent chemotherapy has greatly improved survival rates for patients with localised ESFT from 10 to 70–80% [10, 85, 86]. As with osteosarcoma treatment, incorporation of cytotoxic chemotherapy prior to and following local treatment is standard. The period of induction therapy allows for response assessment and careful multidisciplinary planning of definitive local therapy for site(s) of disease. ESFT is radiosensitive and local therapy may include surgery and/or radiation therapy [87]. When radiation therapy is used, chemotherapy is given concurrently with removal of the anthracycline for 2 cycles to avoid risk of radiation recall. For localised ESFT, our practice is to deliver four to six cycles of neoadjuvant multi-agent chemotherapy induction over 12 weeks prior to definitive local therapy and then consolidation chemotherapy is given post-operatively for a total of fourteen cycles.

The current standard therapy that we utilise is based on a series of trials demonstrating incremental improvements beginning with the first Intergroup Ewing's Sarcoma study (IESS-I). This trial demonstrated that patients with localised primary tumours treated with vincristine-actinomycin-cyclophosphamide (VAC) plus doxorubicin (VAC-D) had superior recurrence free survival (RFS) compared to those treated with VAC plus chest irradiation or VAC alone (5-year RFS; 60% versus 44% versus 22%, respectively) [88]. The subsequent IESS-II study demonstrated that high-dose intermittent 3-weekly dosing was superior to moderate-dose weekly chemotherapy [89]. Further analyses determined that doxorubicin dose-intensity was critical to favourable outcomes and therefore dactinomycin was subsequently removed from further trial regimens, establishing vincristine-doxorubicin-cyclophosphamide (VDC) as the treatment backbone [90]. Further improvement to long-term survival was achieved by adding alternating cycles of ifosfamide/etoposide (VDC-IE) with significantly better five-year RFS compared to VDC alone (69% versus 54%) [91]. An example of the schedule and dosing of VDC-IE is shown below (Fig. 12.2).

Cycle	Week	Treatment
1	1	VDC
2	3	IE
3	5	VDC
4	7	IE
5	9	VDC
6	11	IE
Local therapy		
7	13	VDC
8	15	IE
9	17	VDC
10	19	IE
11	21	VC*
12	23	IE
13	25	VC*
14	27	IE

VDC
- Vincristine 2mg/m2 IV day 1
- Doxorubicin 37.5mg/m2/d IV days 1 and 2
- Cyclophosphamide# 1200mg/m2 IV day 1

IE
- Ifosfamide# 1800mg/m2/d days 1 to 5
- Etoposide 100mg/m2/d days 1 to 5

* Doxorubicin is omitted due to potential accumulative cardiotoxicity
#Concurrent mesna is required given risk of haemorrhagic cystitis

Fig. 12.2 VDC-IE multi-agent regimen for Ewing's sarcoma

Given ESFT's sensitivity to alkylating agents, which have a steep dose–response curve, several approaches have been explored to exploit this dose–response relationship. One such method is treatment with interval-compressed VDC-IE, reducing the interval between treatment courses from 3 to 2 weeks (14 day cycles). The phase III COG AEWS0031 trial demonstrated that 2 weekly VDC-IE was associated with improved 5-year RFS (73% vs. 65%) and with a similar toxicity profile [8]. However, this study was based on a younger patient population with only 10% of patient being aged above 18 years, and tolerability and efficacy are therefore unknown in older individuals. Interval-compressed VDC-IE with granulocyte colony-stimulating factor (G-CSF) support is therefore widely adopted as the standard regimen for front-line treatment of children and adolescents with localised EFT and the schedule is shown below. Conventional 3-weekly VDC-IE is still considered for patients >25 years as safety, feasibility and toxicity data of interval compression is lacking in the adult patient population.

European co-operative groups have employed a different approach utilising risk stratified treatment of localised tumours. As per European EuroEWING-99 and EWING 2008 trials, a different induction backbone was used comprising six three-weekly courses of vincristine-ifosfamide-doxorubicin-etoposide (VIDE) [92, 93]. Following induction chemotherapy and surgery, patients were stratified as standard risk if they had good histological response (>90% tumour necrosis). Patients were stratified as high risk if they had:

- Localised disease and poor histological response at surgery after induction chemotherapy.
- Initial surgery or in whom surgery was not feasible and had large volume tumour (>200 mL) at diagnosis.

Standard risk patients received standard consolidation chemotherapy with eight cycles of vincristine, actinomycin and cyclophosphamide or ifosfamide. Two-hundred and fourteen high-risk patients were then randomised to either seven courses of vincristine-dactinomycin-ifosfamide (VAI) or myeloablative megatherapy with busulfan plus melphalan (BuMel) followed by autologous haematopoietic cell rescue. BuMel autograft was associated with improved 8-year EFS (61% versus 47%) and overall survival (65% versus 56%).

This risk stratified approach can be considered in patients with localised disease. Results are awaited for recent studies comparing VIDE with VDC-IE backbone. Such an approach for patients with high-risk localised disease may result in increased lung and gonadal toxicities and requires careful consideration regarding the interaction between radiation therapy and busulfan. The choice also needs take into account the treating centre's familiarity with the regimen. Furthermore, care must be taken as this study was in patients younger than 50 years and three patients died of treatment-related toxicities [93].

12.4.1 Metastatic Disease

About 20–50% of patients with ESFT will present with primary metastatic disease [94] [95]. Outcomes are poor, with survival rates dropping to 40% for patients with lung only metastases and 6% for other sites [96]. Standard treatment for these patients is unclear given the scarcity of randomised data, therefore enrolment into clinical trials should be considered.

In general, the approach to primary metastatic ESFT is multi-agent chemotherapy combined with definitive local therapy of all sites of disease where possible. Even in cases of disseminated metastatic disease, such an approach may achieve a complete remission and a significant period of disease control beyond therapy. For patients with pulmonary metastases, chemotherapy followed by supplemental whole lung irradiation is recommended for those who achieve a complete response to chemotherapy. Whole lung irradiation has been demonstrated to reduce the rate of pulmonary relapse by 50% and improve EFS [97]. Metastasectomy is reserved for residual pulmonary disease after chemotherapy and radiotherapy.

The same chemotherapy regimens used in localised ESFT is generally employed. VDC-IE is the most widely used but its efficacy over VDC in metastatic disease is unclear. Of 120 patients with metastatic ESFT enrolled in the original trial of alternating IE with VDC, 59 were assigned to VDC-IE and 62 to VDC alone [91]. There was no significant difference in event-free survival between the two treatment groups. The role of HDCT has also been investigated in a subset of patients with primary lung metastases enrolled in the EuroEWING-99 trial [98]. Six cycles of VIDE were completed in 250 patients (89%) and 169 of these patients (60%) subsequently received BuMel autograft. The 3-year OS was 34% demonstrating that such intensive therapy can be tolerated and has clinical activity. However the EuroEWING 99-2pulm trial did not demonstrate any benefit of BuMel autograft compared to seven courses of VAI and lung irradiation (VAI-RT) in patients with primary lung metastases following VIDE [99]. The current EWING 2008 trial (NCT00987636) randomised patients with primary disseminated metastases who completed VIDE induction therapy to VAI consolidation chemotherapy with or without HDCT and results are awaited. Therefore, the place of HDCT in the treatment of primary metastatic disease remains unclear and is usually not recommended outside of clinical trials.

12.4.2 Post-Treatment Surveillance

Consensus-based guidelines recommend physical examination, chest imaging, and local imaging of the primary site every three months for two years, then every six months of years 3 to 5, and annually thereafter [63, 64]. Long-term follow-up for survivors to address complications from combined treatments and risk of secondary malignancies is also vital.

12.4.3 Recurrent and Relapsed Disease

Relapse following primary therapy is associated with poor prognosis, with an estimated 5-year overall survival and event-free survival rates of 10–20% and 5–10%, respectively [100, 101]. Poor prognostic factors are relapse within two years of therapy, recurrence at combined local and distant sites and elevated lactate dehydrogenase at diagnosis [101].

Salvage with systemic therapy and local control, especially in those with late pulmonary relapse can be effective, with long-term survival rates of 40% [102]. The most commonly used chemotherapy regimen is combination of irinotecan and temozolomide (IT) however evidence is based on phase I trials or case series with varying doses and schedules and primarily in paediatric patients. Estimated response rates range from 17 to 55% with median progression-free survival of 3 to 8 months [103–105]. Combination IT with vincristine was explored in a small number of patients, demonstrating response rates of 63% and a 10-month survival rate of 22% [106]. Other options include topotecan plus cyclophosphamide (response rates of 35%), high-dose ifosfamide (34%), oral etoposide (24%) and docetaxel plus gemcitabine (29%) [107–110]. The current rEECur trial (NCT02727387) seeks to compare chemotherapy regimens for relapsed ESFT. As the majority of ESFT patients are young with limited co-morbidities, relapse even if not salvageable may be effectively controlled with serial lines of chemotherapy and radiation therapy if the disease remains chemo-sensitive.

The role of HDCT in the relapse setting is unclear and evidence is based on retrospective series [111]. Further prospective research is needed for relapsed ESFT as all studies to date have been small and the best treatment is still unknown. Enrolment onto open clinical trials is strongly recommended.

12.4.4 Special Considerations

12.4.4.1 Local Therapy

Surgery (with or without post-operative radiotherapy) achieves better local control than radiation alone and so should be the primary consideration [112, 113]. Definitive radiation should be reserved only for patients in which function-preserving surgery is not possible.

Timing of local therapy is critical as significant delays are associated with worse survival. In our centre, local therapy occurs after 12 weeks of neoadjuvant chemotherapy following response assessment and multidisciplinary planning during induction chemotherapy. In one study, 10-year overall survival for patients with localised ESFT was improved in those that received local therapy at 6 to 15 weeks from chemotherapy initiation (70.3%) compared to those delayed to ≥16 weeks (57.1%) [114]. The difference in survival appeared to be compounded in patients receiving radiation therapy alone. Therefore, careful planning to ensure appropriate timing of local therapy is paramount.

12.5 Giant Cell Tumour of Bone

GCTB is rare, non-malignant osteolytic tumours that account for 3–5% of all primary bone cancers [115]. Although usually considered benign, they are often locally aggressive and 2–3% of GCTB cases will develop distant disease, predominantly with pulmonary implants [116, 117]. Spontaneous malignant transformation is also possible but given its rarity, incidence is unknown.

Surgery with *en bloc* excision and intralesional curettage are traditional treatments for resectable disease [118]. The aim of any surgical approach is to remove the tumour whilst preserving functional anatomy. Local recurrence rates vary according to the surgical technique and whether packing of the defect with bone cement or graft is undertaken [119, 120]. Local intra-operative adjuvant therapies with chemical or thermal methods have been used but randomised data supporting their use is lacking [121–123].

The recognition of RANKL (receptor activator of nuclear factor kinase ligand) as an important factor in the pathogenesis of GCTB has led to the use of denosumab, a fully humanised monoclonal antibody against RANKL. Pre-operative denosumab is a reasonable approach in patients who have potentially resectable GCTB but for whom upfront surgery would result in unacceptable functional outcomes or significant morbidity. Denosumab therapy is also associated with improved pain control and function [16]. Pooled analyses have indicated that denosumab therapy is associated with high radiographic response rates of 60–100% and histopathological response rates of 80% [124, 125]. It is also associated with improved recurrence rates of 9–10%, compared to historical controls of 35–45% for curettage alone [126]. However, follow-up for these trials has been short and long-term toxicity data is still immature. Regardless, pre-operative denosumab is approved for use in GCTB. Recommended dosing is 120 mg subcutaneously every 28 days but optimal duration is not well established and in trials, have varied widely from 6 to 153 months [16, 63, 127, 128]. Given the lack of long-term toxicity data, the duration of treatment should be kept as short possible, often 6 months, in order to convert the patient to operable.

The role of adjuvant denosumab is still unclear. There is only limited conflicting data and as such, it is not recommended to use denosumab in the adjuvant setting [129, 130].

12.5.1 Unresectable or Metastatic Disease

Denosumab is recommended in patients with unresectable or metastatic disease. Evidence is drawn from a seminal phase II trial of 37 patients treated with 120 mg of monthly denosumab after loading doses on days 8 and 15 of the first month [16]. Of the 35 assessable patients, 85% had an either radiographic or histological (≥ 90% elimination of giant cells on evaluation) response. Further expansion of this trial involved 282 patients including those with surgically unsalvageable GCTB or in whom surgery was likely to be associated with severe morbidity [128]. After median follow-up of 13 months, 96% of those with unresectable disease had no evidence of disease progression. Of those in whom upfront surgery was deemed unacceptable due to anticipated morbidity, 74% had no surgery and 62% of those that underwent surgery had a less morbid procedure than initially planned. Although a high clinical benefit rate is seen in this young age demographic, limited information is known about its long-term effects including rates of osteonecrosis of the jaw, atypical femoral fractures, malignant transformation and effect on fertility.

Chemotherapy and interferon therapy have been used in GCTB [131–135]. However randomised data is lacking and evidence is mostly based on case series. Interferon alfa-2b is recommended by some guidelines as an alternative when serial embolization, denosumab or radiation therapy is not possible but its poor tolerance must be taken into consideration [63].

12.5.2 Post-Treatment Surveillance

The National Comprehensive Cancer Network (NCCN) has recommended physical examination, imaging of the surgical site when clinically indicated, and chest imaging every 6 months for 2 years then annually thereafter [63].

12.6 Chondrosarcoma

Chondrosarcomas are a heterogeneous group of neoplasms that arise from transformed cells that produce cartilage. It is the third most common primary bone cancer, accounting for 30% of all cases [1]. They are histologically classified into three grades based on nuclear size, pattern of staining, cellularity and mitotic rate [136], and this provides prognostic information [137, 138]. Ten year survival rates for grade I and grade II tumours are greater than 90% and 62–86%, respectively [139–141]. High-grade or grade III tumours have worse prognosis, associated with high metastasis rates and 10-year survival of only 55% [141].

Histologically, chondrosarcomas are divided into several types [3]. The most common, conventional chondrosarcoma, accounts for nearly 85% of all cases and is further subdivided into 1) central, arising from the medullary cavity and usually in the absence of a precursor (commonly referred to as central primary chondrosarcoma) or 2) peripheral, developing from the surface of the bone and transforming from pre-existing benign cartilage lesions such as endochondromas or osteochondromas [13, 142]. A minority (<1%) occurs at the surface of bone, likely of periosteal origin and is referred to as periosteal chondrosarcomas, previously known as juxtacortical [13].

Several other rare subtypes also exist, accounting for 10–15% of chondrosarcomas:

- Clear cell—characterised by numerous cells with abundant clear, vacuolated cytoplasm [143]. Although usually classified as a low-grade variant, recurrence after simple excision and curettage is high [144]. Prognosis is excellent when treated with adequate wide surgical margins with 10 year disease survival rates of 90% [143]. However, it has a tendency for very late recurrence and metastasis even 20 years after initial diagnosis [143, 145]. Therefore, long-term follow-up is mandatory.
- Dedifferentiated—a high-grade, non-cartilaginous sarcoma juxtaposed with a low or intermediate chondrosarcoma with an abrupt interface between the two components [146]. The differentiated component can demonstrate various features such of those found in osteosarcoma, angiosarcoma or leiomyosarcoma. It exhibits aggressive behaviour and has a poor 5-year survival of less than 20% [147].
- Mesenchymal—a rare high-grade variant composed of both undifferentiated small cells and islands of atypical cartilage [148]. Around 22–50% originate in soft tissue, especially within the central nervous system [149, 150]. Mortality rates are also high, estimated at 54% [151]. They also have a tendency toward late local and metastatic recurrence [152]. Given its rarity, standard treatment is unknown.

Wide excision with negative margins is the standard treatment for chondrosarcomas, regardless of grade [63]. In selected cases of low-grade and extremity localised chondrosarcomas, intralesional excision can be considered [63, 153].

Chondrosarcoma, particularly conventional and clear-cell types, are generally considered chemo- and radio-insensitive given their low percentage of dividing cells and poor vascularity [13]. Therefore, adjuvant chemotherapy is not recommended even in intermediate-to-high grade conventional tumours [13, 63]. There is limited evidence for the use of chemotherapy in other subtypes:

- Mesenchymal—there are a number of case series and retrospective studies showing the potential benefit to chemotherapy [154–156]. The optimal timing and

regimens are unclear, with patients receiving a number of agents including dactinomycin, platinum derivatives, anthracyclines, etoposide and methotrexate [154]. In one retrospective study, the addition of chemotherapy to surgery appeared to increase 10-year survival from 46% to 80% [155]. Response rates to chemotherapy of up 31% have been reported [156].
- Dedifferentiated—the evidence is unclear with conflicting conclusions drawn from retrospective studies. One retrospective study of 18 patients concluded adjuvant chemotherapy appeared to offer a survival benefit but this is not consistent with other reviews [14, 157, 158].

Regardless of the histological subtype, further prospective data is needed and enrolment into open clinical trials is recommended.

12.6.1 Metastatic Disease

There is limited evidence to support resection of metastases, particularly of the lungs, but consensus guidelines do recommend excision of all disease sites if possible [63, 159]. A single small prospective trial demonstrated the benefit of combination of cisplatin and doxorubicin with two of six patients with dedifferentiated chondrosarcoma achieving a complete response and two of five patients with mesenchymal chondrosarcoma experiencing stable disease [160]. Another retrospective study of 180 patients with advanced chondrosarcomas treated with mostly anthracycline-based regimens reported response rates of 31% for mesenchymal chondrosarcoma, 20.5% for dedifferentiated, 11.5% for conventional and 0% for clear-cell subtype [156].

12.6.2 Surveillance

Guidelines recommend physical examination, imaging of the primary site and of the chest as clinically indicated every 6 to 12 months for 2 years then yearly as appropriate for low-grade lesions [63].

A more intensive program is recommended for high-grade lesions given the higher propensity for metastases and late recurrences. Physical examination, imaging of the primary site and of the chest every 3 to 6 months for the first 5 years and yearly thereafter for a minimum of 10 years are suggested [63].

12.6.3 Special Consideration

12.6.3.1 Novel Therapies

A greater understanding of the pathogenesis of chondrosarcomas is driving the development of new treatment options for this entity. The most important signalling pathways include *Hedgehog*, *Src*, *PI3K-Akt-mTOR* and angiogenesis [15]. Unfortunately, clinical trials targeting molecular pathways, particularly platelet-derived growth factor receptors (PDGFR), have been relatively disappointing with a lack of clear clinical utility using dasatinib, imatinib and oestrogen receptor blockers [161–163]. A retrospective study of ten patients with unresectable chondrosarcoma treated with combination of sirolimus (an mTOR inhibitor) and cyclophosphamide demonstrated a disease control rate of 70%, however further prospective data is needed [164]. More recently, mutations in isocitrate dehydrogenase (*IDH1/2*) have been identified in 40–50% of primary conventional chondrosarcomas, which opens up the possibility of using IDH inhibitors for this entity [165].

12.7 Chordoma

Chordomas arise from the cellular remnants of the notochord, an embryonic structure of the mesodermal cells that plays an organisational role in nervous system development and later forms part of the vertebral column [166]. As such, they predominantly arise in the axial skeleton, most commonly at the sacrum and base of skull [167].

Chordomas are generally chemo-insensitive so preferred primary treatment is wide excision with adequate margins, with reported local recurrence rates as low as 17% [63, 168]. Radiation therapy, either pre- or post-operatively, is associated with improved local disease control and survival [169, 170].

A greater molecular understanding of chordomas has revealed several potential targets for therapy. These include the *PI3K-Akt-mTOR* signalling pathway, epidermal growth factor receptor (EGFR) and platelet-derived growth factor receptor (PDGFR) [171–173]. This had led to several phase II trials exploring therapies directed at these targets. Imatinib, a tyrosine kinase inhibitor, was studied in a phase II trial of 56 patients with advanced chordoma, resulting in a clinical benefit rate of 64% and a median PFS of 9 months [174]. A second study treated patients resistant to first-line imatinib with combination of imatinib and sirolimus, an mTOR inhibitor [175]. Of the 9 assessable patients, 7 patients had stable disease and 1 had a partial response, resulting in a clinical benefit rate of 89%.

Lapatinib, an EGFR inhibitor, has demonstrated activity in advanced progressing EGFR-positive chordomas [176]. In a phase II study of 18 patients, 38.9% had stable disease with a median PFS of 6 months. Sorafenib, a multi-kinase inhibitor, has also been studied, with response rates of 3.7% and 12-month overall survival of 86.5% [177].

12.7.1 Surveillance

Physical examination, imaging of surgical site and the chest as clinically indicated are recommended for up to 10 years. Chest imaging is recommended every 6 months for 5 years then annually thereafter [63].

12.7.2 Relapsed and Recurrent Disease

Local recurrences are common and up to 40% of patients with local recurrence will also develop distant metastases to lungs, bone, soft tissue, lymph nodes, liver and skin [166]. Patients with recurrent disease should be managed with surgery where possible. Systemic treatment with the previously therapies such as imatinib, sirolimus, lapatinib or sorafenib is recommended if available [63].

References

1. Howlander N et al. SEER Cancer Stat Facts: Bone and Joint Cancer. SEER, [Online]. https://seer.cancer.gov/statfacts/html/bones.html. Accessed 4 July 2019.
2. Australian Institute of Health and Welfare [AIHW]. Cancer Data in Australia; Australian Cancer Incidence and Mortality books. Australian Institute of Health and Welfare (AIHW), 2018. [Online]. Available: https://www.aihw.gov.au/reports/cancer/cancer-data-in-australia. [Accessed 4 July 2019].
3. Fletcher C, et al. WHO classifications of Tumours of soft tissue and bone. Lyon: IARC Press; 2013.
4. Gorlick R et al, Holland-Frei Cancer Medicine. 6th edition, BC Decker Inc. 2003.
5. Nesbit M, et al. Multimodal therapy for the management of primary, non-metastatic Ewing's sarcoma of bone: a long-term follow-up of the First Intergroup study. J Clin Oncol. 1990;8:1667–74.
6. Whelan J, et al. Management of osteosarcoma. Curr Treat Options in Oncol. 2006;7:444–55.
7. Jaffe N, et al. Can cure in patients with osteosarcoma be achieved exclusively with chemotherapy and abrogation of surgery? Cancer. 2002;95(10):2202–10.
8. Womer R, et al. Randomised controlled trial of interval-compressed chemotherapy for the treatment of localised Ewing sarcoma: a report from the Children's oncology group. J Clin Oncol. 2012;30(33):4148–54.
9. Bielack SS, et al. Methotrexate, doxorubicin, and cisplatin (MAP) plus maintenance Pegylated interferon alfa-2b versus MAP alone in patients with Resectable high-grade osteosarcoma and good histologic response to preoperative MAP: first results of the EURAMOS-1 good response randomized controlled trial. J Clin Oncol. 2015;33(20):2279–87.
10. Noone A et al. SEER Cancer Statistics Review, 1975–2015. SEER, April 2018. [Online]. https://seer.cancer.gov/csr/1975_2015/. Accessed 4 July 2019.
11. Beilack SS, et al. Prognostic factors in high-grade osteosarcoma of the extremities or trunk: an analysis of 1,702 patients treated on neoadjuvant cooperative osteosarcoma study group protocols. J Clin Oncol. 2002;20(3):776–90.
12. Kager L, et al. Primary metastatic osteosarcoma: presentation and outcome of patients treated on neoadjuvant cooperative osteosarcoma study group protocols. J Clin Oncol. 2003;21(10):2011–8.
13. Gelderblom H, et al. The clinical approach towards chondrosarcomas. Oncologist. 2008;13(3):320–9.
14. Staals A, et al. Dedifferentiated chondrosarcomas arising in pre-existing osteochondromas. J Bone Joint Surg Am. 2007;89(5):987.
15. Polychronidou G, et al. Novel therapeutic approaches in chondrosarcoma. Future Oncol. 2017;13(7):637–48.
16. Thomas D, et al. Denosumab in patients with giant-cell tumour of bone: an open-label, phase 2 study. The Lancet Oncol. 2010;11(3):275–80.
17. Kratz CP, et al. Cancer screening recommendations for individuals with li-Fraumeni syndrome. Clin Cancer Res. 2017;23(11):38–45.

18. DerKinderen et al. Non-ocular cancer in patients with hereditary retinoblastoma and their relatives. Int J Cancer. 1988;41(4): 499–504.
19. Kasper B, et al. Prognostic factors in adolescents and young adults (AYA) with high risk soft tissue sarcoma treated by adjuvant chemotherapy: a study based on pooled European Organisation for Research and Treatment of Cancer (EORTC) clinical trials 62771 and 62931. Eur J Cancer. 2013;49(2):449–56.
20. Janeway K, et al. Outcome for adolescent and young adult patients with osteosarcoma. Cancer. 2012;118(18):4597–605.
21. Van de Graff WT, et al. Soft tissue sarcomas in adolescents and young adults: a comparison with their paediatric and adult counterparts. Lancet Oncol. 2017;18(3):166–75.
22. White V et al. Management of sarcoma in adolescents and young adults: an Australian population-based study. J Adolescent Young Adult Oncol. 2019; 8(3).
23. Freyer DR, et al. The clinical trials gap for adolescents and young adults with Cancer: recent Progress and conceptual framework for continued research. Current Paediatric Reports. 2015;3(2):137–45.
24. Klenike AM, et al. Adolescents and young adults with cancer: aspects of adherence - a questionnaire study. *Adolescent Health.* Medicine and Therapeutics. 2018;9:77–85.
25. Collins M et al. Benefits and adverse events in younger versus older patients receiving neoadjuvant chemotherapy for osteosarcoma: findings from a meta-analysis. J Clin Oncol 2013;31(18):2303–2312.
26. Casali P et al. Bone sarcomas: ESMO-PaedCan-EURACAN: Clinical Practice Guidelines for diagnosis, treatment and follow-up. Ann Oncol. 2018;29(Suppl 4):79–95.
27. Srikanthan A et al. Fertility preservation in post-pubescent female cancer patients: A practical guideline for clinician. Mol Clin Pathol. 2018; 8(1).
28. Lewin J, et al. Variations of surveillance practice for patients with bone sarcoma: a survey of Australian sarcoma clinicians. Sarcoma. 2017;2017:9.
29. Mulrooney D, et al. Cardiac outcomes in a cohort of adult survivors of childhood and adolescent cancer: retrospective analysis of the childhood Cancer survivor study cohort. BMJ. 2009;339:4606.
30. Ness KK, et al. Physical performance limitations in the childhood cancer survivor cohort. J Clin Oncol. 2009;27(14):2382–9.
31. Tai E, et al. Health status of adolescent and young adult cancer survivors. Cancer. 2012;31(35):4884–91.
32. D'Agostino N, et al. Psychosocial challenges and resource needs of young adult cancer survivors: implications for program development. J Psychosoc Oncol. 2013;31(6):585–600.
33. Ginsberg J, et al. Long-term survivors of childhood Ewing sarcoma: report from the childhood Cancer survivor study. J Natl Cancer Inst. 2010;102(16):1272–83.
34. Youn P, et al. Long-term cause-specific mortality in survivors of adolescent and young adult bone and soft tissue sarcoma. Cancer. 2014;120(5):2334–41.
35. Children's Oncology Group Long-term follow-up guidelines. Children's Oncology Group, Oct 2018. [Online]. www.survivorshipguidelines.org. Accessed 4 July 2019.
36. Hosalkar H, et al. Limb sparing surgery for pediatric musculoskeletal tumors. Paediatric Blood Cancer. 2004;42:295–310.
37. Bishop M, et al. Assess the prognostic significant of histologic response in osteosarcoma: a comparison of outcomes on CCG-782 and INT0133. Paediatr Blood Cancer. 2016;63(10):1737–43.
38. Hanafy E, et al. Tumour histopathological response to neoadjuvant chemotherapy in childhood solid malignancies: is it still impressive. J Investig Med. 2018;66:289–97.
39. Ferrari S, et al. An updated on chemotherapy for osteosarcoma. Expert Opinions in Pharmacotherapy. 2015;16(18):2727–36.
40. Anninga J, et al. Chemotherapeutic adjuvant treatment for osteosarcoma: where do we stand? Eur J Cancer. 2011;47(16):2431–45.
41. Meyers P, et al. Osteosarcomas: a randomised, prospective trial of the addition of ifosfamide and/or muramyl tripeptide to cisplatin, doxorubicin and high-dose methotrexate. J Clin Oncol. 2005;23(9):2004–11.

42. Winkler K, et al. Neoadjuvant chemotherapy of osteoma: results of a randomised co-operative trial (COSS-82) with salvage chemotherapy based on histological tumour response. J Clin Oncol. 1988;6(2):329–37.
43. Whelan J, et al. EURAMOS-1, an international randomised study for osteosarcoma: results from pre-randomisation treatment. Ann Oncol. 2015;26:407–14.
44. Von Hoff D, et al. Risk factors for doxorubicin-induced congestive heart failure. Ann Intern Med. 1979;91:710–7.
45. Bacci G, et al. Neoadjuvant chemotherapy for high-grade central osteosarcoma of the extremity. Histologic response to preoperative chemotherapy correlated with histologic subtype of tumour. Cancer. 2003;97(12):3068.
46. Wagner M, et al. Chemotherapy for bone sarcoma in adults. J Oncol Pract. 2016;12(3):208–16.
47. Provisor A, et al. Treatment of non-metastatic osteosarcoma of the extremity with preoperative and postoperative chemotherapy: a report from Children's Cancer group. J Clinc Oncol. 1997;15:76–84.
48. Imran H, et al. Effect of time to resumption of chemotherapy after definitive surgery on prognosis for non-metastatic osteosarcoma. J Bone Joint Surg Am. 2009;91:604–12.
49. Frampton J, et al. Mifamurtide: a review of its use in the treatment of osteosarcoma. Paediatr Drugs. 2010;12(3):141–53.
50. Meyers P, et al. Osteosarcoma: the addition of muramyl tripeptide to chemotherapy improved overall survival - report from Children's oncology group. J Clin Oncol. 2008;26(4):633.
51. Hunsberger S, et al. Complexities in interpretation of osteosarcoma clinical trial results. J Clin Oncol. 2008;26(3):3103–4.
52. Marko et al. Prevalence of metastasis at diagnosis of osteosarcoma: an international comparison. Pediatr Blood Cancer. 2016; 63(6):1006–1011.
53. Samer S, et al. Osteosarcoma with metastasis at initial diagnosis: current outcomes and prognostic factors in context of a comprehensive cancer Centre. Molecular and clinical oncology. 2014;2(5):811–6.
54. Duranlia AG et al. Outcomes of adolescent and adult patients with lung metastatic osteosarcoma and comparison of synchronous and metachronous lung metastatic groups. PLoS. 2016; 11(5).
55. Jeffree M, et al. The metastatic patterns of osteosarcoma. Br J Cancer. 1975;32(1):87–107.
56. Deboer J, et al. Molecular alterations as target for therapy in metastatic osteosarcoma. Clin Exp Metastasis. 2011;28(5):493–503.
57. Kager L, et al. Primary metastatic osteosarcoma: presentation and outcome of patients treated on neoadjuvant cooperative osteosarcoma study group protocols. J Clinc ONcol. 2003;21:3108–14.
58. Bacci G, et al. Osteogenic sarcoma of the extremity with detectable lung metastases at presentation. Cancer. 1997;79(2):245–54.
59. Aljubra A, et al. Osteosarcoma in adolescent and adults: survival analysis with and without lung metastases. Ann Oncol. 2009;20(6):1136–41.
60. Goorin A, et al. Phase II/III trial of etoposide and high-dose ifosfamide in newly diagnosed metastatic osteosarcoma. J Clinc Oncol. 2002;20:426–33.
61. Meyers P, et al. Osteogenic sarcoma with clinically detectable metastasis at initial presentation. J Clinc Oncol. 1993;11:449–53.
62. Boye K, et al. High-dose chemotherapy with stem cell rescue in the primary treatment of metastatic and pelvic osteosarcoma. Pediatr Blood Cancer. 2014;16:840–5.
63. NCCN NCCN Guidelines for Bone Cancer. J Nat Comprehens Cancer Network. 2017; 15(2).
64. Meyer J, et al. Imaging guidelines for children with Ewing sarcoma and osteosarcoma: a report from the Children's oncology group bone tumour committee. Pediatr Blood Cancer. 2008;51:163.
65. Gelderblom H, et al. Survival after recurrent osteosarcoma: data from 3 European osteosarcoma intergroup (EOI) randomised controlled trials. Eur J Cancer. 2011;47:895–902.
66. Bielack SS, et al. Second and subsequent recurrence of osteosarcoma: presentation, treatment, and outcomes of 249 consecutive cooperative osteosarcoma study group patients. J Clin Oncol. 2008;27:557–65.

67. Gentet J, et al. Ifosfamide and etoposide in childhood osteosarcoma. A phase II study of the French society of Paediatric oncology. Eur J Cancer. 1997;33(2):232–7.
68. Palmerini E, et al. Gemcitabine and docetaxel in relapsed and unresectable high grade osteosarcoma and spindle cell sarcoma of bone. BMC Cancer. 2016;16:280.
69. Berger M, et al. Phase 2 trial of two courses of cyclophosphamide and etoposide for relapsed high-risk osteosarcoma patients. Cancer. 2009;115(13):2980–7.
70. Loeb D, et al. Dose-finding study of 153Sm-EDTMP in patients with poor-prognosis osteosarcoma. Cancer. 2009;115:2514–22.
71. Anderson P, et al. Bone-seeking radiopharmaceuticals as targeted agents of osteosarcoma: samarium-153-EDTMP and radium-223. Adv Exp Med Biol. 2014;804:291–304.
72. Grignani G, et al. A phase II trial of sorafenib in relapsed and unresectable high-grade osteosarcoma after failure of standard multi-modal therapy. Ann Oncol. 2012;23:508–16.
73. Duffaud F, et al. Efficacy and safety of regorafenib in adult patients with metastatic osteosarcoma: a non-comparative, randomised, double-blind, placebo-controlled, phase 2 study. Lancet Oncol. 2019;20(1):120–33.
74. Davis L, et al. Randomized double-blind phase II study of Regorafenib in patients with metastatic osteosarcoma. J Clin Oncol. 2019;37(16):1424–31.
75. Whang-Peng J, et al. Cytogenetic characterization of selected small round cell tumors of childhood. Cancer Genet Cytogenet. 1986;21(3):185–208.
76. Burchill S, et al. Ewing's sarcoma: diagnostic, prognostic and therapeutic implications of molecular abnormalities. J Clinc Pathol. 2003;56(2):96–102.
77. May W, et al. The Ewing's sarcoma EWS/FLI-1 fusion gene encodes a more potent transcriptional activator and is a more powerful transforming gene than FLI-1. Mol Cell Biol. 1993;13(12):7393–8.
78. Gamberi G, et al. Molecular diagnosis in Ewing family tumors. J Mol Diagn. 2011;13(3):313–24.
79. Italiano A, et al. High prevalence of CIC fusion with double-homeobox (DUX4) transcription factors in EWSR1-negative undifferentiated small blue round cell sarcomas. Genes Chromosomes Cancer. 2012;51(3):207–18.
80. Bunda S et al. CIC protein instability contributes to tumorigenesis in glioblastoma. Nat Commun. 2019; 10(661).
81. Specht K, et al. Novel BCOR-MAML3 and ZC3H7B-BCOR gene fusions in undifferentiated small blue round cell sarcomas. Am J Surg Pathol. 2016;40:433–42.
82. Puls F, et al. BCOR-CCNB3 (Ewing-like) sarcoma: a clinicopathologic analysis of 10 cases, in comparison with conventional Ewing sarcoma. Am J Surg Pathol. 2014;38(10):1307–18.
83. Renzi S, et al. Ewing-like sarcoma: an emerging family of round cell sarcomas. J Cell Physiol. 2019;234(6):7999–8007.
84. Wang W et al. Undifferentiated "Round" cell ("Ewing-like") sarcoma: not always so-round nor Ewing-like Virchows Archiv. 2017; 470(4):371–372.
85. Jurgens H, et al. Multidisciplinary treatment of primary of Ewing's sarcoma of bone. A 6-year experience of a European cooperative trial. Cancer. 1988;61:23–32.
86. Cotterill S et al. Prognostic factors in Ewing's tumour of bone: an analysis of 975 patients from European Intergroup Cooperative Ewing's Sarcoma Study Group. J Clin Oncol. 2000;3108–14.
87. Sailer S, et al. The role of radiation therapy in localized Ewing' sarcoma. Semin Radiat Oncol. 1997;7(3):225–35.
88. Nesbit M, et al. Multimodal therapy for the management of primary, non-metastatic Ewing's sarcoma of bone: a long-term follow-up of the first intergroup study. J Clin Oncol. 1990;8:1664.
89. Burgert E, et al. Multimodal therapy for the management of nonpelvic, localised Ewing's sarcoma of bone: intergroup study IESS-II. J Clin Oncol. 1990;8:1514.
90. Smith M, et al. Influence of doxorubicin dose intensity on response and outcome for patients with osteogenic sarcoma and Ewing's sarcoma. J Natl Cancer Inst. 1991;83(20):1460.

91. Grier H, et al. Addition of ifosfamide and etoposide to standard chemotherapy for Ewing's sarcoma and primitive neuroectodermal tumour of bone. N Engl J Med. 2003;348:694–701.
92. Paulussen M, et al. Results of the EICESS-92 study: two randomised trials of Ewing's sarcoma treatment - cyclophosphamide compared with ifosfamide in standard-risk patients and assessment of benefit of etoposide added to standard treatment in high-risk patients. J Clin Oncol. 2008;26:4385–93.
93. Whelan J et al. High-dose chemotherapy and blood autologous stem-cell rescue compared with standard chemotherapy in localised high-risk Ewing Sarcoma: result of EURO--E.W.I.N.G.99 and Ewing-2008. J Clin Oncol. 2018;36(31): 3110–3119.
94. Patrico M, et al. Ewing's sarcoma in children: twenty-five years of experience at the Instituto Portuges de Oncologica de Francisco Gentil. J Surg Oncol. 1991;47:37–40.
95. Cangir A, et al. Ewing's sarcoma metastatic at diagnosis. Results and comparisons of two intergroup Ewing's sarcoma studies. Cancer. 1990;66:887–93.
96. Balamuth N, et al. Ewing's sarcoma. Lancet Oncol. 2011;11:184–92.
97. Paulussen M, et al. Primary metastatic (stage IV) Ewing tumour: survival analysis of 171 patients from the EICESS studies. Ann Oncol. 1998;9(3):275.
98. Ladenstein R, et al. Primary disseminated multifocal Ewing sarcoma: results of the Euro-EWING 99 trial. J Clin Oncol. 2010;28(20):3284–91.
99. Dirken U, et al. Efficacy of busulfan-melphalan high dose chemotherapy consolidation compared to conventional chemotherapy combined with lung irradiation in Ewing sarcoma with primary lung metastases: result of EURO-EWING 99-R2pulm randomised trial. J Clin Oncol. 2016;34(15):110001.
100. Ferrari S, et al. Post-relapse survival in patients with Ewing sarcoma. Paediatr Blood Cancer. 2015;62(6):994–9.
101. Leavey P, et al. Prognostic factors for patients with Ewing sarcoma at first recurrence following multi-modality therapy: a report from Children's oncology group. Pediatr Blood Cancer. 2008;51(3):334–8.
102. Bacci G, et al. Metachronous pulmonary metastases resection in patients with Ewing's sarcoma initially treated with adjuvant or neoadjuvant chemotherapy. Eur J Cancer. 1995;31(6):999.
103. Casey DA, et al. Irinotecan and temozolomide for Ewing sarcoma: the memorial Sloan-Kettering experience. Pediatr Blood Cancer. 2009;53:1029–34.
104. Blanchette P S et al. Irinotecan and temozolomide in adults with recurrent sarcoma. J Solid Tumours. 2015; 5(2)
105. Wagner LM, et al. Phase I trial of temozolomide and protracted irinotecan in pediatric patients with refractory solid tumours. Clin Cancer Res. 2004;10:840–8.
106. Rabciborska A, et al. Vincristine, irinotecan and temozolomide in patients with relapsed and refractory Ewing sarcoma. Pediatr Blood Cancer. 2013;60:1621–5.
107. Saylors R, et al. Cyclophosphamide plus topotecan in children with recurrent or refractory solid tumours: a pediatric oncology group phase II study. J Clin Oncol. 2001;19(15):2463.
108. Navid F, et al. Combination of gemcitabine and docetaxel in treatment for patients with refractory bone sarcoma. Cancer. 2008;113:419–25.
109. Kbudi R, et al. Oral etoposide for recurrent/progression sarcomas of childhood. Pediatr Blood and cancer. 2003;42(4):320–4.
110. Ferrari S, et al. Response to high-dose ifosfamide in patients with advanced/recurrent Ewing sarcoma. Pediatr Blood Cancer. 2009;52(5):581–4.
111. Tenneti P, et al. Role of high-dose chemotherapy and autologous hematopoietic cell transplantation for children and young adults with relapsed Ewing's sarcoma: a systematic review. Blood. 2017;130:2014.
112. Schuck A et al. Local therapy in localised Ewing tumours: results of 1058 patients treated in the CESS 81, CESS 86 and EICESS 92 trials. Int J Radiat Oncol Biol. 55: 168–177.
113. Garcia-Castellano J et al. Histopathologic and radiologic assessment of chemotherapeutic response in Ewing's sarcoma: a review. Sarcoma. 2012; 357–424.
114. Lin T, et al. Timing of local therapy affect survival in Ewing sarcoma. Int J Radiat Oncol Biol Phys. 2019;104(1):127–36.

115. Turcotte R, et al. Giant cell tumour of bone. Orthop Clin A Arm. 2006;37(1):35–51.
116. Viswanathan S, et al. Metastatic giant cell tumour of bone: are there associated factors and best treatment modalities? Clin Orthop Relat Res. 2009;468(3):827–33.
117. Donthineni R, et al. Metastatic behaviour of giant cell tumour of the spine. Int Orthop. 2009;34:384.
118. Sobti A, et al. Giant cell tumor of bone. Arch Bone Jt Surg. 2016;4(1):2–9.
119. Campanacci M, et al. Giant cell tumour of bone. J Bone Joint Surg Am. 1987;69:106–14.
120. Kivioja A, et al. Cement is recommended in intralesional surgery of giant cell tumours: a Scandinavian sarcoma group study of 294 patient followed for a median time of 5 years. Acta Orthop. 2008;79:86.
121. Lewis V, et al. Argon beam coagulation as an adjuvant for local control of giant cell tumour. Clin Orthop. 2007;454:192–7.
122. Durr H, et al. Phenol as an adjuvant for local control in the treatment of giant cell tumour of the bone. Eur J Surg Oncol. 1999;25:610.
123. Malawer M et al. Cryosurgery in the treatment of giant cell tumour. A long-term followup study. Clin Orthop Relat Res. 1999; 176.
124. Luengo-Alonso G, et al. Denosumab treatment for giant-cell tumour of bone: a systematic review of the literature. Arch Orthop Trauma Surg. 2019;139:1339.
125. Khodamorad J, et al. Denosumab in patients with giant cell tumor and its recurrence: a systematic review. Archiv Bone Joint Surg. 2018;6(4):260–8.
126. Marvogenis A et al. Giant cell tumor of bone revisited. SICOT J. 3:54.
127. Rutkowski P, et al. Surgical downstaging in an open-label phase II trial of denosumab in patients with giant cell tumor of bone. Ann Surg Oncol. 2015;22(9):2860–8.
128. Chawla S, et al. Safety and efficacy of denosumab for adults and skeletally mature adolescents with giant cell tumour of bone: interim analysis of an open-label, parallel-group, phase 2 study. Lancet Oncol. 2013;14(9):901–8.
129. Errani C, et al. Denosumab may increase the risk of local recurrence in patients with giant-cell tumour of bone treated with curettage. J Bone Joint Surg Am. 2018;100(6):496–504.
130. Lipplaa A, et al. Adjuvant zoledronic acid in high risk giant cell tumor of bone: a multi-Centre randomised phase II study. Oncologist. 2019;24:1–7.
131. Wei F, et al. Interferon alfa-2b for recurrence and metastatic giant cell tumor of the spine: report of two cases. Spine. 2010;15(35):1418–22.
132. Kaiser U, et al. Generalised giant-cell tumour of bone: successful treatment of pulmonary metastases with interferon-alpha. J Cancer Res Clinc Oncol. 1993;119(5):301.
133. Gonazalez Vela J, et al. Therapy with alpha interferon for advanced and metastatic giant cell tumor of bone. J Clin Oncol. 2005;23(16):9078.
134. Stewart D, et al. Prolonged disease-free survival following surgical debulking and high-dose cisplatin/doxorubicin in a patient with bulky metastases from giant cell tumor of bone refractory to "standard" chemotherapy. Am J Clin Oncol. 1995;18(2):144–8.
135. Mella O, et al. Chemotherapy of a malignant, metastasizing giant cell-tumour of bone: report of an unusual case and the response to combination chemotherapy. Cancer. 1982;50(2):207–11.
136. Evans H, et al. Prognostic factors in chondrosarcoma of bone: a clinicopathologic analysis with emphasis on histologic grading. Cancer. 1977;40(2):818–3.
137. Sjoerd N et al. The identification of prognostic factors and survival statistics of conventional central chondrosarcoma. Sarcoma. 2015;11.
138. Andreou D, et al. Survival and prognostic factors in chondrosarcoma. Acta Orthop. 2011;82(6):749–55.
139. Andreou G, et al. Metastatic potential of grade I chondrosarcoma of bone: results of a multi-institutional study. Ann Surg Oncol. 2016;23:120–5.
140. Van Praag V, et al. Incidence, outcomes and prognostic factors during 25 years of treatment of chondrosarcoma. Surg Oncol. 2018;27(3):402–8.
141. Angelini A, et al. Clinical outcome of central, conventional chondrosarcoma. J Surg Oncol. 2012;106(8):929–37.

142. Reiedel R, et al. The clinical management of chondrosarcoma. Curr Treat Options in Oncol. 2009;10:94–106.
143. Unni K, et al. Chondrosarcoma: clear-cell variant. A report of sixteen cases. J Bone Joint Surg Am. 1976;58:676–832.
144. Bjornsoon J, et al. Clear cell chondrosarcoma of bone. Observation in 47 cases. Am J Surg Pathol. 1984;8:223–30.
145. Present D, et al. Clear cell chondrosarcoma of bone. A report of 8 cases. Skelet Radiol. 1991;20(3):187–91.
146. Dahlin D, et al. Dedifferentiation of low-grade chondrosarcoma. Cancer. 1971;28(2):461 6.
147. Staals E, et al. Dedifferentiated central chondrosarcoma. Cancer. 2006;106(12):2682–91.
148. Nussbeck W, et al. Mesenchymal chondrosarcoma: an immunohistochemical study of 10 cases examining prognostic significance of proliferative activity and cellular differentiated. Pathology. 2004;36(3):230–3.
149. Huvos A, et al. Mesenchymal chondrosarcoma. A clinicopathological analysis of 35 patients with emphasis on treatment. Cancer. 1983;51(7):1230–7.
150. Salvati M et al. Central nervous system mesenchymal chondrosarcoma. 2005; 24(2): 317–323.
151. Nakashmia Y, et al. Mesenchymal chondrosarcoma of bone and soft tissue. A review of 111 cases. Cancer. 1986;57(12):2444–53.
152. J Xu J et al. Mesenchymal chondrosarcoma of bone and soft tissue. A systemic review of 107 patients in the past 20 years. PLoS ONe. 2015;10(4).
153. Hanna S, et al. Outcome of intralesional curettage for low-grade chondrosarcoma of long bones. Eur J Surg Oncol. 2009;35(12):1343–7.
154. Dantonello T, et al. Mesenchymal chondrosarcoma of soft tissue and bone in children, adolescent and young adults. Cancer. 2008;112(11):2424–31.
155. Frezzia AM, et al. Mesenchymal chondrosarcoma: prognostic factors and outcome in 113 patients. A European musculoskeletal oncology society study. Eur J Cancer. 2015;51(3):374–81.
156. Italiano A, et al. Advanced chondrosarcoma: role of chemotherapy and survival. Ann Oncol. 2013;24(11):2916–22.
157. Dickey I, et al. Dedifferentiated chondrosarcoma: the role of chemotherapy with updated outcomes. J Bone Joint Surg Am. 2004;86(11):2412–8.
158. Grimer R, et al. Dedifferentiated chondrosarcoma: prognostic factors and outcome from a European group. Eur J Cancer. 2007;43(14):2060–5.
159. Nakamura T, et al. Oncological outcome after lung metastasis in patients presenting with localized chondrosarcoma at extremities: Tokai musculoskeletal oncology consortium study. Onco Targets Ther. 2016;9:4747–51.
160. Nooji M, et al. Doxorubicin and cisplatin chemotherapy in high-grade spindle cell sarcomas of the bone, other than osteosarcoma or malignant fibrous histiocytoma: a European osteosarcoma intergroup study. Eur J Cancer. 2005;41(2):225.
161. Schuetze S, et al. Phase 2 study of dasatinib in patients with previously treated, high grade advanced sarcoma. Cancer. 2016;122(6):868–74.
162. Grigani G, et al. A phase 2 trial of imatinib mesylate in patients with recurrent non-resectable chondrosarcomas expressing platelet-derived growth factor receptor-alpha or -beta: an Italian sarcoma group study. Cancer. 2011;117(4):826–31.
163. Mejier D et al. Expression of aromatase and estrogen receptor alpha in chondrosarcoma, but no beneficial effect of inhibiting estrogen signalling in vitro and in vivo. Clin Sarcoma Res. 2011;1(5).
164. Bernstein-Molho R, et al. Clinical activity of mTOR inhibition in combination with cyclophosphamide in the treatment of recurrent unresectable chondrosarcomas. Cancer Chemother Pharmacol. 2012;70(6):855–60.
165. Amary M et al. central and periosteal chondromas but not in other mesenchymal tumours. J Pathol. 2011; 224(3): 334–343.

166. Wasserman J, et al. Chordoma of the head and neck: a review. Head Neck Pathol. 2018;12(2):261–8.
167. Stacchiotti S, et al. Building a global consensus approach to chordoma: a position paper from the medical and patient community. Lancet Oncol. 2015;16:71–83.
168. Ruggieri P, et al. Surgical margins and local control in resection of sacral chordomas. Clin Orthop Relat Res. 2010;468(11):2939–47.
169. Amchietti M et al. The treatment of chordoma and chondrosarcoma of the skull base with particular attention to radiotherapy. Clin Oncol. 2017; 2: 1195.
170. Moojen V, et al. Long-term results: adjuvant radiotherapy in en bloc resection of sacrococcygeal chordoma is advisable. Spine. 2011;36:656–61.
171. Presneau N, et al. Potential therapeutic targets for chordoma: PI3K/AKT/TSC1/TSC2/mTOR pathway. Br J Cancer. 2009;100(9):1406–14.
172. Shalaby A, et al. The role of epidermal growth factor receptor in chordoma pathogenesis: a potential therapeutic target. J Pathol. 2011;233(3):336–46.
173. Tamborini E, et al. Molecular and biochemical analyses of platelet-derived growth factor receptor (PDGFR) B, PDGFRA and KIT receptors in chordomas. Clin Cancer Res. 2006;12:6920–8.
174. Stacchioti S, et al. Phase II study of imatinib in advanced chordoma. J Clinc Oncol. 2012;30(9):914–20.
175. Stacchiotti S, et al. Response to imatinib plus sirolimus in advanced chordoma. Ann Oncol. 2009;20(11):1886–94.
176. Stacchiotti S, et al. Phase II study on lapatinib in advanced EGFR-positive chordoma. Ann Oncol. 2013;24(7):1931–6.
177. Bompas E. Sorafenib in patients with locally advanced and metastatic chordomas: a phase II trial of the French sarcoma group (GSF/GETO). Ann Oncol. 2015;26(10):2168–73.

The Importance of Margins in Sarcoma Surgery

13

Peter F. M. Choong and Claudia Di Bella

13.1 Introduction

Sarcoma was first used as a term [1] to describe a tumour based on its fleshy feel and gross appearance almost 200 years ago by the London surgeon, John Abernethy, whose name sarcoma first bore (Abernethy's sarcoma). 75 years after that Samuel Gross, another renowned surgeon, described it as a highly aggressive tumour second only to carcinoma by the way it "infected" the surrounding tissues. He recommended amputation, despite the 30% operative mortality at that time because of his observations that any attempt at local resection was almost uniformly met with local recurrence, metastasis and death [2]. Presumably, what Gross was describing was the highly invasive, locally recurrent and systemically aggressive nature of sarcoma which treatment at the time was hampered by the lack of clear knowledge of surgical margins or availability of adjuvant treatment. Gross had erroneously attributed the locally recurrent nature of the tumour to its biological aggressiveness rather than the inadequacy of surgical resection.

It was almost 150 years later, before William Enneking published a body of work [3–7] which reflected for the first time a better understanding of the nature of sarcoma growth, its relationship to surrounding tissues and, therefore, what was required to excise the tumour completely. His concept of surgical margins was the basis of the development of his surgical staging system [4] which was subsequently adopted by the American Musculoskeletal Tumour Society (MSTS). This was a preoperative anatomic-based approach to surgical planning that aimed to resect tumour with the best local control rate while preserving limb function where

P. F. M. Choong (✉) · C. Di Bella
Department of Surgery, University of Melbourne, Melbourne, VIC, Australia

Department of Orthopaedics, St. Vincent's Hospital, Melbourne, VIC, Australia

Bone & Soft Tissue Tumour Service, Peter MacCallum Cancer Centre, Melbourne, VIC, Australia
e-mail: pchoong@unimelb.edu.au; claudia.dibella@unimelb.edu.au

P. F. M. Choong (ed.), *Sarcoma*, https://doi.org/10.1007/978-981-15-9414-4_13

possible. Today, surgery with adequate surgical margins is the mainstay of treatment with curative intent.

The basis of the MSTS system was that sarcomas (bone and soft tissue) were surrounded by specific anatomic layers and the ability to control local recurrence was predicated on the characteristics of the anatomic layers that were left intact around a tumour at the time of its removal. Four distinct surgical margins were described [4], including intralesional, marginal, wide and radical, each sequentially providing a stronger barrier to invasion and hence lower incidence of local recurrence of tumour (Figs. 13.1 and 13.2).

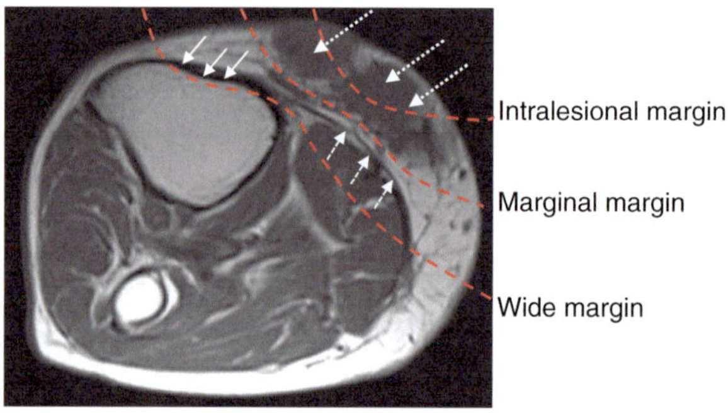

Fig. 13.1 Axial T1-weighted MRI of subcutaneous soft tissue sarcoma in lower leg (dotted arrows). Intralesional margin passes through subcutaneous tumour. Marginal margin passes through inflammatory pseudocapsule. Wide margin passes deep to periosteum of tibia, under deep fascia and includes layer of gastrocnemius. Periosteum (solid white arrows). Deep fascia (dashed white arrows). Margins (dashed red line)

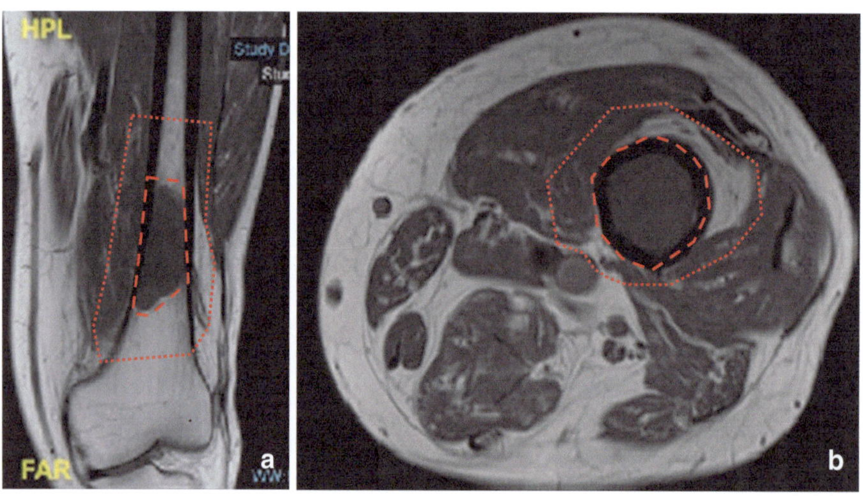

Fig. 13.2 (**a**) Coronal and (**b**) axial T1-weighted MRI of femoral bone sarcoma. Intralesional margin passes through tumour, for example, if treated with intramedullary rod fixation or curettage. Marginal margin passes immediately adjacent to tumour and subperiosteally (dashed red line). Wide margin passes includes periosteum and a cuff of surrounding muscle or fascia (dotted red line). The proximal and distal bone margin is at least 2 cm but may be as wide as 5 cm from the tumour depending on the response to chemotherapy

At the time that Enneking was first developing his concepts, imaging modalities were few, and quality was limited. Soft tissue imaging was restricted to early generations of computed tomography [8]. Positron emission tomography was experimental, and the response to neoadjuvant treatment was inferred by indirect information from ancillary tests. For example, the loss of neovascularisation on angiography [9], the appearance of cystic change within tumours or the appearance of calcification on plain radiographs and reduction of bone and soft tissue nuclear activity after neoadjuvant treatment [10, 11] were correlated with tumour response. Because of the reliance on indirect evidence and to ensure the highest quality of margins, surgeons often took far wider margins than may have been necessary.

With the advent of magnetic resonance imaging [12], more sophisticated computed tomography and PET scanning [13], greater detail about the tissues surrounding a tumour and more information regarding the responsiveness of the tumour to neoadjuvant treatment have allowed the surgical margins to be tailored to individual situations, and the size of surgical margins has decreased over time (Fig. 13.3). It is important to note, however, that tumour margins are classified according to the narrowest margin obtained, because tumour behaviour with regard to local recurrence is related to the narrowest margin achieved [14].

Since the development of the MSTS system, the heterogeneity of published classification systems has made defining adequacy of surgical margins challenging. A recent comparison of surgical margins classified by the American Joint Committee on Cancer (AJCC) R, MSTS categories and metric distance was undertaken on 166

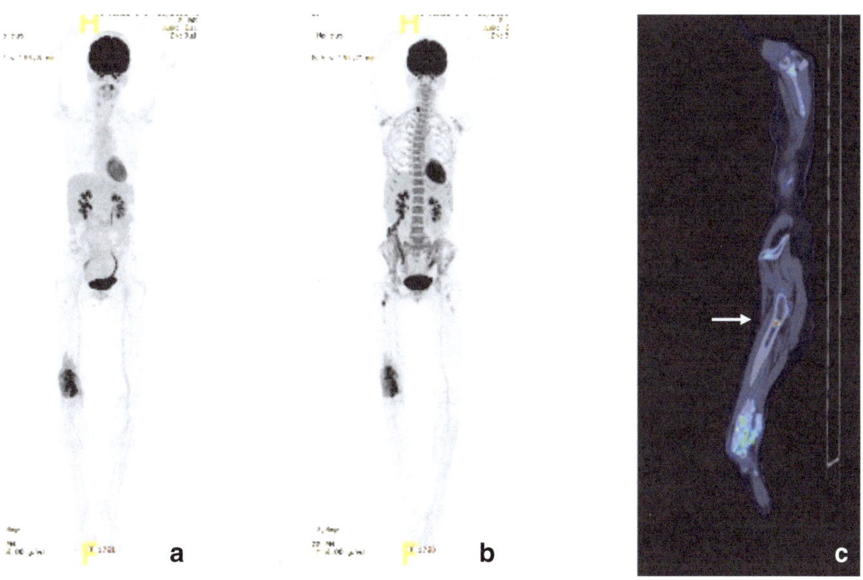

Fig. 13.3 PET scan (**a**) on diagnosis (**b**) after neoadjuvant chemotherapy. Note ipsilateral proximal femoral tracer uptake (**b**) and (**c**) (white arrow) indicating poor response to chemotherapy and development of skip metastasis. This was treated with total femoral resection

primary high-grade sarcomas which had not received neoadjuvant therapy [15]. The comparison reported that the MSTS system and metric distance showed higher sensitivity and negative predictive value in comparison to the AJCC R classification. The authors recommended that the MSTS system or metric distance be used and reported that "Musculoskeletal Tumor Society wide/radical margins or tumor clearances of 5 mm (without adjuvant radiotherapy) or 1 mm (with adjuvant radiotherapy) appear to define the minimum safe surgical resection margins necessary to decrease the likelihood of local recurrence of high-grade pleomorphic sarcomas of the extremity or trunk" [15]. In comparison to the R system, the MSTS and metric distance is a preoperative planning system for surgery where specific anatomical structures are identified, measured and included in the operative plan. The AJCC R system, however, is a post hoc finding reported by the pathologists and does not give any indication as to the preoperative planning involved in the resection.

13.2 Special Considerations

13.2.1 Response to Neoadjuvant Treatment

The responsiveness of sarcoma to neoadjuvant therapy has been shown to have an inverse relationship to local recurrence of disease [16–18]. Moreover, this may be accentuated if margins less than wide margins are achieved [18]. For example, the risk of local failure is three times higher with poor responders to chemotherapy when adequate margins are used. The risk is five times higher when good responders are treated with inadequate margins. However, when poor responders are treated with inadequate margins, the risk of local recurrence is 50 times greater.

13.2.2 Tumour Grade

Higher-grade tumours are more susceptible to local recurrence of disease [19–21]. This may be a manifestation of biological aggressiveness with satellite lesions existing well outside the inflammatory pseudocapsule and acting as local metastases. Moreover, the operative site may also behave as a *locus minoris resistentiae* attracting circulating tumour cells to attach and multiply locally. These mechanisms may explain the unexpected local recurrences in association with tumours that have been resected with wide surgical margins. It is recommended that high-grade tumours be resected with generous margins to mitigate against the incidence of unexpected local recurrences and adjuvant therapy be employed.

Low-grade tumours, such as low-grade myxoid tumours or well-differentiated lipoma-like liposarcomas, are often excised with a belief that the same level of fastidiousness to surgical margins that apply to higher-grade tumours may not apply to low-grade varieties. However, studies continue to show that the incidence of local recurrence is related to the quality of the surgical margin. In this regard, consideration should be made of the context in which low-grade tumours are treated. Studies

[22] have reported that low-grade tumours that are less than 5 cm may be resected with wide margins without requiring neoadjuvant radiotherapy. Larger tumours (>5 cm) or those where marginal margins are anticipated, however, have been shown to benefit from local radiotherapy. This suggests that judicious use of radiotherapy may be considered if a decision mandates that a narrow margin is to be used or if surgery is to be performed in a large >5 cm tumour.

13.2.3 Unplanned Excision

Despite information regarding the appropriate management of sarcoma that promotes multidisciplinary tumour centre-based care being publicised in the literature, inadvertent surgery and inexpert care continue to be delivered even in cities where tumour centres exist. Almost one third of all sarcoma presentations to a tumour centre are following inadvertent resection [23–25]. The incidence of inadequate margins is significantly higher with advertent resection than as planned resections. Even when sarcoma is suspected and treated in non-tumour centres [26], the incidence of inadequate excisions is higher than if the tumour was treated at a tumour centre. The consequence is commonly more extensive re-excisions, higher rates of amputation, more complex reconstructions, higher local recurrence rates and a greater risk of death from disease [23, 24].

13.2.4 Histotype and Depth

Local recurrence of sarcoma is often a direct result of the quality of the surgical margin. However, in certain circumstances, the biological characteristics of the tumour may impart a greater risk of local recurrence because of the tendency for local regional metastases (angiosarcoma) [27], infiltrative invasive behaviour (dermatofibrosarcoma protuberans DFSP) [28], and significant inflammatory pseudocapsule (myxofibrosarcoma) [29]. Tumour depth has been found to be an independent prognostic indicator for local recurrence [19]. Whether deeper tumours are associated with greater surgical complexity and therefore more difficult margin attainment remains unclear.

13.3 MSTS Classification of Surgical Margins

13.3.1 Intralesional Margin

Any incision that passed through the capsule of the tumour is regarded as an intralesional margin. The potential outcome of this is spillage of tumour cells outside the tumour with subsequent contamination of the surrounding tissue during the procedure or post-operative haematoma. Intralesional surgery usually occurs in association with inadvertent excisions of sarcoma. This is to be avoided at all cost as the consequence of contamination of the surrounding tissue may be a complex re-excision and reconstruction, amputation or worse still an increased risk of death from disease (local recurrence and/or metastasis). The only time that intralesional surgery may be contemplated is when it is part of an open biopsy. Because of the attendant risks, this should only be performed by a sarcoma expert.

13.3.2 Marginal Margin

The centrifugal nature of sarcoma growth with expansion outward compresses surrounding tissue that abuts the tumour. In addition, the cytokines released by the tumour invoke an inflammatory response around the tumour margin which together with the compressed tissue form an inflammatory pseudocapsule. The inflammatory nature around the tumour is associated with localised oedema, and this allows easy dissection of the pseudocapsule. When tumours are removed by dissection through the inflammatory pseudocapsule, it is often described as "shelling out". This gives the surgeon a false sense of security that the tumour has been removed in its entirety. Unfortunately, the pseudocapsule, being inflamed and hypervascular, contains satellite lesions which are not grossly visible but when left behind by surgery that transgresses the pseudocapsule has a very high risk of reappearing as a local recurrence of tumour.

Application of marginal margins is sometimes required in order to preserve adjacent neurovascular or other vital structures. For example, the flexor fossae (axilla, femoral triangle, cubital fossa) are not well compartmentalised, and sarcomas arising within these spaces frequently abut against the neurovascular structures that pass through it. In order to preserve these structures, dissection of the adventitia of the vessel or the epineurium is required to preserve an anatomic structure between the tumour and the vital structure. The quality of the margin can be upgraded with the application of preoperative radiotherapy in these situations. In this regard, marginal margins and radiotherapy can give local control rates equivalent to wide margins alone.

13.3.3 Wide Margin

Wide surgical margins are those that leave a cuff of normal tissue around the tumour and are associated with a low risk of recurrence of disease. When Enneking first developed the concept of surgical margins, it was recommended that normal tissue was divided at least 5 cm from the proximal and distal extent of the tumour in the longitudinal directions and that a normal named anatomic layer be included in radial direction from the tumour. Using this margin, a considerable amount of normal tissue was removed with the tumour. Over time, this has been modified such that lesser amounts of tissue are removed while still being true to the concept of removal with a cuff of normal tissue.

The early Scandinavian experience suggested that instead of excising a tumour with a normal named anatomic layer of tissue around it, the amount of normal tissue could be reduced in the excision by just including the tissue in which the tumour arose [30]. For example, a tumour arising from a muscle could be excised simply by myectomy of that muscle, rather than excising the tumour, the muscle in which it arose and another layer outside the muscle. This was popularised, but in the absence of radiotherapy, the results later demonstrated that the amount of residual tissue around the tumour may not be sufficient to provide good local control and the risk of recurrence approached that of a marginal margin [25, 31].

In the mid-1990s, the Japanese experience promoted a better understanding of the physical barrier that certain tissues provided against tumour invasion, and this led to an emphasis on the quality of the surgical margin rather than just the quantity [32]. It was felt that some tissues were of sufficient robustness as to be a strong barrier against tumour invasion despite being only millimetres thick. For example, the articular cartilage seemed to be a natural barrier to tumour invasion despite being only millimetres thick and in the face of bone tumours that could invade through thick cortical bone. The fascia lata may also be a few millimetres thick and yet was a strong barrier against invasion from a sarcoma arising from the quadriceps muscle.

Researchers in the field were able to compare different tissues and assign to them relative thicknesses (in cm) that allowed surgeons to plan margins that complied with the principles of wide margin surgery. For example, a thick fascia (2–3 mm), e.g. facia lata, was found to be equivalent to 3 cm of muscle. Therefore, if this covered a quadriceps tumour, then this was all the tissue that was required to be excised with the tumour to achieve a wide margin on that aspect of the tumour. In comparison, muscle alone was a poor barrier to tumour, so the thickness of muscle around a tumour to be included with the resected tumour that would be equivalent to the fascia lata was 3 cm.

A practical definition of a wide margin is that the tumour had a cuff of normal tissue around it that extended more than 2 cm to the tumour in the longitudinal plane and included one named anatomic layer in the radial plane that in quality was equivalent to 3 cm of muscle.

13.3.4 Radical Margin

A radical margin is employed when the contents of the entire tumour-bearing compartment is removed. The body is divided into multiple anatomic compartments. For example, the quadriceps muscle lies within the anterior compartment of the thigh, the hamstring musculature lie within the posterior compartment of the thigh and the adductor muscles lie within the adductor compartment. Each compartment is separated from the other by intermuscular septae (e.g. medial, lateral), and each compartment has a major neurovascular structure running through it. Resection of the entire quadriceps from its origin to insertion is referred to as a radical resection as there are no other muscles left within that compartment. The vessels in that compartment are surrounded by a thick adventitia which may be dissected and left between the vessel and the tumour as a defined boundary/margin. In certain circumstances, this characteristic of the vessel may permit its preservation. Other times, if the tumour surrounds the vessel, then it would have to be sacrificed and reconstructed as part of the radical resection. With better imaging and the use of radiotherapy, fewer radical resections are now performed, as planning of surgical margins can be undertaken with considerable accuracy because of the high definition of both MRI and CT scans these days. Radical resections are now usually preserved for situations where there has been intracompartmental contamination due to prior surgery.

13.3.5 Adequacy of Surgical Margins

Radical and wide margin surgery are often classified as adequate, while intralesional and marginal margins are classified as inadequate for local control of disease if no other modality of treatment is applied. The addition of radiotherapy in soft tissue sarcoma and chemotherapy in bone sarcoma has the potential to upgrade the quality of the margin. In special circumstances radiotherapy may also be employed in bone sarcoma (Ewing's), and chemotherapy is employed in certain centres for soft tissue sarcoma. In both of these cases, the use of these modalities in a neoadjuvant setting has been shown to provide local control benefit.

Margin	Adequacy
Radical	Adequate
Wide	
Marginal + radiotherapy	
Marginal	Inadequate
Intralesional	

13.3.6 Amputation

It is often misconceived that an amputation provides better local control of tumour than attempts at local excision. In fact, it is the adequacy of the surgical margin that correlates to the incidence of local recurrence not the type of procedure. A marginal margin amputation is no better than a local excision with the same margin. Similarly, a wide or radical margin amputation is as good as a similar margin used for local excision. The choice of whether an amputation is used or not will depend on whether the limb is deemed to be functional following local excision, whether the defect created after a local excision is reconstructable, whether a local excision creates too great a risk to the ongoing treatment of the individual, whether the patient chooses amputation or not as the primary procedure or whether the procedures is for palliative or curative intent.

References

1. Abernethy J. Attempts to form a classification of tumours according to their anatomical structures. London: Longman and Rees; 1817.
2. Gross S. Sarcoma of the long bones: based on a study of one hundred sixty-five cases. Am J Med Sci. 1879;8:338–77.
3. Enneking WF. Advances and treatment of primary bone tumors. J Fla Med Assoc. 1979;66(1):28–30.
4. Enneking WF, Spanier SS, Goodman MA. A system for the surgical staging of musculoskeletal sarcoma. Clin Orthop Relat Res. 1980;(153):106–20.
5. Enneking WF, Springfield DS. Osteosarcoma. Orthop Clin North Am. 1977;8(4):785–803.
6. Simon MA, Enneking WF. The management of soft-tissue sarcomas of the extremities. J Bone Joint Surg Am. 1976;58(3):317–27.
7. Simon MA, Spanier SS, Enneking WF. Management of adult soft-tissue sarcomas of the extremities. Surg Annu. 1979;11:363–402.
8. Hudson TM, Schiebler M, Springfield DS, Hawkins IF Jr, Enneking WF, Spanier SS. Radiologic imaging of osteosarcoma: role in planning surgical treatment. Skelet Radiol. 1983;10(3):137–46.
9. Hudson TM, Enneking WF, Hawkins IF Jr. The value of angiography in planning surgical treatment of bone tumors. Radiology. 1981;138(2):283–92.
10. Enneking WF, Chew FS, Springfield DS, Hudson TM, Spanier SS. The role of radionuclide bone-scanning in determining the resectability of soft-tissue sarcomas. J Bone Joint Surg Am. 1981;63(2):249–57.
11. Chew FS, Hudson TM, Enneking WF. Radionuclide imaging of soft tissue neoplasms. Semin Nucl Med. 1981;11(4):266–76.
12. Iwata S, Araki A, Funatsu H, Yonemoto T, Kamoda H, Itami M, et al. Optimal surgical margin for infiltrative soft tissue sarcomas: assessing the efficacy of excising beyond the infiltration. J Surg Oncol. 2018;118(3):525–31.
13. Kandathil A, Subramaniam RM. PET/computed tomography and precision medicine. Musculoskeletal Sarcoma PET Clin. 2017;12(4):475–88.
14. Virkus WW, Marshall D, Enneking WF, Scarborough MT. The effect of contaminated surgical margins revisited. Clin Orthop Relat Res. 2002;397:89–94.
15. Cates MM, Cates JMM. Surgical resection margin classifications for high-grade pleomorphic soft tissue sarcomas of the extremity or trunk: definitions of adequate resection margins and recommendations for sampling margins from primary resection specimens. Mod Pathol. 2019;
16. Andreou D, Bielack SS, Carrle D, Kevric M, Kotz R, Winkelmann W, et al. The influence of tumor- and treatment-related factors on the development of local recurrence in osteosarcoma after adequate surgery. An analysis of 1355 patients treated on neoadjuvant cooperative osteosarcoma study group protocols. Ann Oncol. 2011;22(5):1228–35.
17. Bacci G, Forni C, Longhi A, Ferrari S, Mercuri M, Bertoni F, et al. Local recurrence and local control of non-metastatic osteosarcoma of the extremities: a 27-year experience in a single institution. J Surg Oncol. 2007;96(2):118–23.
18. Picci P, Sangiorgi L, Rougraff BT, Neff JR, Casadei R, Campanacci M. Relationship of chemotherapy-induced necrosis and surgical margins to local recurrence in osteosarcoma. J Clin Oncol. 1994;12(12):2699–705.
19. Liu CY, Yen CC, Chen WM, Chen TH, Chen PC, Wu HT, et al. Soft tissue sarcoma of extremities: the prognostic significance of adequate surgical margins in primary operation and reoperation after recurrence. Ann Surg Oncol. 2010;17(8):2102–11.
20. Sabolch A, Feng M, Griffith K, Rzasa C, Gadzala L, Feng F, et al. Risk factors for local recurrence and metastasis in soft tissue sarcomas of the extremity. Am J Clin Oncol. 2012;35(2):151–7.

21. Posch F, Leitner L, Bergovec M, Bezan A, Stotz M, Gerger A, et al. Can multistate modeling of local recurrence, distant metastasis, and death improve the prediction of outcome in patients with soft tissue sarcomas? Clin Orthop Relat Res. 2017;475(5):1427–35.
22. Choong PF, Petersen IA, Nascimento AG, Sim FH. Is radiotherapy important for low-grade soft tissue sarcoma of the extremity? Clin Orthop Relat Res. 2001;387:191–9.
23. Bianchi G, Sambri A, Cammelli S, Galuppi A, Cortesi A, Righi A, et al. Impact of residual disease after "unplanned excision" of primary localized adult soft tissue sarcoma of the extremities: evaluation of 452 cases at a single institution. Musculoskelet Surg. 2017;101(3):243–8.
24. Charoenlap C, Imanishi J, Tanaka T, Slavin J, Ngan SY, Chander S, et al. Outcomes of unplanned sarcoma excision: impact of residual disease. Cancer Med. 2016;5(6):980–8.
25. Trovik CS. Scandinavian sarcoma group P. local recurrence of soft tissue sarcoma. A Scandinavian sarcoma group project. Acta Orthop Scand Suppl. 2001;72:300):1–31.
26. Choong PF, Gustafson P, Rydholm A. Size and timing of local recurrence predicts metastasis in soft tissue sarcoma. Growth rate index retrospectively analyzed in 134 patients. Acta Orthop Scand. 1995;66(2):147–52.
27. Salas S, Stoeckle E, Collin F, Bui B, Terrier P, Guillou L, et al. Superficial soft tissue sarcomas (S-STS): a study of 367 patients from the French sarcoma group (FSG) database. Eur J Cancer. 2009;45(12):2091–102.
28. Llombart B, Monteagudo C, Sanmartin O, Lopez-Guerrero JA, Serra-Guillen C, Poveda A, et al. Dermatofibrosarcoma protuberans: a clinicopathological, immunohistochemical, genetic (COL1A1-PDGFB), and therapeutic study of low-grade versus high-grade (fibrosarcomatous) tumors. J Am Acad Dermatol. 2011;65(3):564–75.
29. Imanishi J, Slavin J, Pianta M, Jackett L, Ngan SY, Tanaka T, et al. Tail of superficial Myxofibrosarcoma and undifferentiated pleomorphic sarcoma after preoperative radiotherapy. Anticancer Res. 2016;36(5):2339–44.
30. Rydholm A, Rooser B, Persson BM. Primary myectomy for sarcoma. J Bone Joint Surg Am. 1986;68(4):586–9.
31. Trovik CS, Bauer HC, Berlin O, Tukiainen E, Erlanson M, Gustafson P, et al. Local recurrence of deep-seated, high-grade, soft tissue sarcoma: 459 patients from the Scandinavian sarcoma group register. Acta Orthop Scand. 2001;72(2):160–6.
32. Kawaguchi N, Ahmed AR, Matsumoto S, Manabe J, Matsushita Y. The concept of curative margin in surgery for bone and soft tissue sarcoma. Clin Orthop Relat Res. 2004;419:165–72.

Surgical Management of Lower Limb Sarcomas

14

Peter F. M. Choong and Grant Pang

The commonest location for both bone and soft tissue sarcomas is the lower limb. The proximal soft tissue of the lower limb sees the highest frequency of soft tissue sarcomas, while the knee joint (distal femur and proximal tibia) is the commonest location for bone sarcomas, in particular, osteosarcoma. The femoral diaphysis is one of the most common sites for the development of Ewing's sarcoma. Chondrosarcomas are one of the commoner primary bone tumours and arise either as a solitary lesion, part of malignant transformation from an osteochondroma or transformation from a constitutional condition such as multiple enchondromatosis (Ollier's disease). Tumours of the lower limb have their greatest functional impact on the mobility of patients. In this regard, limb sparing surgery aims to resect tumours with adequate oncologic margins while preserving sufficient tissue to allow the reconstruction of a functional limb. A functional limb is one that is able to bear weight, allow locomotion and, if possible, remain sensate.

The modern management of lower limb sarcomas is a multidisciplinary approach delivered at an expert tumour centre. Here specialist clinicians include surgical, medical and radiation oncologists, who are supported by a team of pathologists, radiologists, nuclear physicians and cyto- and molecular geneticists. Deliberations occur in a multidisciplinary setting, and a consensus opinion is developed which guides specific treatment.

P. F. M. Choong (✉)
Department of Surgery, University of Melbourne, Melbourne, VIC, Australia

Department of Orthopaedics, St. Vincent's Hospital, Melbourne, VIC, Australia

Bone & Soft Tissue Tumour Service, Peter MacCallum Cancer Centre, Melbourne, VIC, Australia
e-mail: pchoong@unimelb.edu.au

G. Pang
Department of Orthopaedics, St. Vincent's Hospital, Melbourne, VIC, Australia

Bone & Soft Tissue Tumour Service, Peter MacCallum Cancer Centre, Melbourne, VIC, Australia

P. F. M. Choong (ed.), *Sarcoma*, https://doi.org/10.1007/978-981-15-9414-4_14

14.1 Anatomical Considerations

14.1.1 Soft Tissue Sarcomas

14.1.1.1 Buttock Tumours (Fig. 14.1)

Tumours of the buttock are challenging for a number of reasons [1, 2]. First, depending on the depth of the tumour within the gluteal musculature, the functional impact of resection can be significant. Resection of gluteus maximus, the main extensor of the hip and an important antigravity muscle may result in weakness of ascending stairs, rising from chairs and moving quickly across ground. Patients may be left with an extensor lurch from loss of the gluteus maximus.

Resection of the gluteus medius will result in a typical Trendelenburg gait. This is characterised by a drop of the contralateral pelvis and listing of the torso towards the affected side when patient bears weight through the operated side. Superficial buttock tumours may result in sparing of the gluteus medius, but deep buttock tumours almost always result in sacrifice of both the gluteus maximus and medius in an effort to maintain wide margins of resection.

A second challenge of buttock tumours, particularly those which are deep and central in the buttock is the potential to involve the inferior gluteal vasculature. This system of vessels supplies the gluteus maximus. Resection of the tumour in this location will potentially devascularised the gluteus maximus and overlying skin.

A third challenge of buttock tumours is where the tumour has extended to the level of the sciatic notch. Several important named structures emerge from the pelvis through the sciatic notch. These include the sciatic nerve, the superior and

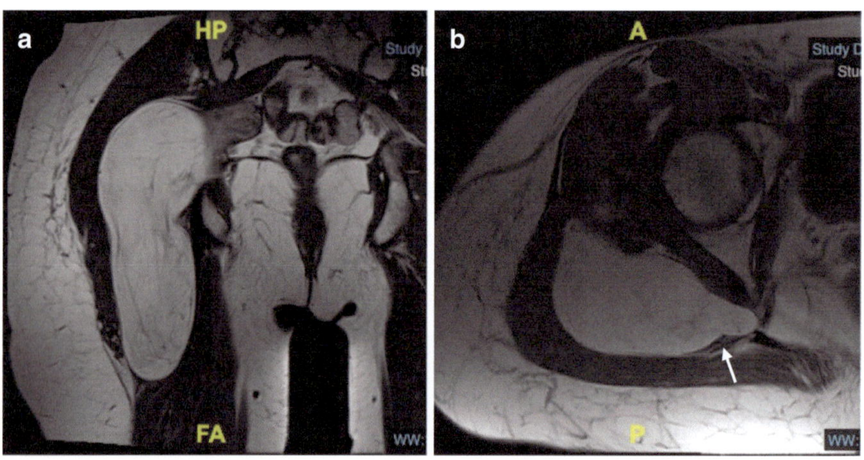

Fig. 14.1 T1-weighted (**a**) coronal and (**b**) axial MRI images of a well-differentiated lipoma-like liposarcoma. Note involvement of the sciatic notch, which contains the emerging inferior and superior gluteal vessels and the sciatic (solid arrow) and pudendal nerves

inferior gluteal vessels (main branches from the internal iliac system) and the pudendal nerve and vessels (Fig. 14.1b). Dissection around the notch may result in injury to these structures. Occasionally, the tumour is so deep within the sciatic notch or even arising from the contents of the notch, e.g. sciatic nerve tumour, that securing vascular control of the issuing vessels is not possible without ligating and dividing the branches as they divide from the internal iliac system, or even resorting to ligating the main internal iliac vessels themselves. Before surgery is attempted for buttock tumours, it is imperative that the question as to whether the notch can be "secured" is answered. The answer to this question will help to define the approach to the surgery of the buttock tumour.

14.1.1.2 Quadriceps Tumours (Fig. 14.2)

The quadriceps is by far the most common site for soft tissue sarcomas. Because of the size of the muscle group, the vastus lateralis is perhaps more commonly affected. Resection of the quadriceps will result in varying degrees of weakness depending on whether the femoral nerve branches are involved in the resection or the quantity of muscle resected [3–7]. As the quadriceps are an important antigravity muscle, rising from a seated position or ascending an incline or steps may be problematic afterwards.

Several considerations need to be held when resecting quadriceps tumours.

First, proximal quadriceps tumours are more likely to involve the femoral nerve and its branches, and, therefore, special attention should be entertained to reconstructing the divided nerves or by neurotising free vascularised muscle flaps [3, 6,

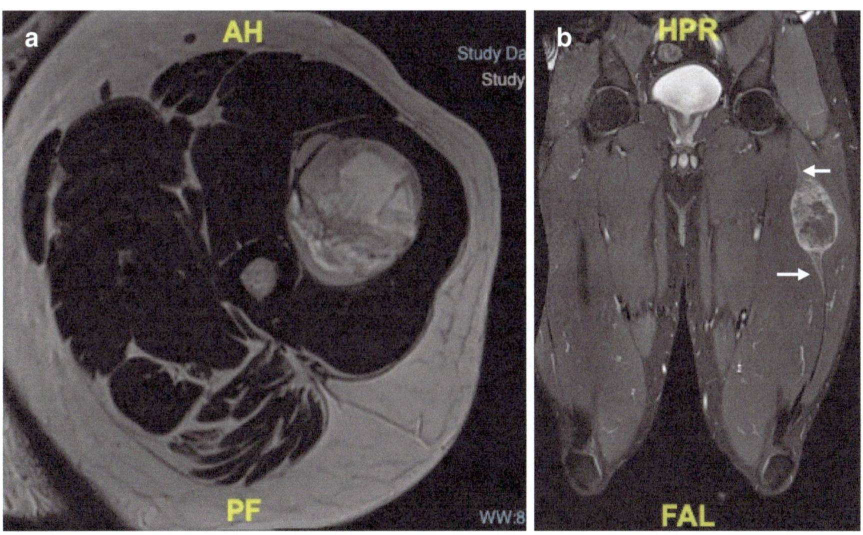

Fig. 14.2 (**a**) T2-weighted axial MRI image of a myxoid liposarcoma involving the vastus lateralis muscle. (**b**) T1-weighted fat-saturated coronal post-gadolinium contrast image demonstrating a "tail" of interfascial oedema (arrow)

8–10]. However, evidence that point to an evidence-based preference is lacking with many techniques succeeding in achieving extensor activity after composite functional flap reconstructions [5].

Second, the femoral vessels lie medial to the quadriceps and may be compromised in particularly large quadriceps tumours. The profunda femoris is an important vessel that needs to be secured during the resection as inadvertent division may result in considerable haemorrhage that can be difficult to control in the setting of an adjacent tumour that may be obstructing its optimal visualisation and therefore ligation. In this regard, special interrogation of the preoperative staging images is required to delineate the course of the vessel and its relationship to the tumour. More importantly, preoperative planning as to whether inclusion of the femoral vessels is required as part of wide resectional limb sparing surgery with vascular reconstruction or amputation [11–13].

Occasionally, the proximity of the tumour to the vessels is so close as to be difficult to differentiate one from the other. In this circumstance, consideration should be given to sacrifice of a segment of the vessels as part of the en bloc resection of the tumour [11]. Radiotherapy for soft tissue sarcomas may cause the tumour to shrink away from the vessels allowing preservation of the latter. Post radiotherapy restaging studies are critical for assessing response to neoadjuvant therapy. Leiomyosarcomas that arise from the femoral vein often surround the artery as well as extending into the quadriceps compartment. This is one scenario when vascular resection and reconstruction is mandatory during limb salvage surgery. A multidisciplinary approach will provide the best outcomes.

Special attention must always be paid when dealing with more distal quadriceps tumours as they may compromise the passage of the femoral vessels from Hunter's canal through the adductor hiatus in adductor magnus into the popliteal fossa. Careful dissection is always required here as the tightness of the adductor hiatus may distort the vessels, particularly if they are being compressed by a large adjacent tumour. Injury to the femoral vessels at this point may be very difficult to control in the presence of a large and obstructing tumour. Dividing the tendon of insertion of the adductor magnus into the adductor tubercle may help to relieve the tension within the adductor hiatus and more freedom to dissect and secure the vessels.

Third, large soft tissue sarcomas which are closely applied to the femoral diaphysis may require inclusion of the femoral diaphyseal periosteum as the deep margin of the tumour (Fig. 14.3). Including this structure increases the risk of devascularising the femoral shaft and this is amplified by the pre- or post-operative irradiation of the operative field which will include the femoral shaft. In such a circumstance, devascularisation may lead to femoral shaft fracture [14, 15]. This is one time where prevention is far better than cure should a femoral shaft fracture arise. Often, pathologic fractures after surgery and radiotherapy lead to non-union and will require complex grafting and other reconstructive procedures that continue to be at high risk of failure. It is best to prophylactically support the femur with an intramedullary rod which can be placed either at the same time or shortly afterwards (~ 6 weeks) [15].

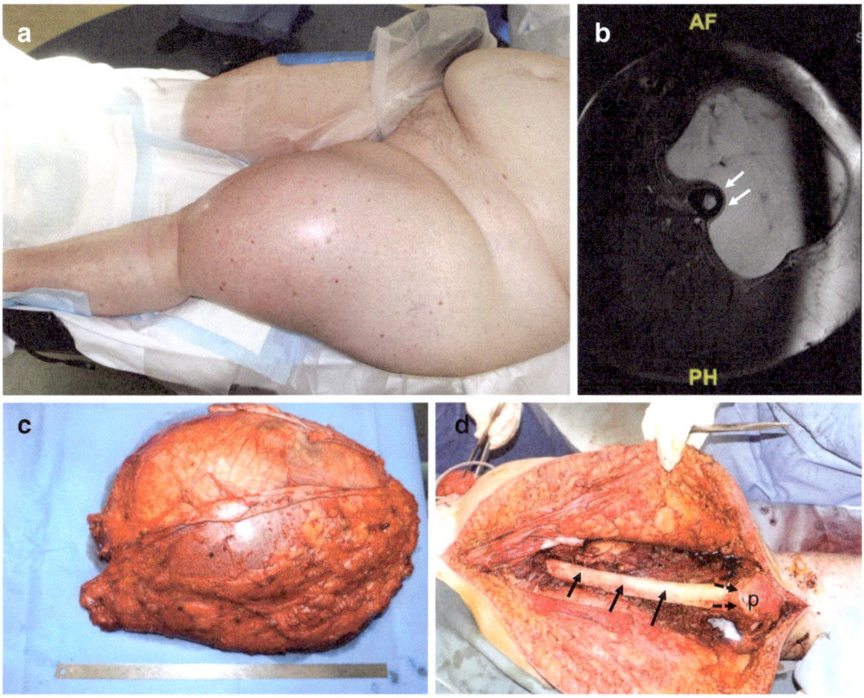

Fig. 14.3 (**a**) Massive left quadriceps sarcoma. (**b**) T2-weighted fat suppressed axial MRI image of a myxoid liposarcoma involving almost the whole quadriceps muscle. Note the close proximity to the femur (arrows) (**c**) Quadriceps resection from origin to insertion into patella. (**d**) Femoral shaft on view denuded of periosteum which is the deep margin of the resection (solid arrows). Note patella (P) with resection ending at the quadriceps tendon insertion into the patella (dashed arrows)

Fourth, resection of large tumours may sometimes lead to creation of considerable dead spaces. These may sometimes lead to large seromas which drain chronically through the operative wound. Recurrent attempts at aspiration of such seromas may lead to infection which can be quite problematic. It is best to avoid dead space formation by filling the defect by the use of vascularised tissue transfers. Bringing fresh vascularised tissues into the operative defect has the added advantage not only of reducing the space for seroma formation but also of allowing more healthy healing of the wound which has been traumatised not only by the surgical dissection but also the effects of radiotherapy [16]. Myo-cutaneous flaps help to close the defect while reducing tension across the suture lines. Early planning discussions are recommended between resectional and reconstructive teams [17–20].

Fifth, resection of distal quadriceps tumours may compromise the extensor mechanism at a number of levels including the quadriceps tendon, patella insertion of the tendon and the patella tendon. Adequate repair of this will require careful consideration of the role of autogenous and allograft material to reconstruct the continuity of the quadriceps mechanism [21–29].

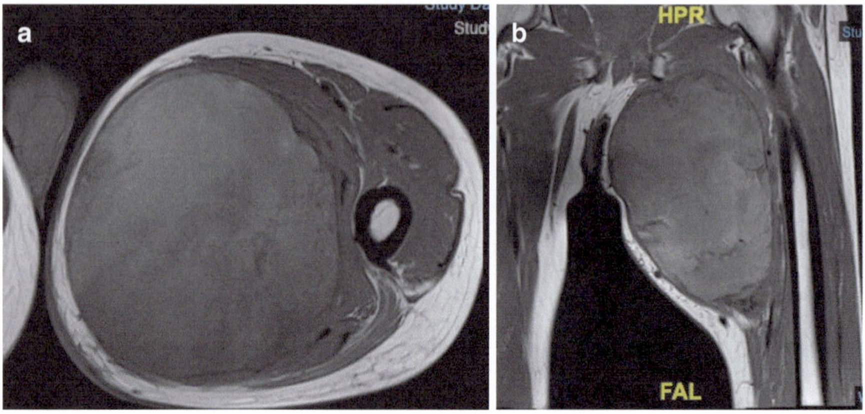

Fig. 14.4 T1-weighted (**a**) axial and (**b**) coronal MRI images of massive adductor compartment undifferentiated pleomorphic sarcoma

14.1.1.3 Adductor Compartment Tumour

Adductor compartment tumours are a particular challenge because they may grow to considerable sizes before the patient seeks medical attention (Fig. 14.4). The adductor compartment can be thought of as a pyramidal space with the base against the obturator foramen of the pelvis with the point at the adductor hiatus. Its anterior and posterior walls converge along the femur, and its medial wall is contained by the gracilis muscle. Once removed, the dead space left behind can be quite substantial. Free vascularised or transpositional flaps have been used to obliterate the dead space [30–35].

Proximally, the obturator nerve and vessels emerge from the obturator foramen and may be a source of challenge for haemostasis when dissecting at the level of the anterior pelvis. The adductor longus proximally and the adductor magnus distally is the bed on which the femoral vessels lie, and these need to be carefully dissected and protected when lifting them free from the adductor muscles. The adductor canal is a confined space and the tightest part is often proximally.

Once the tumour is removed, the pyramidal space is more easily appreciated, and this space will not collapse into itself as it is held open by the relatively rigid structures of the quadriceps anteriorly, the femoral shaft laterally and the anterior pelvis proximally. In this regard, there is a very high risk of perpetuating a dead space with subsequent seroma formation. Filling of this defect with a vascularised soft tissue flap is highly recommended [30–35].

14.1.1.4 Hamstring Compartment

The posterior compartment of the thigh is filled with the four hamstring muscles and the sciatic nerve. Tumours within the hamstring compartment can usually be excised while preserving the sciatic nerve [36–40]. The sciatic nerve is often the deepest structure within the compartment, and excision of the entire hamstring musculature can be performed while retaining the sciatic nerve. As with the other compartment of the thigh, the surgical defect will require filling with soft tissue flaps to obliterate the dead space and to prevent seroma formation. If the nerves to the various hamstrings are identified, these may be considered for neurotisation to muscle transfers that are brought into the field.

14.1.1.5 Popliteal Tumours

Popliteal tumours are poorly confined because the flexor fossae have few boundaries that separate the tumour from the vital neurovascular structures [41, 42]. The sciatic nerve has usually divided into its tibial and common peroneal components at the proximal apex of the rhomboid space defined by the medial and lateral hamstrings and the medial and lateral gastrocnemii. More often the common peroneal nerve has been compressed laterally under the tendon of biceps, and the tibial nerve and popliteal vessels have been pushed either deeply against the capsule or medially as they emerge into the popliteal fossa through the adductor hiatus. Historically, popliteal fossa tumours were considered for amputation because of the poor containment of the tumour and the sentiment that high-grade tumours would be poorly controlled with surgery. However, with the increasing role of preoperative radiotherapy, the induction of a fibrous rind around the tumour has allowed a marginal resection which when combined with the beneficial effects of radiotherapy gives results equivalent to wide margins alone. Moreover, it is now becoming clear that it is the size rather than the grade of the tumour which determines its operability [41, 42]. In this regard, all popliteal tumours should be considered as potential candidates for limb sparing surgery.

14.1.1.6 Calf Tumours

Superficial calf tumours may be resected easily with good prospect of local control of disease. Only in the lateral and proximal aspect of the lower leg should concern be given to potential sacrifice of the common peroneal nerve. This nerve and its branches, however, are amenable to reconstruction. Deep calf tumours, however, can be challenging because the important neurovascular supply to the foot passes primarily through the deep compartment of the calf (Fig. 14.5). Protecting this is paramount. Should sacrifice of the deep neurovascular structures of the calf be considered, then plans for either vascular or neural reconstruction should be made, or if this is deemed too difficult, then amputation should be entertained from the outset. Reconstruction of the neurovascular structures if successful will give protective sensation to the foot. Claw toes is often a sequel of surgery to deep tumours of the calf.

14.1.1.7 Anterior Lower Leg Tumours

Like calf tumours, superficial tumours are easier to treat. Deep tumours, however, may compromise the deep nerve and vessel supply. Moreover, resection of the anterior musculature of the lower leg will almost always leave the leg with a drop foot abnormality. Nerve injury within the anterior calf will exacerbate a foot drop but leave only a patch of numbness on the dorsum of the foot. Vascular injury however may result in muscle injury and clawing of the toes or compromise of the circulation

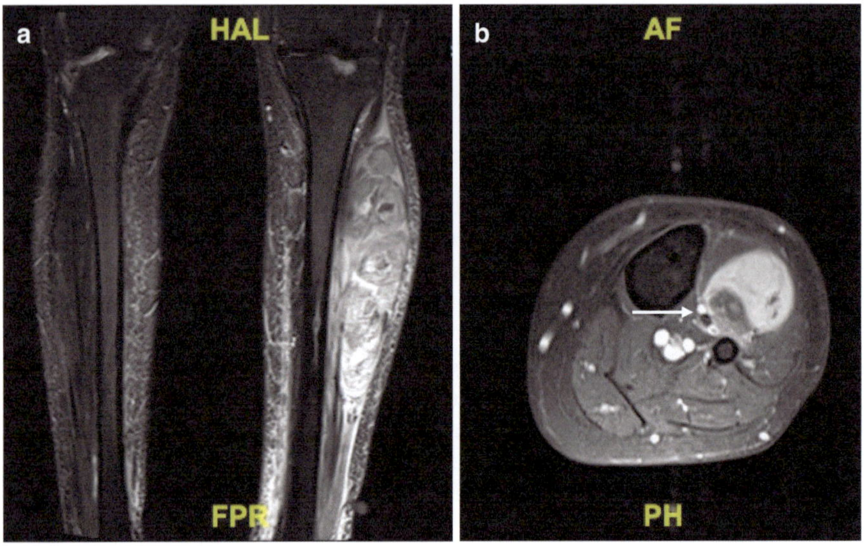

Fig. 14.5 (**a**) Post-contrast coronal STIR and (**b**) axial T1-weighted fat-saturated MRI images of anterior lower leg undifferentiated pleomorphic sarcoma. Note proximity to anterior compartment neurovascular structures (arrow)

to the foot. It is critical that lower leg tumours are carefully investigated with regard to the vascular supply of the lower limb, so that appropriate revascularisation procedures are undertaken where appropriate.

14.1.1.8 Foot Tumours

Foot tumours are notoriously difficult to treat for a number of reasons. The foot is poorly compartmentalised and containment of the tumour or post-operative haematoma after inadvertent prior excision can be difficult [43]. In this regard extension of the tumour or spread of the contaminated haematoma means that the risk of tumour spread is high and surgical resection is likely to sacrifice considerable tissue. Resections that require sacrifice of the bone of the foot may also compromise the integrity of the tripod that the skeleton of the foot creates that allows normal weight bearing and balanced tread pattern. Upsetting the balanced structure of the foot may result in abnormal shifts in weight bearing patterns such that pressure ulceration or other deformities may develop. Moreover, soft tissue sacrifice with subsequent soft tissue reconstruction may result in insensate skin which when placed under weight bearing stress may lead to pressure ulceration. Should foot surgery be contemplated, then, special attention to foot orthoses and footwear is mandatory. It is always interesting how well patients can cope after very complex resectional surgery of the foot. If surgery and reconstruction of the foot is likely to be highly complex, then consideration should be given to undertaking amputation in the first instance as the functional outcome of a below-knee amputation is exceptionally good.

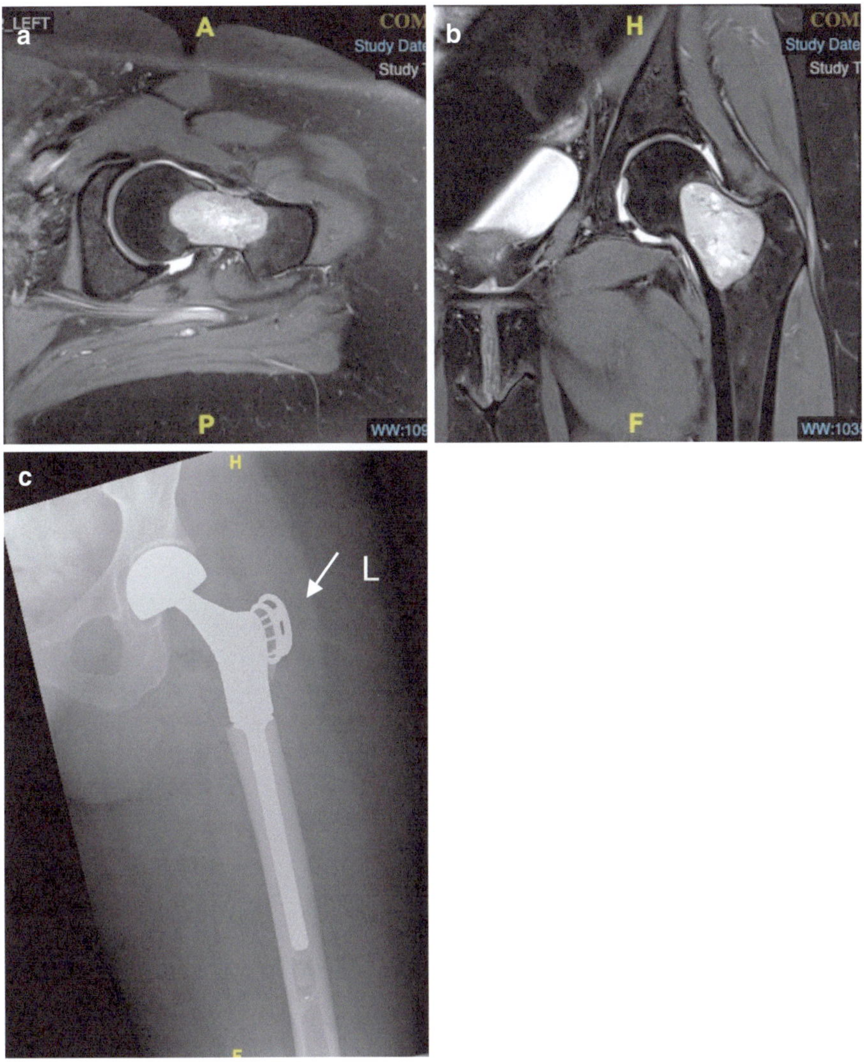

Fig. 14.6 Proton density fat-saturated (**a**) axial and (**b**) coronal MRI images of proximal femoral tumour. (**c**) Sliver of greater trochanter with attached gluteus medius was preserved and reattached to the proximal femoral tumour endoprosthesis (arrow)

14.1.2 Bone Sarcomas

14.1.2.1 Proximal Femoral Tumours

Resection of the proximal femur may result in abductor dysfunction if the greater trochanter requires sacrifice. If the greater trochanter can be preserved together with the attached gluteus medius muscle, then reconstruction of the abductor mechanism onto the shoulder of the proximal femoral tumour endoprosthesis will allow return of abductor function (Fig. 14.6).

If proximal femoral resection is performed through an intra-articular approach, the labrum and part of the capsule of the hip joint may be saved and later repaired in an encircling manner around the neck/head of the endoprosthesis to improve stability.

14.1.2.2 Distal Femoral Tumours

The synovium and articular cartilage are anatomic boundaries to the extension of intraosseous tumours. These are most often intact with distal femoral tumours, but careful scrutiny of the anatomic imaging, particularly MRI, is required to ensure that intra-articular extension of tumour has not occurred (Fig. 14.7). A joint effusion may occur sympathetically, but if blood stained then intra-articular extension needs to be suspected and an extra-articular resection may be required. If intra-articular extension is suspected, then aspiration of the joint prior to any arthrotomy may be undertaken.

The cruciate ligaments are conduits by which tumour may extend into the knee joint. Careful examination of preoperative imaging (MRI) is mandatory to establish whether invasion of the cruciate ligaments have occurred or not. The collateral

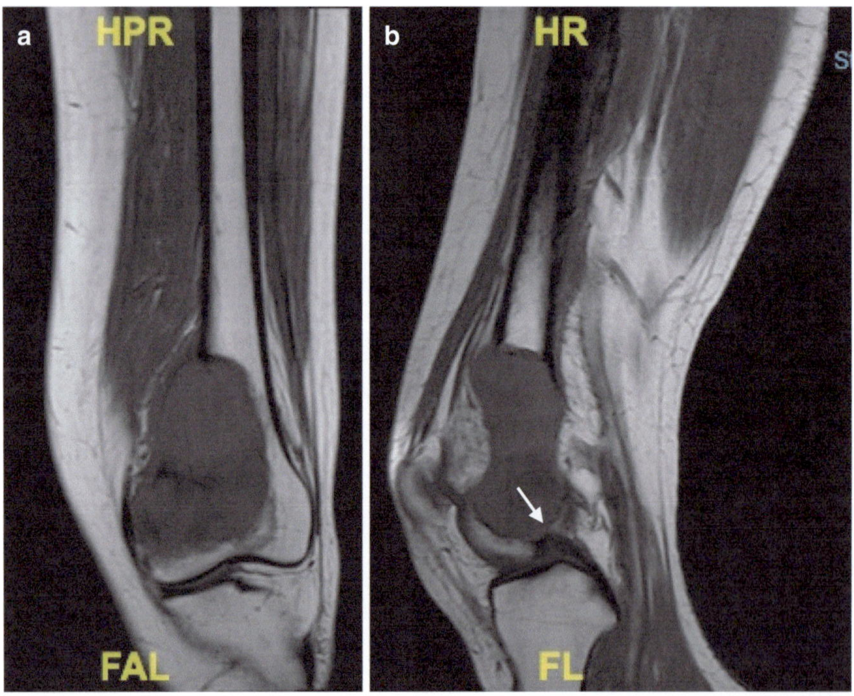

Fig. 14.7 T1-weighted (**a**) coronal and (**b**) axial MRI images of distal femoral tumour. No effusion to suggest intra-articular involvement. Tumour is close to the posterior cruciate ligament (arrow). While an intra-articular resection is preferred, careful division of the cruciate ligaments at the tibial attachment is required to ensure no contamination should tumour extend along the cruciate ligaments

ligaments are extracapsular, and these should pose no difficulty if involved, and resection at their distal extent can be performed without compromising the resection or reconstruction.

14.1.2.3 Proximal Tibial Tumours

Proximal tibial sarcomas may involve the tibial tuberosity and the insertion of the patella tendon. If so, then sacrifice of the patellar tendon mechanism is required, and formal reconstruction by a variety of techniques may be required [21, 44–47]. Care should also be taken to delineate if the superior tibio-fibular joint is affected or not. Should this joint be involved, then sacrifice of the fibular head en bloc with the tibia must be performed. The region of the tibio-fibular joint has significant anatomical importance. The anterior tibial vessels pass under the joint and should be protected where possible when the joint is sacrificed. The common peroneal nerve passes around the neck of the fibular nearby, and this should also be identified and carefully protected. The anterior branch that innervates the anterior tibial musculature should also be identified and protected.

14.1.2.4 Distal Tibial Sarcomas

Distal tibial sarcomas are uncommon. The anterior and posterior tibial vessels pass in close proximity to the distal tibia, and care should be taken to ensure that they are not compromised by the tumour. The tendons around the ankle are surrounded by thick synovial sheaths. The tendons can be sharply dissected out of these sheaths, and continuity may thus be preserved. Specifically, the posterior and anterior tibial tendons and peroneus longus should be spared if possible, to maintain the arch of the foot.

14.1.3 Investigations

14.1.3.1 Plain Radiographs

Standard orthogonal radiographs are mandatory to allow an assessment of the condition of the affected bone. This will clarify if the abnormality is related to other conditions of bone, e.g. enchondroma, avascular necrosis, fibrous dysplasia, Paget's disease, chronic osteomyelitis, etc. Plain radiographs may also highlight soft tissue abnormalities including soft tissue oedema, calcification and joint effusion. Plain radiographs are important for templating the bone when planning the choice of tumour endoprosthesis.

14.1.3.2 Anatomic Imaging

Magnetic resonance imaging (MRI) is the imaging modality of choice for both soft tissue and bone sarcomas because of its unsurpassed contrast. This allows excellent soft tissue and intramedullary delineation of tumour extent. It is important that sequences include at least T1 images that demonstrate anatomy, T2 images that demonstrate pathology, fat suppression images (with and without contrast enhancement) and orientations that include axial, coronal and sagittal images. The entire tumour-bearing compartment should be imaged to ensure that the entire extent of the tumour is visualised and also to ensure that any skip lesions are identified should they be present. In areas where clear delineation of anatomy is required such as where neurovascular structures may be affected, e.g. popliteal fossa and sciatic notch, behind the ankle, MRI is a critical investigation that should be deployed.

Computed tomography (CT) provides excellent bone imaging. Fine slice images are able to delineate tumour involvement of cortical and trabecular bone. While CT is able to provide good information on soft tissue abnormalities, particularly with the addition of contrast, it is not as good as MRI for soft tissue or intramedullary bone imaging, and it is recommended that MRI is the modality of choice for examining both bone and soft tissue sarcoma.

14.1.3.3 Functional Imaging

Functional imaging provides information on the biologic activity of the tumour and whether this activity is uniform or limited to specific parts of the tumour. This will help to guide biopsy, assess response to preoperative therapies, establish unifocal or multifocal disease and also assist in planning surgical margins. Functional imaging includes whole body ^{99}technetium methylene diphosphonate (MDP) bone or ^{201}thallium scintigraphy and flourodeoxyglucose positron emission tomography (PET).

14.1.3.4 Systemic Imaging

The purpose of systemic imaging (pulmonary CT, PET) is to identify if metastasis has occurred. The presence of metastasis will alter the strategic approach to treatment and whether metastases have occurred or not needs to be established prior to the commencement of treatment. In the presence of metastases, treatment more often than not adopts a palliative approach, while a curative strategy is usually employed when no metastasis is seen. A palliative approach may also include definitive limb sparing surgery.

14.1.4 Biopsy

Biopsy is critical for diagnosing the tumour. This has important implications for appropriate preoperative adjuvant treatment and subsequent surgery. Biopsy like the definitive surgery also requires planning to ensure that the most representative site is targeted, the safest approach is employed and that the entry site is placed within the line of the incision to allow subsequent inclusion in the resection specimen without compromising the approach or extent of the surgery. All biopsies should be image guided, and for greatest accuracy, this should be CT-guided.

Biopsy of proximal femoral tumours should be from a lateral approach as the incision for definitive surgery is usually through a lateral portal. Most femoral head, neck and intertrochanteric lesions may be accessed via a lateral approach. Variation to this may be if the greater trochanter can be salvaged, and, therefore, efforts should be made to avoid transgressing this structure if at all possible.

Biopsy of diaphyseal lesions should also be accessed from a lateral position as the surgical approach to the diaphysis is also from the lateral side.

Biopsy of distal femoral lesions can be challenging as one should avoid transgressing the joint capsule. The joint capsule rises above the patella and extends medially and laterally towards the lateral and medial epicondyles. Biopsy tracks should be planned according to information from MRI of the distal femur.

Tibial biopsy is often performed from an anterior approach. The subcutaneous nature of the bone anteriorly makes most part of the bone accessible for biopsy. Care should be taken to avoid involvement of the tibial tuberosity and patella tendon where possible by angling the approach from the medial or lateral directions.

Biopsy of the proximal fibular also requires caution because of the adjacent common peroneal nerve. CT-guided biopsy from an anterior or anterolateral approach is recommended to avoid the nerve.

Biopsy of soft tissue sarcomas of the lower limb will depend on the site of the tumour. Most superficial tumours may be biopsied directly from the vertex of the tumour as this is the thinnest portion of overlying skin which will most likely be included as an ellipse with the resection. Deeper tumours, however, pose challenges as care should be taken of surrounding neurovascular structures.

Quadriceps compartment tumours are usually approached from a lateral or anterior approach taking care to avoid the femoral vessels in Hunter's canal.

Adductor compartment muscles are usually approached from the medial side.

Hamstring compartment muscles are usually approached posteriorly. For tumours of the biceps, it is critical to know if the sciatic nerve has a high division as the peroneal branch of the nerve is closely related to the deep surface of the biceps as it passes distally and laterally towards the fibular head.

Anterior and peroneal compartment lower leg soft tissue sarcomas are usually approached directly from infront. Calf compartment tumours are approached from behind, but depending on whether the tumour is deep or in the gastrocnemeii, the approach is either midline or overlying the specific gastrocnemius.

14.1.5 Preoperative Preparation

General medical assessment must be carried out to ensure that the patient is fit for surgery. Particular attention must be paid to the patient's cardiovascular function. If the patient has received preoperative chemotherapy, there may be compromise of cardiac function. This needs to be clarified and delineated prior to surgery and the results of cardiac function tests known to the perioperative medical, anaesthetic and surgical teams. The extent to which cardiac function is compromised may dictate the nature of mitigating efforts.

Patients on chemotherapy may suffer marrow suppression prior to surgery. It is critical that the platelet levels are above 50, white cell count above 1.0 and haemoglobin above 8. Surgery planned for 2 weeks after the last dose of chemotherapy should provide sufficient time for the patient to have recovered from the haematological nadir of chemotherapy. Care may need to be individualised between patients, and the decision to proceed with surgery should occur after multidisciplinary consensus has been achieved.

Restaging studies include MRI of the entire tumour-bearing compartment (from joint above to joint below), functional scans (thallium or PET) and pulmonary CT. In addition, plain radiographs and CT scans should be included for bone tumours. Ideally, restaging studies should be performed within 6 weeks of definitive surgery. If there is a delay beyond 8 weeks, it may be prudent to repeat these to ensure that there has been no local or systemic progression of disease.

14.1.6 Operative Preparation

14.1.6.1 Anaesthetic

Modern combination regional/general anaesthetic may assist in achieving good intraoperative anaesthesia with appropriate and adequate post-operative analgesia.

14.1.6.2 Antibiotics

Prophylactic antibiotics should be delivered prior to the incision because of the potential for immunosuppression with preoperative adjuvant local or systemic therapy. Antibiotic regimes should follow institutional preferences.

Example of prophylactic antibiotics include cefazolin 2 g (continued every 8 h) and vancomycin 1 g intravenously (continued every 12 h) prior to the operative incision. To avoid the "red man" syndrome which is an idiosyncratic peripheral vasodilation following administration of vancomycin, it is recommended that the dose be titrated over 30 min prior to surgery. Antibiotics should be continued at the discretion of the treating team.

14.1.6.3 Urinary Catheter

Surgery may be prolonged and post-operatively, and patients may require an epidural anaesthetic or be on high dose narcotic analgesics. These may result in urinary retention that can be distressing to the patient. A urinary catheter should be inserted prior to surgery and removed once the patient is independently mobile.

14.1.7 Positioning for Soft Tissue Sarcoma Resection

Patients should be positioned in a way that allows the most practical approach to tumour resection. Recognising that there may be a need for soft tissue plastic reconstructive surgery with either a pedicled or free vacularised flap, the final positioning and draping of the patient will need to take into consideration the needs of the resecting and reconstructing teams, as well as the anaesthetic team. As these procedures may be prolonged, particularly if including soft tissue reconstruction, careful padding of all prominences should be undertaken to prevent pressure injuries. Sequential calf or foot compression devices may be applied to the unoperated limb as a prophylaxis measure against deep vein thrombosis.

14.1.7.1 Buttock Tumours

Buttock resections are best performed with the patient in the lateral position.

Resection of quadriceps, adductor compartment and anterior lower leg tumours is best performed with the patient in the supine position.

Hamstring and calf compartment tumours are best resected with the patient in the prone position.

14.1.8 Positioning for Bone Sarcoma Resection

Unlike soft tissue sarcomas, positioning for bone sarcomas may need greater stability to ensure accurate intraoperative assessment of joint position and leg length. The use of specially designed supports as per total hip or total knee replacement surgery is adequate. Like soft tissue resections, careful protection of all prominences should be undertaken to prevent pressure injuries, and sequential calf or foot compression devices should be applied to reduce the risk of deep vein thrombosis. Very occasionally, bone or soft tissue grafts may be required. This should be anticipated and planned for ahead of time to allow appropriate draping to occur.

14.1.8.1 Proximal and Total Femoral Tumours

Patients should be positioned in the lateral position if proximal femoral resection is planned. The same position can also adopted for total femoral resections as external rotation of the lower limb while extending or flexing the knee can be performed after the hip is dislocated. This manoeuvre should easily allow dissection of the distal femur and knee. Once the proximal femur (or total femur) has been reconstructed, the lateral position allows on table assessment of length. The lateral position also allows assessment of cup and neck version prior to final seating of the prosthesis.

Some surgeons choose to perform a total femoral resection with the patient in the supine position. In this position, the surgeon may have a better approach to the preparation of the knee. This can also be performed with a sand bag under the buttock to elevate this to allow easier visualisation and dissection around the posterior part of the hip joint without the operating table obstructing the approach.

14.1.8.2 Knee Tumours

Patients should be positioned as per a total knee replacement. This allows the correct draping to exclude unnecessary parts from the sterile field while also benefitting from the use of side supports and foot holders to maintain the knee in varying degrees of flexion during the dissection and preparation of the cut surfaces. Care should be taken to ensure that the stocking around the foot (if one is used) provides sufficient exposure to allow more distal extension of the operative wound should the need arise.

14.1.8.3 Foot Tumours

Patients should be draped in the supine position with an occlusive drape placed at least to the level of the knee in case proximal extension of the surgery is required. The foot should be positioned at the end of the table so that any plantar or heel surgery may be performed in an unobstructed way by elevation above the table.

14.2 Surgical Technique

14.2.1 Key Points for Resection of Soft Tissue Sarcomas

The surface marking of the tumour should be displayed with an indelible ink pen. If this is a virgin tumour, then a decision should be made if an ellipse of overlying skin should be sacrificed en bloc with the tumour. This is to contain the biopsy site and tract, as well as to remove any skin from the beginning that may ultimately be prone to ischaemic necrosis.

For subcutaneous tumours or those that have been previously inadvertently operated on, a much wider area of tissue around the tumour should be excised to encompass satellite or seeded lesions. This margin should also be marked prior to the surgery for inclusion in the resection.

The incision should be placed longitudinally along the line of the long axis of the limb and include the biopsy site and tract.

The resecting team should not aim to reduce the resection margin for aesthetic reasons as this may ultimately compromise local control of disease.

The aim of soft tissue dissection is to isolate the tumour with a cuff of normal tissue. For a wide margin, a named normal anatomical layer must be included in the radial direction from the tumour and at least 2 cm proximally and distally to the tumour in the longitudinal axis.

Occasionally, a closer margin is required, particularly if large tumours lie adjacent to vital neurovascular structures. In such circumstances, careful dissection of the nerve and vessels leaving their sheath or the periosteum from adjacent bone in continuity with the tumour may increase the quality of the margin.

The use of coagulating/incising forceps or metal ligatures may allow expeditious haemostasis and division of soft tissue from around the tumour. To assist in subsequent anastomosis of free vascularised flaps, arterial and vein branches should be handled carefully and ligated and divided with adequate length to allow a healthy anastomosis without tension.

It is highly recommended that resections of deep tumours which may leave a dead space be filled with donor tissue either as a pedicled or free vascularised flap. This is to obliterate the dead space to minimise the formation of a seroma that may either lead to chronic drainage or infection. Additionally, the placement of healthy flaps into the dead space may also include a cutaneous component which will reduce the tension of wound closure and subsequent surgical site complications.

14.2.2 Key Points for Resection of Bone Sarcomas

14.2.2.1 Proximal Femoral Resection

The most important surgical point to remember when resecting the proximal femur is the high risk of instability afterwards. Care should be taken to mitigate this as much as possible.

Preserve the labrum and as much hip capsule as possible if hemiarthroplasty reconstruction is to be employed. After repair with the hip prosthesis reduced into position, these soft tissue structures will help to increase the stability of the joint.

Preserve the greater trochanter with abductor musculature attached if possible. This will allow reattachment of the abductor mechanism on completion of implantation of proximal femoral prosthesis. It is easier to reattach the greater trochanter when the hip is dislocated as it will allow more accurate placement and fixation of the trochanter. In order to gauge the position of the trochanter on the prosthesis, reduce the hip, and then lay the greater trochanter in position under some tension. Mark on the prosthesis where the trochanter will be placed. Dislocate the hip, and position the greater trochanter on the shoulder of the prosthesis as marked. Fix the trochanter into place with an internal fixation device (often a trochanteric claw device held with screws or cables).

Ensure that the version of the prosthesis is appropriate prior to final seating. It is recommended that the prosthesis is anteverted between 10 and 15°.

Because of the significant release or resection of soft tissue around the proximal femur, it is likely that the prosthesis will be longer than the resection length in order to achieve appropriate soft tissue tension and, therefore, stability. The patient must be forewarned of this possibility. In addition, the offset of the device may vary considerably depending on the prosthesis choice.

If proximal resection of the femur includes the greater trochanter with or without some length of abductor muscle, the abductor muscle attachment may be reconstructed using synthetic mesh or tape. Post-operatively, repairs of the abductor mechanism should be protected with a hip abduction brace, and weight bearing on the reconstructed side should be protected (touch weight bearing) at the discretion of the surgeon.

14.2.2.2 Distal Femoral Resection

There are several key surgical checkpoints to remember when performing a distal femoral resection. These include the vascular anatomy, the level of the femoral osteotomy, and the relationship of the patellofemoral joint.

The femoral artery is at risk of injury as it passes from Hunter's canal into the popliteal fossa. Early identification of the adductor magnus tendon and releasing this will help to increase the safety of the femoral vessels at the level of the hiatus.

The penetrating branch of the popliteal artery which passes forward to the posterior cruciate ligament and capsule is at risk of avulsion if the joint is not handled carefully. Once the femoral artery and vein are released from the adductor hiatus, they can be carefully dissected away from the posterior knee capsule under direct vision. The forward-passing branches can then be ligated and divided safely.

The popliteal artery has a trifurcation as it divides into the posterior tibial, anterior tibial and peroneal branches. The bifurcation into the anterior and posterior tibial vessels has to be respected during dissection, as injury to the anterior tibial branch may result in ischemia and a post-operative compartment syndrome.

The diameter of the shaft of the distal femoral component must sit on cortical bone. If the host prosthesis junction is in trabecular bone, the prosthesis may subside leading to femoral fracture or early loosening. To prevent this, additional amount of metaphyseal bone may need to be resected to allow the diaphyseal component of the prosthesis to sit against cortical bone of the diaphysis.

It is important to ensure that the distal femoral component is seated in the correct rotation to avoid patella subluxation or dislocation. Often the femoral component is misplaced in internal rotation as the proximal femur tends to externally rotate once the femoral osteotomy has been performed. The linea aspera is a useful landmark to align the prosthesis and a sagittal plane passing through the linea aspera should represent the antero-posterior alignment of the prosthesis. The linea aspera is only palpable in the diaphyseal portion of the femur. If a lower femoral osteotomy is made where the linea aspera is not well defined, then flexing the knee to 90° on completion of the proximal tibial preparation with the femoral and tibial components in position and gently rotating (internally/externally) until the patella is observed to be sitting centrally in the sulcus should ensure a stable patellofemoral articulation post-operatively.

It is important that the tibial component is not internally rotated. Moreover, it is important to ensure that the tibial component is centred over the tibial intramedullary canal to avoid impingement of the tibial stem of the component which will tilt the tibial component into valgus or varus.

In order to achieve the best patella-femoral alignment and quadriceps function, care should be taken to ensure that the femoral and tibial segments are of appropriate lengths. Over lengthening or shortening of the reconstruction may lead to prothesis dislocation, restricted range of flexion or nerve palsy.

14.2.2.3 Total Femoral Resection (Fig. 14.8)

Total femoral resection invokes the same key points as for resection of the proximal and distal femur combined.

The surgical approach may be a longitudinal lateral incision from knee to hip or a midline knee incision curving laterally and posteriorly to become a lateral incision above the middle of the thing. The decision for which incision will depend on surgeon preference and tumour mandates.

The total femoral component rotates about an axis that passes from the hip joint to the knee joint. In unique circumstances and depending on the type of hinge mechanism at the knee, the total femoral component may flip through 180° around this axis of rotation. To prevent this from happening, it is important to ensure that there is adequate tension in the soft tissues and also that the prosthesis is anchored to the surrounding soft tissues. A technique to anchor the prosthesis is to surround the diaphyseal component with synthetic mesh and then stitch the various accessible components of the quadriceps musculature to this. If possible, the abductor

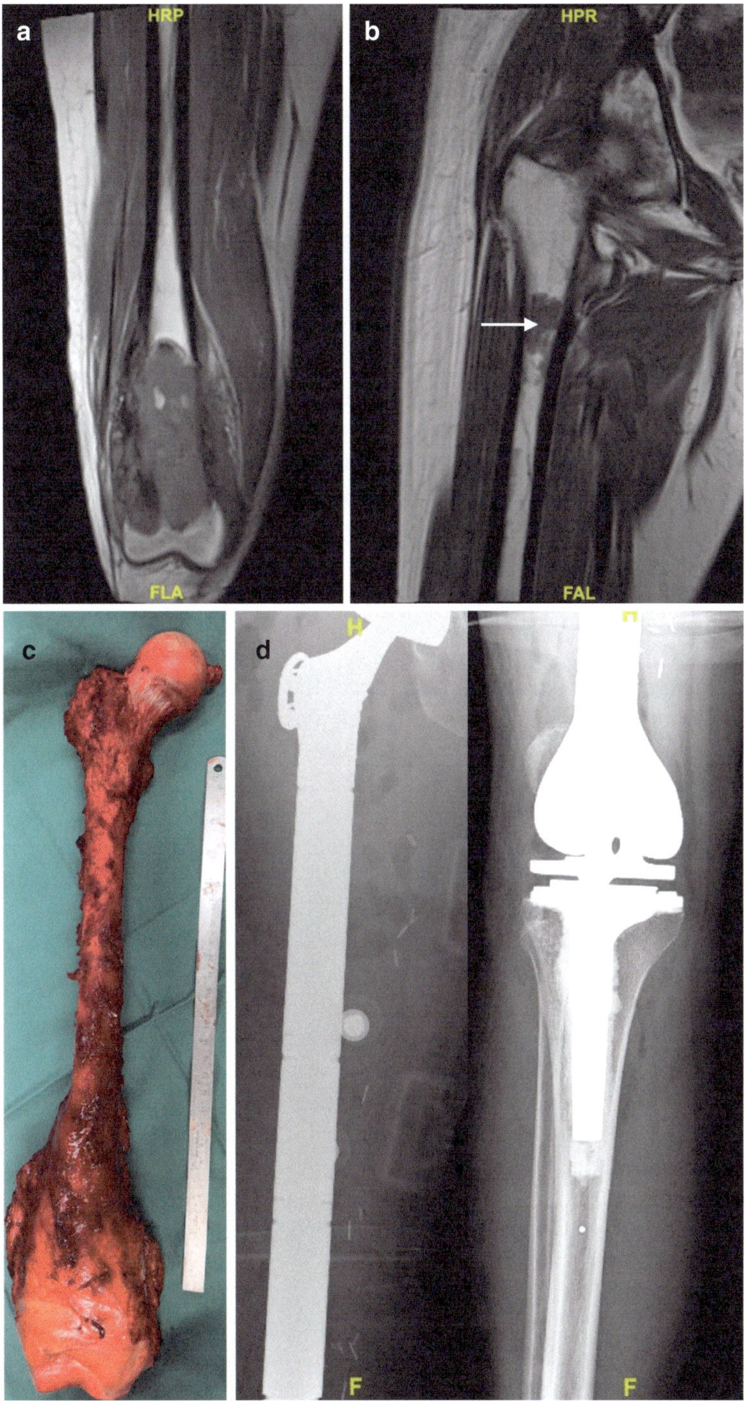

Fig. 14.8 T1-weighted coronal MRI images of (**a**) distal femoral tumour and (**b**) proximal skip lesion (arrow). This tumour was treated with (**c**) total femoral resection and (**d**) reconstruction with a total femoral tumour endoprosthesis

mechanism should be reconstructed back to the shoulder of the prosthesis to provide added stability.

Some prostheses have design features at the knee to prevent rotation beyond a certain amount or any rotation at all. Knowledge of the prosthetic design and rationale may help to prevent an unnecessary complication.

14.2.2.4 Proximal Tibial Resection

Resections of the proximal tibia are challenging because of the tibial tuberosity and patella tendon, the superior tibio-fibular joint, the common peroneal nerve and the bifurcation of the popliteal vessels into anterior and posterior tibial vessels.

If possible, the patella tendon should be preserved and reconstructed. There are a variety of techniques available including biologic and synthetic reconstructions. Biologic reconstructions that are purely muscle, e.g. gastrocnemius flap, are relatively easy to perform and function well. However, due to the stretching forces passing through the extensor mechanism, attenuation of the reconstruction is common and may give rise to patella alta and patella instability. This should be borne in mind when employing muscle flap reconstructions. Synthetic material may be used to reconstruct the patella tendon mechanism with good effect. However, surgeons should be mindful that synthetic material if abrasive and prominent may erode through overlying soft tissue.

Involvement of the superior tibio-fibular joint by tumour will determine if it needs to be resected en bloc with the tibia or not. If it is not involved, then dissection of the superior tibio-fibular joint is relatively easy and can be performed without injury to the common peroneal nerve or the anterior tibial vessels as they pass forward over the top of tibialis posterior and the interosseous membrane. If the tibio-fibular joint is involved, then resection of the fibular at the neck of the fibular should allow inclusion of the superior tibio-fibular joint with the operative specimen. Prior to transecting the neck of the fibular, careful dissection and protection of the common peroneal nerve and its branches need to be performed.

Reconstruction of the proximal tibia may be biological (allograft, autograft), prosthetic or a combination consisting of an allograft-prosthetic composite. The choice will depend on indications, availability of device and surgeon preference. The proximal tibial region is subcutaneous anteriorly. Following reconstruction, the wound may not be able to be closed because of the prominence of the reconstruction, or closure brings thin skin directly onto the underlying reconstruction. A simple method of protecting the overlying skin and underlying reconstruction is by rotating a gastrocnemius flap over the reconstruction. The exposed gastrocnemius can then be covered with a split skin graft. Harvesting the gastrocnemius flap can be easily done after the resected proximal tibia has been delivered from the wound.

14.2.2.5 Distal Tibial Resection

Other than the flexor hallucis longus, distal tibial tumours are generally surrounded by tendons rather than muscle belly. The tendons may be sharp dissected out of their sheaths to protect them. If possible, an epiphyseal sparing resection of the distal tibia is likely to allow ankle mobility. In this regard, an intercalary resection with either autogenous (fibular) or allograft reconstruction may be employed. If the epiphyseal cannot be spared, then an intercalary arthrodesis between tibia and talus can be considered. If the talus has to be included in the distal tibial resection, an intercalary resection between tibia and calcaneus may be considered. If there is an extraosseous extension that makes limb preservation challenging or dangerous, then a below-knee amputation is recommended. With modern prosthetics, a below-knee amputation provides an excellent solution for distal tibial tumours and near normal function of the limb may be expected.

14.2.2.6 Amputation

Amputations are considered when the planned resection of the lower limb is predicted to result in a non-functional limb. Occasionally, amputation is also performed as a palliative procedure to provide local control of tumour, e.g. ulceration or pathologic fracture. Amputations should also be planned and performed with the same levels of care to ensure that appropriate margins of surgery are employed. Picking the right level for amputation is critical for ensuring a strong lever arm for the use of a lower limb amputation prosthesis [48]. Post-operative rehabilitation is essential if a lower limb amputation prosthesis is being considered. Prevention of flexion contractures, optimising stump mobility and strength and maintaining balance during gait and standing are the key goals of post-operative rehabilitation. Newer modalities for movement and function are now being considered including the use of virtual reality for optimising mobility training [49]. Pain control may be a prolonged problem for those with phantom pain, and the management of this should be considered as part of the multidisciplinary approach to care [50].

References

1. Soyfer V, Corn BW, Bickels J, Merimsky O. Primary high-grade soft-tissue sarcoma of the buttock: a rare but distinct clinical entity. Br J Radiol. 2016;89(1062):20151017.
2. Behranwala KA, Barry P, A'Hern R, Thomas JM. Buttock soft tissue sarcoma: clinical features, treatment, and prognosis. Ann Surg Oncol. 2003;10(8):961–71.
3. Walley KC, Taylor EM, Anderson M, Lozano-Calderon S, Iorio ML. Reconstruction of quadriceps function with composite free tissue transfers following sarcoma resection. J Surg Oncol. 2017;115(7):878–82.
4. Muramatsu K, Ihara K, Miyoshi T, Yoshida K, Hashimoto T, Taguchi T. Transfer of latissimus dorsi muscle for the functional reconstruction of quadriceps femoris muscle following oncological resection of sarcoma in the thigh. J Plast Reconstr Aesthet Surg. 2011;64(8):1068–74.
5. Ek EW, Rozen WM, Ek ET, Rudiger HA. Surgical options for reconstruction of the extensor mechanism of the knee after limb-sparing sarcoma surgery: an evidence-based review. Arch Orthop Trauma Surg. 2011;131(4):487–95.
6. Innocenti M, Abed YY, Beltrami G, Delcroix L, Balatri A, Capanna R. Quadriceps muscle reconstruction with free functioning latissimus dorsi muscle flap after oncological resection. Microsurgery. 2009;29(3):189–98.
7. Willcox TM, Smith AA, Beauchamp C, Meland NB. Functional free latissimus dorsi muscle flap to the proximal lower extremity. Clin Orthop Relat Res. 2003;410:285–8.
8. Grinsell D, Di Bella C, Choong PF. Functional reconstruction of sarcoma defects utilising innervated free flaps. Sarcoma. 2012;2012:315190.

9. Grinsell D, Lonie S, Wilson KC, Choong PFM. The innervated rectus abdominis flap for quadriceps reconstruction. J Plast Reconstr Aesthet Surg. 2019;72(6):941–5.
10. Stranix JT, Lee ZH, Lam G, Mirrer J, Rapp T, Saadeh PB. Limb-sparing sarcoma reconstruction with functional composite thigh flaps. Microsurgery. 2018;38(5):466–72.
11. Adelani MA, Holt GE, Dittus RS, Passman MA, Schwartz HS. Revascularization after segmental resection of lower extremity soft tissue sarcomas. J Surg Oncol. 2007;95(6):455–60.
12. Bertoldo U, Brach del Prever EM, Gino G, Mellano D, Albertini U, Piana R, et al. The integration of vascular surgical techniques with oncological surgical protocols in the treatment of soft tissue sarcomas of the limbs. Chir Organi Mov. 2003;88(2):217–23.
13. Bonardelli S, Nodari F, Maffeis R, Ippolito V, Saccalani M, Lussardi L, et al. Limb salvage in lower-extremity sarcomas and technical details about vascular reconstruction. J Orthop Sci. 2000;5(6):555–60.
14. Bishop AJ, Zagars GK, Allen PK, Moon BS, Lin PP, Lewis VO, et al. Treatment-related fractures after combined modality therapy for soft tissue sarcomas of the proximal lower extremity: can the risk be mitigated? Pract Radiat Oncol. 2016;6(3):194–200.
15. Lin PP, Schupak KD, Boland PJ, Brennan MF, Healey JH. Pathologic femoral fracture after periosteal excision and radiation for the treatment of soft tissue sarcoma. Cancer. 1998;82(12):2356–65.
16. Chan LWM, Imanishi J, Grinsell DG, Choong P. Preoperative radiotherapy and wide resection for soft tissue sarcomas: achieving a low rate of major wound complications with the use of flaps. Results of a single surgical team. Front Surg. 2017;4:79.
17. Abbott DE, Halverson AL, Wayne JD, Kim JY, Talamonti MS, Dumanian GA. The oblique rectus abdominal myocutaneous flap for complex pelvic wound reconstruction. Dis Colon Rectum. 2008;51(8):1237–41.
18. Langstein HN, Robb GL. Reconstructive approaches in soft tissue sarcoma. Semin Surg Oncol. 1999;17(1):52–65.
19. Ogura K, Miyamoto S, Sakuraba M, Chuman H, Fujiwara T, Kawai A. Immediate soft-tissue reconstruction using a rectus abdominis myocutaneous flap following wide resection of malignant bone tumours of the pelvis. Bone Joint J. 2014;96-B(2):270–3.
20. Scaglioni MF, Giunta G, Barth AA, Giovanoli P. A pedicled split extended vertical deep inferior epigastric (s-vDIEP) flap and an adipo-dermal thigh local flap for the reconstruction of the medial thigh compartment after sarcoma resection: a case report. Microsurgery. 2020;40(1):65–9.
21. Imanishi J, Grinsell D, Choong PF. Bone-patellar tendon-bone allograft reconstruction for peri-patellar tendon sarcomas: case series. Springerplus. 2015;4:740.
22. Babu NV, Chittaranjan S, Abraham G, Bhattacharjee S, Prem H, Korula RJ. Reconstruction of the quadriceps apparatus following open injuries to the knee joint using pedicled gastrocnemius musculotendinous unit as bridge graft. Br J Plast Surg. 1994;47(3):190–3.
23. Bates MD, Springer BD. Extensor mechanism disruption after total knee arthroplasty. J Am Acad Orthop Surg. 2015;23(2):95–106.
24. Bonnin M, Lustig S, Huten D. Extensor tendon ruptures after total knee arthroplasty. Orthop Traumatol Surg Res. 2016;102(1 Suppl):S21–31.
25. Leung KS, Yip KM, Shen WY, Leung PC. Reconstruction of extensor mechanism after trauma and infection by transposition of the Achilles tendon: report of technique and four cases. J Orthop Trauma. 1994;8(1):40–4.
26. Rosenberg AG. Management of extensor mechanism rupture after TKA. J Bone Joint Surg Br. 2012;94(11 Suppl A):116–9.
27. Shi SM, Shi GG, Laurent EM, Ninomiya JT. Modified V-Y turndown flap augmentation for quadriceps tendon rupture following Total knee Arthroplasty: a retrospective study. J Bone Joint Surg Am. 2019;101(11):1010–5.
28. Warrier SK, Mah E, Morrison WA. Extended medial gastrocnemius myocutaneous flap in repair of the quadriceps extension mechanism. ANZ J Surg. 2006;76(12):1110–4.
29. Ziran BH, Goodfellow DB, Deluca LS, Heiple KG. Knee function after patellectomy and cruciform repair of the extensor mechanism. Clin Orthop Relat Res. 1994;(302):138-46.

30. Grainger MF, Grimer RJ, Carter SR, Tillman RM. Wound complications following resection of adductor compartment tumours. Sarcoma. 2001;5(4):203–7.
31. Kito M, Ae K, Koyanagi H, Gokita T, Furuoka H, Okamoto M, et al. Risk factor for wound complications following wide resection of soft tissue sarcoma in the adductor compartment of the thigh. Jpn J Clin Oncol. 2019;49(10):932–7.
32. Moore J, Isler M, Barry J, Mottard S. Major wound complication risk factors following soft tissue sarcoma resection. Eur J Surg Oncol. 2014;40(12):1671–6.
33. Nakamura T, Nakamura K, Hagi T, Asanuma K, Sudo A. Soft tissue sarcoma at the adductor compartment of the thigh may have a greater risk of tumor-associated events and wound complications. J Orthop Surg (Hong Kong). 2019;27(2):2309499019840813.
34. Pradhan A, Cheung YC, Grimer RJ, Abudu A, Peake D, Ferguson PC, et al. Does the method of treatment affect the outcome in soft-tissue sarcomas of the adductor compartment? J Bone Joint Surg Br. 2006;88(11):1480–6.
35. Rudiger HA, Ngan SY, Choong PF. Surgical outcome of soft tissue sarcomas of the adductor compartment. J Orthop Surg (Hong Kong). 2009;17(3):284–7.
36. Aiba H, Hayashi K, Yamada S, Okamoto H, Kimura H, Miwa S, et al. Treatment of a malignant soft tissue tumor arising in the vicinity of the sciatic nerve with an in-situ preparation technique and intensive multidisciplinary therapy. Cancers (Basel). 2019;11(4)
37. Korah MP, Deyrup AT, Monson DK, Oskouei SV, Weiss SW, Landry J, et al. Anatomic tumor location influences the success of contemporary limb-sparing surgery and radiation among adults with soft tissue sarcomas of the extremities. Int J Radiat Oncol Biol Phys. 2012;82(2):933–9.
38. Kulaylat MN, King B, Karakousis CP. Posterior compartment resection of the thigh for soft-tissue sarcomas. J Surg Oncol. 1999;71(4):243–5.
39. Moschella F, D'Arpa S, Pirrello R, Cordova A. Posterior compartment of the lower leg reconstruction with free functional rectus femoris transfer after sarcoma resection. J Plast Reconstr Aesthet Surg. 2010;63(3):e269–72.
40. Rimner A, Brennan MF, Zhang Z, Singer S, Alektiar KM. Influence of compartmental involvement on the patterns of morbidity in soft tissue sarcoma of the thigh. Cancer. 2009;115(1):149–57.
41. Yang RS, Lane JM, Eilber FR, Dorey FJ, al-Shaikh R, Schumacher LY, et al. High grade soft tissue sarcoma of the flexor fossae. Size rather than compartmental status determine prognosis. Cancer. 1995;76(8):1398–405.
42. Eilber FC, Eckardt JJ, Rosen G, Nelson SD, Selch M, Eilber FR. Large, deep, high-grade extremity sarcomas: treating tumors of the flexor fossae. Surg Oncol. 1999;8(4):211–4.
43. Salipas A, Dowsey MM, May D, Choong PF. 'Beware the lump in the foot!': predictors of recurrence and survival in bone and soft-tissue sarcomas of the foot and ankle. ANZ J Surg. 2014;84(7–8):533–8.
44. Fukui N, Cho N, Tashiro T, Nakamura K. Anatomical reconstruction of the patellar tendon: a new technique with hamstring tendons and iliotibial tract. J Orthop Trauma. 1999;13(5):375–9.
45. Kawashima H, Ogose A, Ariizumi T, Yamagishi T, Oike N, Aoyama H, et al. Reconstruction of knee extensor with patellar tendon autograft following intraoperative radiotherapy. Knee. 2020;27(1):257–62.
46. Nakashima H, Yoshida M, Miyamoto K. Anatomical reconstruction of the patellar tendon using the fascia lata attached to the iliac bone following resection for soft tissue sarcoma: a case report. Ups J Med Sci. 2012;117(4):460–4.
47. Titus V, Clayer M. Protecting a patellar ligament reconstruction after proximal tibial resection: a simplified approach. Clin Orthop Relat Res. 2008;466(7):1749–54.
48. Geertzen JHB, de Beus MC, Jutte PC, Otten E, Dekker R. What is the optimal femur length in a trans-femoral amputation? A mixed method study: scoping review, expert opinions and biomechanical analysis. Med Hypotheses. 2019;129:109238.
49. Ulger O, Yildirim Sahan T, Celik SE. A systematic literature review of physiotherapy and rehabilitation approaches to lower-limb amputation. Physiother Theory Pract. 2018;34(11):821–34.
50. Isaacs-Itua A, Sedki I. Management of lower limb amputations. Br J Hosp Med (Lond). 2018;79(4):205–10.

Surgical Management of Upper Limb Sarcomas

15

Peter F. M. Choong and Gerard Powell

15.1 Introduction

The upper limb is the second most common site for sarcomas to arise after the lower limb. The region from the shoulder to the elbow is the commonest location for upper limb sarcomas whether soft tissue or bone. Sarcomas of the upper limb may lead to functional deficits that specifically degrade independence because of the loss of dexterity, strength, coordination and the ability to perform activities of daily living. Depending on whether the sarcoma is primarily bone or soft tissue will lead to very specific surgical strategies. Surgery to the upper limb is complex because of the instability of the shoulder joint, the convergence of important neurovascular structures at the axilla and the close proximity of these to the humerus. Because of the paucity of tissue on the upper limb, even soft tissue sarcomas may compromise the major neurovascular structures. Treatment is a multimodality challenge and best provided at an expert centre.

P. F. M. Choong (✉)
Department of Surgery, University of Melbourne, Melbourne, VIC, Australia

Department of Orthopaedics, St. Vincent's Hospital, Melbourne, VIC, Australia

Bone & Soft Tissue Tumour Service, Peter MacCallum Cancer Centre, Melbourne, VIC, Australia
e-mail: pchoong@unimelb.edu.au

G. Powell
Department of Orthopaedics, St. Vincent's Hospital, Melbourne, VIC, Australia

Bone & Soft Tissue Tumour Service, Peter MacCallum Cancer Centre, Melbourne, VIC, Australia

P. F. M. Choong (ed.), *Sarcoma*, https://doi.org/10.1007/978-981-15-9414-4_15

15.2 Soft Tissue Sarcomas

15.2.1 Anatomic Considerations

The upper limb may be divided into three regions: the upper arm and shoulder (shoulder girdle), the forearm and the wrist and hand. The shoulder joint, elbow joint and wrist are primarily the fulcrums of movement and are important in maintaining the functionality of the upper limb. Soft tissue sarcomas in these regions impact very specific muscle groups depending on their anatomic sites and, by doing so, leave the limb with very specific deficits. Moreover, the close proximity of important neurovascular structures that typically wend their way around all compartments of the upper limb implies that deep-seated sarcomas are more likely to involve these neurovascular structures, or in the effort to protect vulnerable neurovascular structures, substantial parts of muscle bellies may be sacrificed leading to functional deficits from muscle loss alone.

15.2.2 Shoulder Girdle Tumours

Upper arm soft tissue sarcomas may affect the parascapular muscles, the deltoid, the biceps and triceps muscle groups [1–3]. Depending on which parascapular muscle is affected, rotation of the glenohumeral joint may or may not be affected. Involvement of the supraspinatus muscle will have the largest potential impact on upper limb abduction, as it is the main stabiliser of the humeral head on abduction (Fig. 15.1). With its loss, the humeral head cannot be held down after the first 30 degrees of arm abduction, and the continuing action of the deltoid causes the shoulder on the affected side to shrug instead.

Sarcomas affecting the deltoid will lead to weakness of abduction. Depending on the extent of deltoid sacrifice, abductor loss may be minor or complete. A deep-seated deltoid sarcoma will usually require sacrifice of the full thickness and

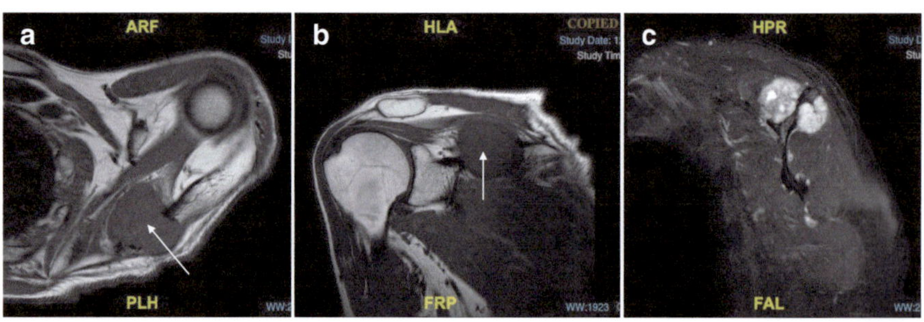

Fig. 15.1 T1-weighted, (**a**) axial, (**b**) coronal and (**c**) sagittal T2 fat-suppressed MRI images demonstrating high-grade chondrosarcoma (arrow) of the supraspinatus fossa and spine of the scapula. Resection will include part of the supraspinatus and infraspinatus muscles

occasionally the entire deltoid. If the axillary nerve is included with the resection, then complete loss of abduction can be expected. Deep-seated deltoid tumours of the posterior deltoid are more likely to result in total abductor loss because the axillary nerve that gives motor innervation to the deltoid enters its deep surface posteriorly and therefore is most vulnerable to injury. In contrast, resection of anterior deltoid tumours has the potential to retain some deltoid function because the posterior origin of the axillary nerve is protected. Superficial sarcomas overlying the deltoid which necessitate only partial thickness resection of the deltoid usually leave the deltoid with good to acceptable function. The axillary nerve can usually be preserved as it is well protected within its epineurium on the deep surface of the deltoid.

15.2.3 Upper Arm Tumours

Upper arm tumours primarily affect flexion and extension of the elbow [4, 5]. Triceps resection will leave the upper limb weak to elbow extension. Depending on the extent of the triceps resection, weakness may vary from mild to complete. Tricipital function is mainly called upon for actions that move against gravity (reaching above the head) or when pushing objects away from the body or reaching outward for something. Most often extension of the elbow is easily achieved under the action of gravity alone for daily activities that do not require significant speed or strength.

Biceps resection will lead to significant functional loss if complete. Patients will not be able to draw their hand towards their mouth or lift objects towards themselves. Partial loss may be compensated to a small degree by action of the muscles that arise from the extensor origin of the forearm and lateral epicondyle of the humerus (brachioradialis, extensor wad).

Tumours of the lower half of the upper arm are liable to involve the major nervous structures of the arm. If laterally placed, tumours may impinge on the radial and posterior interosseous nerves. If medially placed, tumours may impinge on the ulnar and median nerves (Fig. 15.2).

15.2.4 Forearm Tumours (Fig. 15.3)

Forearm soft tissue sarcomas may affect the flexor or extensor compartment of the forearm either by their position or because of the required margins of resection [6–8]. Proximal forearm tumours are more likely to affect the muscle bellies of the forearm musculature, while more distal forearm tumours are more likely to involve the tendons. This has specific impact on the function of the affected muscles because the loss of muscle bellies usually includes the nerve supply. Preservation of the muscle belly with distal tumours, however, affords a greater likelihood of functional preservation through reconstruction of the tendons. Because the flexor digitorum superficialis and profundus have important actions on the movement of the fingers,

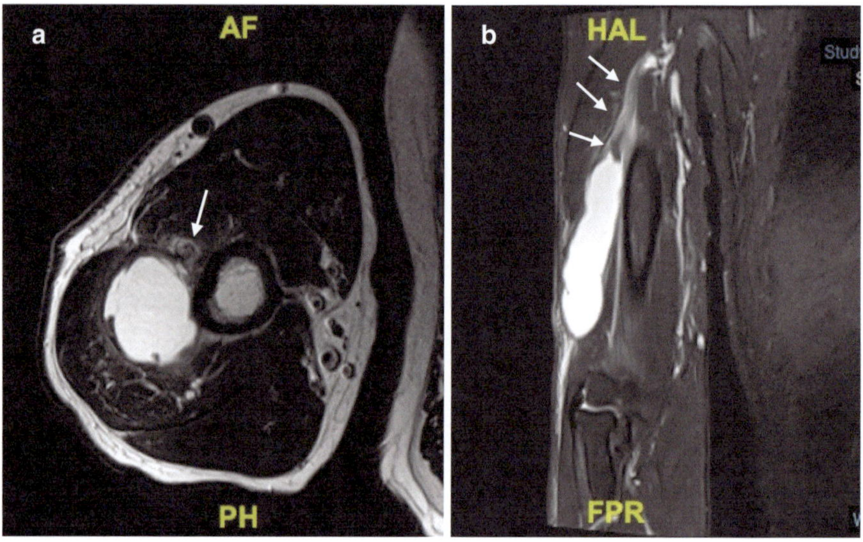

Fig. 15.2 T2-weighted, (**a**) axial, (**b**) coronal T2 contrast-enhanced fat-suppressed MRI images demonstrating high-grade tumour of the upper arm. Note the course of the radial nerve (arrows)

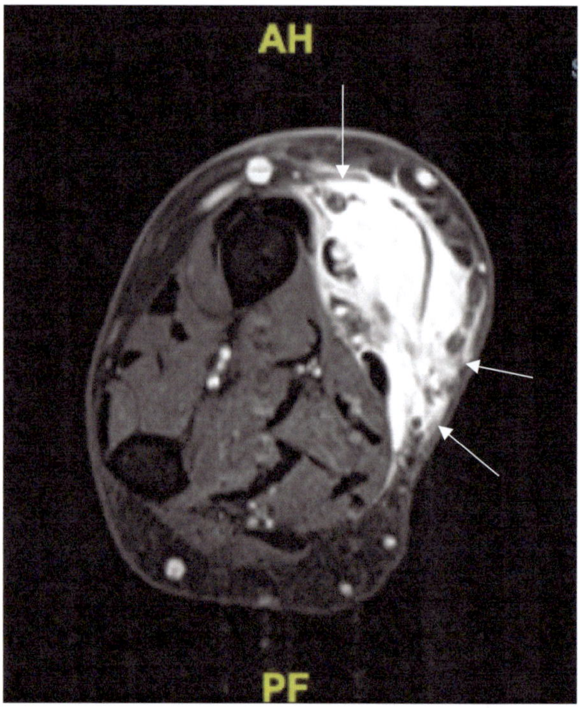

Fig. 15.3 Contrast-enhanced T1-weighted fat-suppressed MRI images demonstrating high-grade tumour of the volar aspect of the forearm. Note the considerable oedema pattern associated with the tumour (arrows). Careful preoperative planning will be required to ensure that the "tail" of oedema is also included in the resection as this is known to be associated with recurrent disease if ignored

flexor compartment tumours are more likely to give rise to greater functional deficits of the hand. Loss of the flexor carpi radialis is usually associated with minimal deficits presumably because of the flexor power of the remaining forearm musculature. Loss of flexor carpi ulnaris, however, is associated with weakness of the movement of ulnar deviation and flexion (wielding a hammer).

Resection of the extensors of the wrist (extensor carpi radialis brevis, longus) or the extensors of the fingers will leave the typical finger or wrist drop. Salvage of function will depend on whether the resection is at the muscle or tendon level.

15.2.5 Wrist and Hand Tumours

Hand tumours are particularly challenging [9–12]. If deep on the palmar side, the potential involvement of the palmar arches and the median and ulnar nerves may make reconstruction extremely difficult. Hypothenar tumours are usually associated with minimal functional loss unless the deep branch of the ulnar nerve is affected whereupon there will be weakness of the intrinsics of the hand and numbness of the ulnar-supplied fingers. The ulnar may be protected within Guyon's canal, so assumption of the need for its sacrifice in all cases may not be valid. Thenar eminence tumours will result in the loss of thumb opposition and abduction.

Sarcomas of the dorsum of the hand may be problematic because of the involvement of the extensor tendons and also the metacarpals. The extent to which there is functional impairment will depend on the extent of the tumour and the associated resection.

Tumours situated in the flexor fossae are particularly problematic as the axilla and the cubital fossa host the convergence of the major neurovascular structures of the upper limb. Potential sacrifice of relevant structures may be required to ensure adequate surgical margins for tumours arising in these two fossae. Tumours on the medial aspect of the upper arm and over the head of the radius are also at risk of compromising vital brachial neurovascular structures.

15.3 Bone Sarcomas

15.3.1 Anatomic Considerations

In comparison to the lower limb, resections of bone sarcomas of the upper limb are associated with greater instability, more challenging reconstructions and potential sacrifice of soft tissue structures (nerves, vessels, tendons, ligaments) because of the greater proportion of bone to soft tissue in the upper limb. Because of this, bone tumour resections are more likely to cause greater functional deficits.

Tumours of the proximal humerus or glenoid are particularly challenging because resection with adequate margins is more often than not associated with resection not only of the capsule of the shoulder but also the rotator cuff musculature. Both these structures are critical to the stability and function of the glenohumeral joint. Because of the multiple extensions of the bursae around the shoulder joint and their frequent communication with the joint, and also the intraarticular nature of the long head of biceps tendon, proximal humeral sarcomas are characterised by the early involvement of the shoulder joint. In this regard, extra-articular resection of tumours involving the proximal humerus and periarticular scapula needs always to be considered.

Tumours of the distal humerus or proximal ulnar always require sacrifice of the elbow joint. In order to maintain mobility of the joint, prosthetic replacement is almost always required if limb salvage surgery is considered.

Involvement of either ulnar or radial shaft usually requires sacrifice with a cuff of forearm muscle, and the deficit will be dependent on which bone is involved. Distal tumours are associated with less functional deficits than more proximal tumours because tendons are often protected by their synovial sheaths, the preservation of muscle bellies usually means protection of innervation of the muscle, and should resection of the tendons be required, reconstruction is usually easily possible.

Resection of the distal radius can be easily treated with wrist arthrodesis via a number of techniques.

Bone sarcomas of the hand are rare. Should they occur, considerable functional deficits may be expected. Limb-sparing surgery is challenging, and oftentimes, attempts will be associated with a poor functional and cosmetic result. Amputation of the hand or ray amputations are more often required to achieve adequate surgical margins.

15.4 Preoperative Staging

Preoperative imaging is essential for assessing the local and systemic extent of tumours of the upper limb. This is particularly critical because of the close proximity of neurovascular structures in the flexor fossae, the medial aspect of the upper arm, and in the proximal forearm. High-definition imaging is critical for planning surgery that achieves adequate surgical margins and appropriate reconstructions when considering limb-sparing surgery. In this regard, imaging of the entire bone or soft tissue compartment is important to ensure that any potential skip lesions or regional lymphadenopathy is identified.

15.5 Anatomic Imaging

Magnetic resonance imaging (MRI) is the imaging modality of choice for both soft tissue and bone sarcomas because of its unsurpassed contrast. This allows excellent soft tissue and intramedullary delineation of tumour extent. It is important that sequences include at least T1 images that demonstrate anatomy, T2 images that demonstrate pathology, fat suppression images (with and without contrast enhancement) and orientations that include axial, coronal and sagittal images.

Computed tomography (CT) provides excellent bone imaging. Fine slice images are able to delineate tumour involvement of cortical and trabecular bone.

Plain orthogonal radiography is mandatory for bone sarcomas as these allow appropriate templating of bone for prosthetic sizing, appreciation of any bone or joint deformities or abnormalities.

15.6 Functional Imaging

Functional imaging provides information on the biologic activity of the tumour and whether this activity is uniform or limited to specific parts of the tumour. This will help to guide biopsy, assess response to preoperative therapies, establish unifocal or multifocal disease and also assist in planning surgical margins.

Functional imaging includes whole body technetium bone or thallium scintigraphy and glucose positron emission tomography (PET).

15.7 Biopsy

Biopsy is critical for diagnosing the tumour. This has important implications for appropriate preoperative adjuvant treatment and subsequent surgery. Biopsy like the definitive surgery also requires planning to ensure that the most representative site is targeted, the safest approach is employed and that the entry site is placed within the line of the incision to allow subsequent inclusion in the resection specimen without compromising the approach or extent of the surgery.

15.8 Systemic Imaging

The purpose of systemic imaging (pulmonary CT, PET) is to identify if metastasis has occurred. The presence of metastasis will alter the strategic approach to treatment, and whether metastases have occurred or not needs to be established prior to the commencement of treatment. In the presence of metastases, treatment more often than not adopts a palliative approach, while a curative strategy is usually employed when no metastasis is seen. A palliative approach may also include definitive limb-sparing surgery.

15.9 Surgery

15.9.1 Soft Tissue Sarcomas

A direct approach to resection is recommended for soft tissue sarcomas. Inclusion of an ellipse of overlying skin oriented with its long axis in line with the long axis of the limb is often required for a number of reasons: first, to minimise the creation of thin skin flaps with subsequent risk of tissue necrosis particularly in patients who have received preoperative adjuvant therapy; second, to avoid dissecting close to the tumour capsule of subcutaneous or large tumours; third, as 1/3 of sarcoma presentations occur after inadvertent resection elsewhere, to ensure that the entire skin incision and previous operative footprint are resected for good local control; and, fourth, to minimise impact on lymphatic drainage by reducing an encircling scar.

It is important that preoperative planning includes a close collaboration with the plastic surgical reconstructive team to optimise the best soft tissue reconstruction that does not compromise the surgical margin. Moreover, as soft tissue surgery to the upper limb is often associated with functional deficits afterwards, reconstructive options to preserve function is an important consideration prior to surgery to ensure appropriate surgery is undertaken and patient/surgeon expectations of the outcome are met.

Functional reconstructions of the upper limb are complex procedures and require the support of expert plastic and reconstructive surgeons. Defects may require multilayered transposition, rotational or free vascularised flaps [13]. Reconstruction of deltoid, triceps and biceps musculature after resection may be achieved through neurotised free muscle flaps or pedicled transposition flaps.

There are a number of strategies for the reconstruction of tumours of the forearm and hand [7, 14]. Reconstruction of finger flexion and extension is more difficult. If resection is limited to one compartment of the forearm, e.g. extensor, then tendon transfers from the flexor side may be employed to power extensor tendons of the wrist and hand, e.g. Jones transfer.

Reconstruction of flexor compartment musculature is a little more difficult because of the differential actions of the flexor digitorum superficialis and profundus tendons. Free vascularised innervated flaps may be employed to revitalise finger and thumb flexion. Innervated flaps or nerve repair may assist in providing protective sensation to the palmar surface of the hand and fingers.

15.9.2 Bone Sarcomas

15.9.3 *Humerus* (Fig. 15.4)

Proximal humeral resections may be reconstructed by a variety of different ways. These include prosthetic reconstructions (proximal humeral tumour endoprosthesis, reverse shoulder tumour endoprosthesis), biologic reconstructions (proximal humeral total condylar allograft, allograft arthrodesis, vascularised autogenous arthrodesis, claviculo-pro-humero reconstruction) and allograft prosthetic composite reconstructions.

The main challenge for any reconstruction following proximal humeral resection is joint stability. Almost all reconstructions other than the reverse shoulder arthroplasty requires a stabilising procedure to prevent subluxation of the proximal humerus that involves either soft tissue transfer [15] or reinforcement with a variety of non-resorbable synthetic meshes [16]. Surrounding the proximal humerus with such synthetic material not only incites a fibrotic reaction which reinforces the stabilising effect of the mesh but also allows a reliable framework to which adjacent musculature may be attached (e.g. rotator cuff, deltoid insertion).

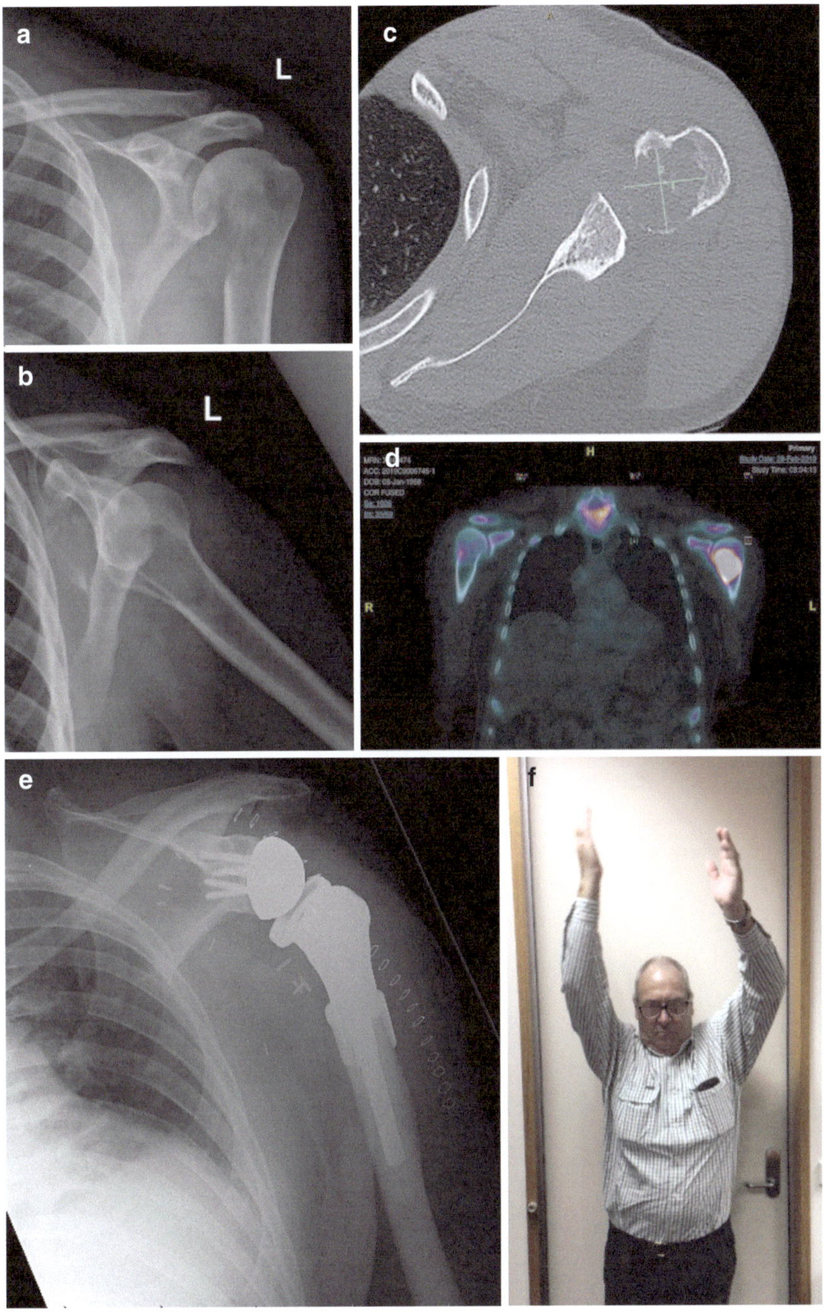

Fig. 15.4 (**a**) Anteroposterior and (**b**) axillary lateral plain radiographs of the shoulder demonstrating a large lytic lesion of the proximal humerus. (**c**) CT scan of the shoulder demonstrating destructive changes extending into the humeral head. (**d**) Thallium scan demonstrating local hypermetabolic tumour. (**e**) Following resection, the proximal humerus was reconstructed with a reverse shoulder tumour endoprosthesis. (**f**) Despite the loss of the supraspinatus tendon, the reverse shoulder mechanism permits a reasonable level of post-operative arm abduction

Occasionally an extra-articular resection of the shoulder joint (Tikhoff-Linberg) is required [17, 18]. Reconstruction of the scapula may sometimes be omitted with reconstruction of the proximal humerus occurring as a hanging arthroplasty where the proximal humerus is either lashed to the rib cage or suspended between the remaining scapula and clavicle [19].

If reconstruction of the scapula is required, for example, to act as a suspensory structure for the arm, then a prosthetic device may be fashioned out of polymethylmethacrylate acetate (PMMA) or a patient-specific metallic implant manufactured to which the parascapular musculature (trapezius, rhomboids, deltoid, serratus anterior) may be attached. It is uncommon for such soft tissue reconstruction around a prosthetic scapula to perform normally through an arc of movement, and at best it provides a structure to which the shoulder reconstruction may be stabilised through stiffness.

Resection of the humeral diaphysis can be reconstructed by direct shortening of the humerus and osteosynthesis, intercalary autogenous (vascularised or non-vascularised) or allograft bone reconstruction or an intercalary prosthetic spacer [20–24].

15.9.4 Elbow

Distal humeral resections are almost always reconstructed with a total elbow tumour endoprosthesis [25, 26]. A number of modularised prosthetic devices are available, and as long as the ulnar is not affected by the tumour, such endoprostheses perform well (Fig. 15.5). The main challenge with reconstructions about the elbow is

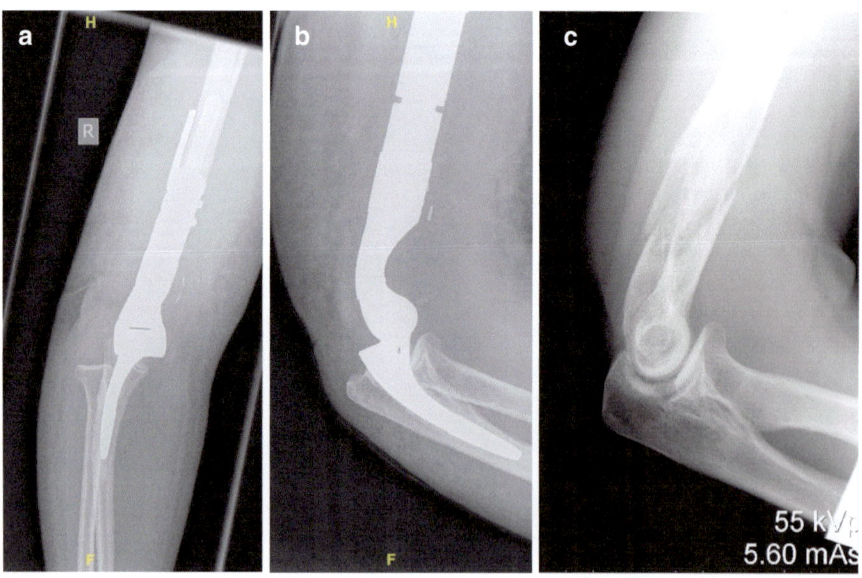

Fig. 15.5 (**a**) Anteroposterior and (**b**) lateral plain radiographs of a distal humeral tumour endoprosthesis following resection of (**c**) a distal humeral tumour

identifying, isolating and protecting the median, ulnar and radial nerves which lie immediately adjacent to the elbow on its medial, lateral and posterior aspects. The ulnar nerve is particularly vulnerable to post-operative neuritis because of its course over the posterior aspect of the elbow. Therefore, surgeons may choose to transpose the ulnar nerve onto the anterior aspect of the elbow. It is important that this manoeuvre is recalled later should reoperation around the elbow is required.

If a distal humeral tumour requires extra-articular resection of the elbow either by involving the joint or the proximal ulnar, then a patient-specific implant will be required. Such a reconstruction is important to match the ulnar component of the tumour endoprosthesis to the intramedullary canal of the recipient's ulnar.

15.9.5 Forearm

Forearm sarcomas account for less than 1% of all sites of sarcoma. Despite this, the challenges for reconstruction are significant because of the importance of the distal extremity. Surgery needs to be carefully planned not only for the resection but also the reconstruction [27] (Fig. 15.6).

Distal ulnar resections do not necessarily require reconstruction. Weakness of pronation, however, may result from this. Some argue that reconstruction of the distal may be required to provide stability to the wrist joint in ulnar deviation. The theory is that a significant ulnar minus deformity may cause the carpus to bear

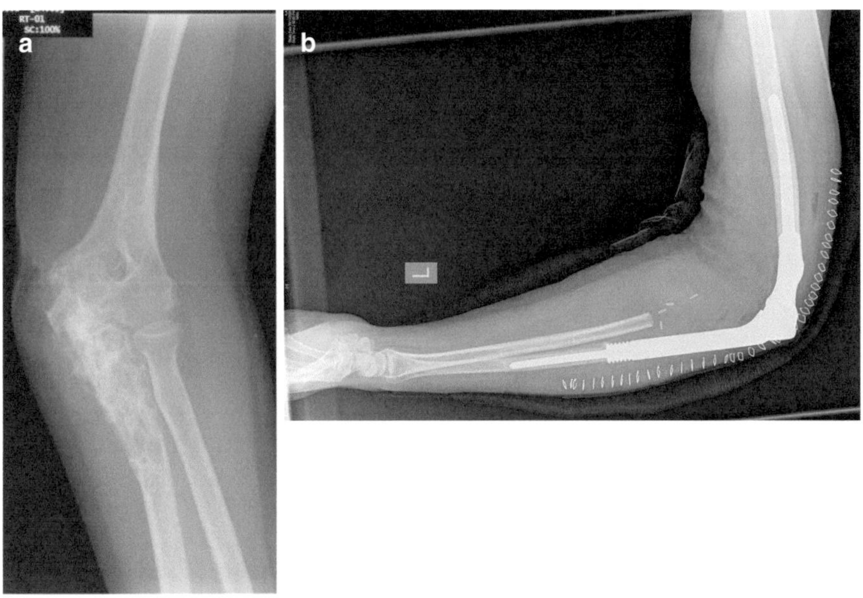

Fig. 15.6 (**a**) Chondrosarcoma of the proximal ulna. (**b**) Resection of the proximal ulnar tumour including the radius and reconstruction with a patient-specific proximal ulnar and elbow tumour endoprosthesis

heavily on the ulnar corner of the distal radius leading to lunate pathology or carpal arthritis. The extent to which this actually occurs remains unknown.

Resection of the distal radius is best treated with wrist arthrodesis (Fig. 15.7). There are several techniques for this procedure, and both allograft and autograft bone may be employed. Internal fixation with standard or arthrodesis plates may be used to support the arthrodesis.

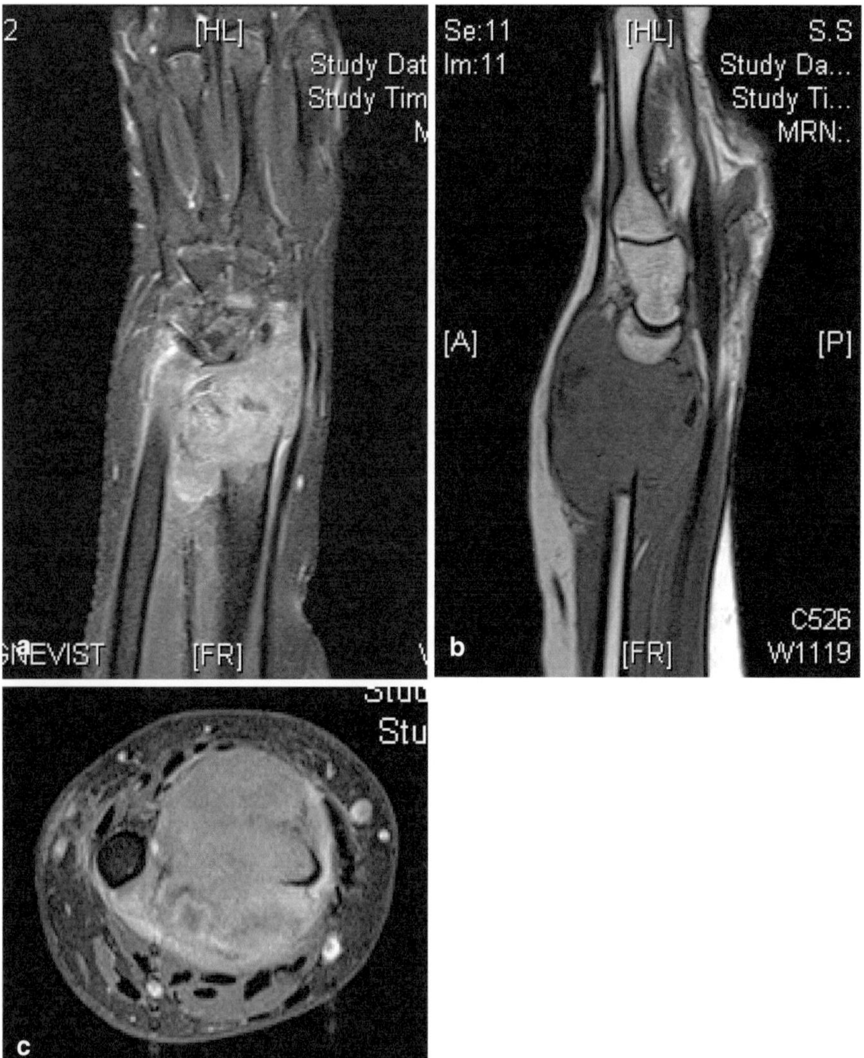

Fig. 15.7 (**a**) Coronal T2-weighted fat-suppressed contrast-enhanced, (**b**) sagittal T1-weighted and (**c**) T2-weighted fat-suppressed contrast-enhanced MRI images of a grade 3 giant cell tumour of the distal radius. (**d**) En bloc resection of the tumour and reconstruction with an autograft fibular arthrodesis. (**e**) Anteroposterior plain radiograph of the reconstruction with autologous fibula supplemented with a spanning plate

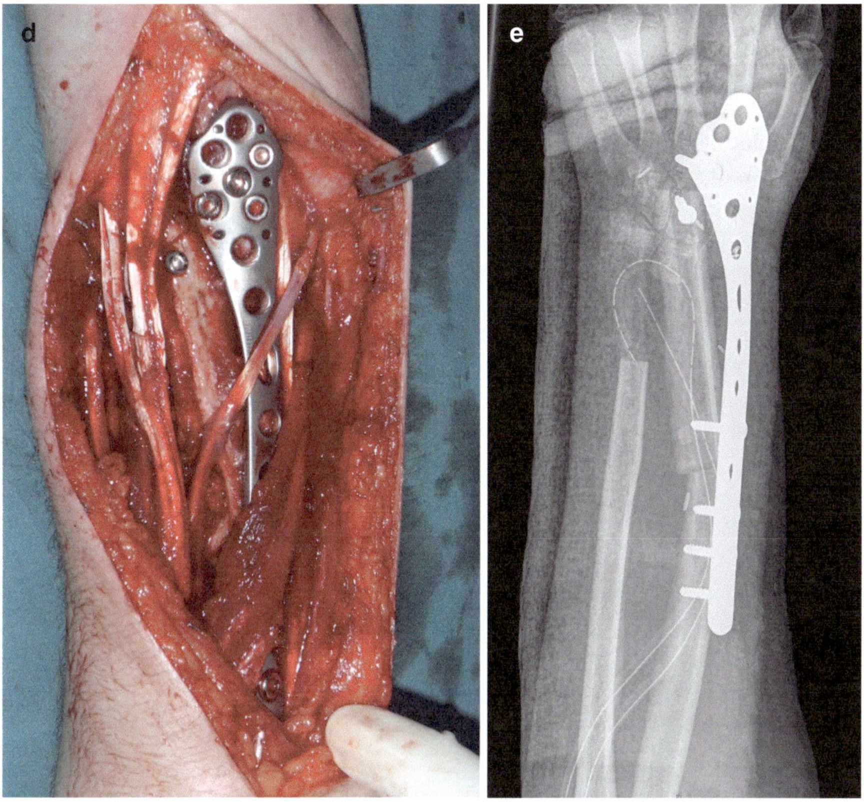

Fig. 15.7 (continued)

Mobile reconstructions of the wrist have been attempted in the past. In this circumstance, the proximal fibular head has been used as the articulating surface. Gaining stability of this mobile reconstruction has proven a challenge with the risk of carpal subluxation ever present.

15.9.6 Amputation

In the setting of a bone or soft tissue sarcoma that is characterised by invasion of vital neurovascular structures where resection is unlikely to result in a functional limb despite reconstruction, amputation should be considered [28, 29]. Large soft tissue tumours of the axilla, medial arm or elbow or deep-seated soft tissue tumours of the forearm are such tumours.

A further circumstance where amputation should be considered is when a tumour is inadvertently excised with wide contamination of neurovascular structures such that the resection of the operative footprint is so wide as to make functional reconstruction and limb preservation unlikely.

If the decision to amputate is made, amputation should be far enough away to ensure good local control of disease. Amputations for forearm sarcomas are usually performed at the level above the elbow. This is to ensure adequate skin flaps are available for closure. Furthermore, with inadvertent excision of forearm sarcomas, the potential for the deep forearm bursae (radial bursa and common flexor sheath) to be contaminated is ever present, and this may give rise to a high risk of local recurrence in the hand and forearm.

High amputation of the upper limb may be at the thoraco-scapular level (forequarter amputation), through the glenohumeral joint (shoulder disarticulation) or within the proximal third of the humerus. For such proximal resections, it is critical to elaborate on whether axillary lymph node involvement is present. This may necessitate reconsideration of the treatment strategy. PET scanning and MRI are highly recommended for determining the presence or absence of axillary involvement.

References

1. Lesensky J, Mavrogenis AF, Igoumenou VG, Matejovsky Z Jr, Nemec K, Papagelopoulos PJ, et al. Complex surgery for locally advanced bone and soft tissue sarcomas of the shoulder girdle. Eur J Orthop Surg Traumatol. 2017;27(6):777–86.
2. Volpe CM, Pell M, Doerr RJ, Karakousis CP. Radical scapulectomy with limb salvage for shoulder girdle soft tissue sarcoma. Surg Oncol. 1996;5(1):43–8.
3. Wodajo FM, Bickels J, Wittig J, Malawer M. Complex reconstruction in the management of extremity sarcomas. Curr Opin Oncol. 2003;15(4):304–12.
4. Koulaxouzidis G, Simunovic F, Bannasch H. Soft tissue sarcomas of the arm - Oncosurgical and reconstructive principles within a multimodal, interdisciplinary setting. Front Surg. 2016;3:12.
5. Murray PM. Soft tissue sarcoma of the upper extremity. Hand Clin. 2004;20(3):325–33. vii
6. Baroudi MR, Ferguson PC, Wunder JS, Isler MH, Mottard S, Werier JA, et al. Forearm soft tissue sarcoma: tumors characteristics and oncologic outcomes following limb salvage surgery. J Surg Oncol. 2014;110(6):676–81.
7. Muramatsu K, Ihara K, Doi K, Hashimoto T, Taguchi T. Sarcoma in the forearm and hand: clinical outcomes and microsurgical reconstruction for limb salvage. Ann Plast Surg. 2009;62(1):28–33.
8. Lazerges C. Soft tissue sarcomas of the forearm, wrist and hand. 2017;Hand Surg Rehabil:233–243.
9. Houdek M, Walczak B, Wilke B, Kakar S, Rose P, AY S. What factors influence the outcomes of surgically treated soft tissue sarcomas of the hand and wrist. Hand. 2017;12:493–500.
10. Mirous MP, Coulet B, Chammas M, Cupissol D, Lazerges C. Extensive limb-sparing surgery with reconstruction for sarcoma of the hand and wrist. Orthop Traumatol Surg Res. 2016;102(4):467–72.
11. Nicholson S, Milner RH, Ragbir M. Soft tissue sarcoma of the hand and wrist: epidemiology and management challenges. J Hand Microsurg. 2018;10(2):86–92.
12. Buecker P, Villafuerte J, Hornicek F, Gebhardt M, Mankin H. Improved survival for sarcomas of the wrist and hand. J Hand Surg Am. 2006;31:452–5.
13. Martin E, Dullaart MJ, van de Sande MAJ, van Houdt WJ, Schellekens PPA, Coert JH. Resuscitating extremities after soft tissue sarcoma resections: are functional reconstructions an overlooked option in limb salvage? A systematic review. Eur J Surg Oncol. 2019;45(10):1762–9.

14. Vetter M, Germann G, Bickert B, Sauerbier M. Current strategies for sarcoma reconstruction at the forearm and hand. J Reconstr Microsurg. 2010;26(7):455–60.
15. van de Sande MA, Cosker T, McDonnell SM, Gibbons CL, Giele H. Use of the composite pedicled pectoralis minor flap after resection of soft tissue sarcoma in reconstruction of the glenohumeral joint. Case Rep Orthop. 2014;2014:937342.
16. Tang X, Guo W, Yang R, Tang S, Ji T. Synthetic mesh improves shoulder function after intraarticular resection and prosthetic replacement of proximal humerus. Clin Orthop Relat Res. 2015;473(4):1464–71.
17. Linberg BE. Interscapulo-thoracic resection for malignant tumors of thc shoulder joint region. Clin Orthop Relat Res. 1928;1999(358):3–7.
18. Malawer MM, Meller I, Dunham WK. A new surgical classification system for shoulder-girdle resections. Analysis of 38 patients. Clin Orthop Relat Res. 1991;267:33–44.
19. Biazzo A, De Paolis M, Donati DM. Scapular reconstructions after resection for bone tumors: a single-institution experience and review of the literature. Acta Biomed. 2018;89(3):415–22.
20. Ayvaz M, Bekmez S, Yucekul A, Mermerkaya MU, Tokgozoglu AM. Titanium mesh cage as an alternative reconstruction method for epiphyseal-sparing tumour resections in children. J Pediatr Orthop B. 2018;27(4):350–5.
21. Gupta S, Kafchinski LA, Gundle KR, Saidi K, Griffin AM, Wunder JS, et al. Intercalary allograft augmented with intramedullary cement and plate fixation is a reliable solution after resection of a diaphyseal tumour. Bone Joint J. 2017.;99-B;99-B(7):973–8.
22. McGrath A, Sewell MD, Hanna SA, Pollock RC, Skinner JA, Cannon SR, et al. Custom endoprosthetic reconstruction for malignant bone disease in the humeral diaphysis. Acta Orthop Belg. 2011;77(2):171–9.
23. Puri A, Gulia A, Jambhekar N, Laskar S. The outcome of the treatment of diaphyseal primary bone sarcoma by resection, irradiation and re-implantation of the host bone: extracorporeal irradiation as an option for reconstruction in diaphyseal bone sarcomas. J Bone Joint Surg Br. 2012;94(7):982–8.
24. Zheng K, Yu XC, Hu YC, Shao ZW, Xu M, Wang BC, et al. Outcome of segmental prosthesis reconstruction for diaphyseal bone tumors: a multi-center retrospective study. BMC Cancer. 2019;19(1):638.
25. Casadei R, De Paolis M, Drago G, Romagnoli C, Donati D. Total elbow arthroplasty for primary and metastatic tumor. Orthop Traumatol Surg Res. 2016;102(4):459–65.
26. Henrichs MP, Liem D, Gosheger G, Streitbuerger A, Nottrott M, Andreou D, et al. Megaprosthetic replacement of the distal humerus: still a challenge in limb salvage. J Shoulder Elb Surg. 2019;28(5):908–14.
27. Muramatsu K, Ihara K, Yoshida K, Tominaga Y, Hashimoto T, Taguchi T. Musculoskeletal sarcomas in the forearm and hand: standard treatment and microsurgical reconstruction for limb salvage. Anticancer Res. 2013;33(10):4175–82.
28. Huayllani M, Restrepo D, Bczar D, Sisti A, Spaulding A, Parker A, et al. What factors define limb salvage or amputation in osteosarcoma of the upper extremities. Anticancer Res. 2019;39:6807–11.
29. Puhaindran ME, Chou J, Forsberg JA, Athanasian EA. Major upper-limb amputations for malignant tumors. J Hand Surg Am. 2012;37(6):1235–41.

Surgical Management of Pelvic Sarcomas

16

Peter F. M. Choong

16.1 Introduction

Tumours of the pelvis account for a sixth of all sarcomas. The pelvis is a challenging area to manage surgically because of the neurovascular structures and viscera within its cavity, the limb girdle musculature which arise from its inner and outer surface and vital structures that course from within to outside the cavity. Moreover, the large volume for expansion within the confines of the pelvic and abdominal cavity and the bulk of the muscle and fat that drape the proximal limb girdle allows tumours both soft tissue and bone to attain considerable sizes before detection.

The pelvis is also important because it provides a structural connection between the lower limb and the rest of the body. Specifically, it connects the lower limb to the spine through the hip joint and sacroiliac joint and to the contralateral side via the anterior pelvis (pubic rami and pubic symphysis) and the sacrum. Resection of any of these parts has the potential to destabilise the pelvic ring and impair the structural integrity of the locomotor mechanism [1, 2].

The pelvic ring and the musculoskeletal system of the pelvic girdle can sustain considerable disruption while still being able to bear weight and contribute to locomotor function [1, 2]. Numerous reconstructive strategies have been developed to rebuild the pelvis after tumour resection with the purpose of providing stability of the pelvic ring, articulation between femur and pelvis and satisfactory functional outcomes [3].

P. F. M. Choong (✉)
Department of Surgery, University of Melbourne, Melbourne, VIC, Australia

Department of Orthopaedics, St. Vincent's Hospital, Melbourne, VIC, Australia

Bone & Soft Tissue Tumour Service, Peter MacCallum Cancer Centre, Melbourne, VIC, Australia
e-mail: pchoong@unimelb.edu.au

P. F. M. Choong (ed.), *Sarcoma*, https://doi.org/10.1007/978-981-15-9414-4_16

16.2 Bone Tumours

Common benign bone tumours of the pelvis include but are not limited to osteochondromas, enchondromas, fibrous dysplasia, aneurysmal bone cysts and simple bone cysts.

Malignant bone tumours more commonly include chondrosarcoma, osteosarcoma and Ewing's sarcoma and lymphoma. However, rarer malignancies may also occur.

16.2.1 Soft Tissue Tumours

Lipoma, schwannoma and myxoma are the commonest benign soft tissue tumours encountered around the pelvis.

Malignant soft tissue tumours are many, but the more common that affect the pelvis include undifferentiated pleomorphic sarcoma, liposarcoma, fibromyxoid sarcoma and synovial sarcoma.

16.2.2 Presenting Symptoms and Signs

Benign bone tumours usually present incidentally or as a painless prominence. Malignant bone tumours, however, often present with deep-seated pain that is unremitting and not responsive to simple analgesics. Nocturnal pain is a feature of malignant bone tumours. If the periacetabular area is affected, then referred pain down the thigh and to the knee may also occur.

Benign soft tissue tumours present with a painless soft lump or incidentally on imaging. A schwannoma may present with deep-seated pelvic discomfort or referred pain if a sensory nerve is affected. Malignant soft tissue tumours present as hard or firm masses often fixed to underlying structures. They may grow to substantial sizes prior to presentation. Compression or impingement on adjacent viscera, for example, the bladder or liver, may give rise to symptoms that herald the presence of the tumour.

16.2.3 Investigations

Because of the complexity of the anatomy and contents of the pelvis, it is crucial that careful and thorough imaging is employed. As many tumours of the pelvis can reach substantial sizes, the risk of metastasis is high if the tumour is malignant. Therefore, systemic imaging should also be employed. All local and systemic investigations lead ultimately to biopsy which should be targeted, planned and image guided.

16.2.3.1 Plain Radiography

Plain radiograph of the pelvis should be performed to give an initial assessment of the extent of bone involvement and the encroachment of tumour on the periacetabulum or the sacroiliac area [4–7]. The internal characteristics of the tumour (e.g. lysis, calcification, fluid levels, mixed lytic sclerotic, bone-in-bone) may give an indication as to the diagnosis. Special attention should also be paid to the types of periosteal elevation (sunray, Codman's triangle, onion skin) which are associated with different types of primary bone tumours [8]. Soft tissue tumours may be noted by asymmetry of soft tissue outlines [9].

16.2.3.2 Computed Tomography

Computed tomography (CT) is an ideal method for imaging the characteristics of bone. It is able to clearly delineate cortical and trabecular destruction and is very useful for identifying breaches in the cortex to signal extraosseous extension [10]. CT is also an important modality in more advanced approaches to image-guided surgery. CT may be used to characterise a pelvic soft tissue mass, but magnetic resonance imaging (MRI) is a better modality for this. CT is mandatory of the lungs to detect the presence of pulmonary metastases.

16.2.3.3 Magnetic Resonance Imaging

Magnetic resonance imaging is perfectly placed to image a pelvic tumour [5, 11–14]. Its unsurpassed soft tissue contrast is invaluable for separating tumour from adjacent structures including vessels, nerves, viscera and bone. Moreover, the fat content of the pelvic marrow space provides excellent contrast for estimating the extent of intraosseous tumours. MRI is mandatory for all cases of pelvic sarcoma whether of bone or soft tissue. T1 sequences allow a nice portrayal of anatomy, while T2 sequences highlight pathology particularly when combined with contrast and suppression of the fat signal. T1 imaging is very useful for identifying the fat layers between the anatomic structures to help define the tumour margins and the surgical margins. It is important that investigation of a posterior pelvic tumour includes examination of the lumbar spine as some tumours of the pelvis may rise high up in the spinal canal or paraspinal space.

16.2.3.4 Functional Imaging

Functional imaging is an important addition to the investigatory armamentarium. The ability to demonstrate metabolic activity is very useful for helping to target biopsies, for pretreatment baseline assessment and for assessing post-treatment response. Various modalities have been described including FDG-PET [15–20], thallium-201 [21–23] and DMSA(V) [22, 23]. These markers target the metabolic machinery of cells to highlight their inherent and post-treatment activity. A reduction in activity is an indication of tumour response to treatment, while an ongoing high signal indicates that the tumour remains viable or has not responded to treatment. The characteristics of the signal pattern, for example, whether the uptake is peripheral or central may indicate where the viable or necrotic tumour is. It is important to note that some tumours show little uptake because of extensive tumour necrosis. This is an indication of the high-grade nature of the tumour rather than one without activity because it is low grade. Careful interpretation with an expert in nuclear medicine is recommended. If there is a poor response to neoadjuvant therapy as predicted by functional imaging, then a careful assessment of the margins should be undertaken with a view to employing the pretreatment tumour dimensions and position as the benchmark for planning surgical margins.

16.2.3.5 Angiography

Angiography is seldom done unless consideration is being given to vascular resection and reconstruction [24–32]. Large pelvic tumours with overhanging protuberances may entrap vessels between themselves and the pelvis, and if suspected angiography would be helpful to delineate the nature and extent of the impingement.

16.2.3.6 Ureterogram/Cystogram

Tumours of the lesser pelvis may impinge on the base of the bladder and compromise the function of the ureters as they enter the bladder. Similarly, anterior pelvic tumours may endanger the urethra as it courses under the pubic arch. Men with previous surgery to the prostate or benign prostatic hypertrophy may be susceptible to urethral damage with dissection because of the tethering of the urethra.

16.2.4 Biopsy

Biopsy of pelvic tumours is essential for appropriate multidisciplinary care because of the wide variations in treatment [33, 34]. Because of the anatomic complexities of the pelvis, biopsies should be carefully planned and performed in a centre expert at managing bone and soft tissue tumours. Image-guided biopsy (CT) allows the proper execution of this plan with reliable diagnostic accuracy which can also be recorded [34]. The entry point of biopsy, the passage of the biopsy instrument and the tissue harvest can be confirmed providing important information for planning the subsequent surgical approach.

Iliac tumours are best biopsied with an entry point that stays close to the iliac crest and a trajectory which passes along the plane of the iliac wing. Tumours of the sacrum should be approached from directly posteriorly. Anterior pelvic tumours may also be biopsied from a direct anterior approach while avoiding the contents of the femoral triangle. Tumours of the periacetabulum are notoriously difficult to biopsy because access to the medial wall may be obstructed anteriorly by the femoral vessels, posteriorly by the contents of the sciatic notch and laterally by the hip joint. In such a situation, an open biopsy may be necessary to allow absolute control of the biopsy process and protection of vital structures while ensuring minimal contamination of the operative field for a subsequent definitive procedure. This is a time where clinical judgement and experience becomes extremely valuable. This is most available at centre expert in the management of bone and soft tissue tumours.

16.3 Preoperative Preparation

Preoperative preparation of the patient is vital to ensure their safety during and after surgery. Pelvic surgery may be accompanied by considerable physiological upset over a long duration of time, and neoadjuvant therapies may compromise numerous bodily systems, so careful testing and preoperative optimisation is necessary.

Anaemia, neutropenia and thrombocytopenia are common with patients undergoing chemotherapy. A nadir of haematological function is usually reached within the first week after delivery of the final pre-operative dose, and most patients' indices have returned to pre-chemotherapy levels by 2 weeks of the final dose. Even patients undergoing radiotherapy may suffer idiosyncratic blood dyscrasias. Large soft tissue tumours may give rise to anaemia because of haemorrhagic necrosis, and tumour-related fevers are not uncommon. Relevant transfusions should be prescribed to ensure that the appropriate levels that are safe for surgery are reached. Considerable blood loss is common, and this may trigger coagulopathies which may be best treated by mitigation in the first instance. Planning of surgery should be timed with optimisation of the haematological status.

Cardiac and renal function are often impacted by the types of agents used for preoperative chemotherapy. Appropriate preoperative cardiac and renal testing is mandatory because of the considerable physiological stress associated with extensive and prolonged pelvic resectional and reconstructive surgery. Intraoperative cardiac monitoring may also be employed using transoesophageal echocardiograms for particularly fragile patients.

Nutritional status is important as many patients stand to lose significant amounts of weight prior to surgery. Wound complications, infection and healing are related to the nutritional state of the individual prior to and after surgery. Engagement of appropriate dietetic advice and support is valuable.

Anaesthetic screening prior to surgery is essential so that the patient and anaesthetist may be aware of possible contingencies leading up to and including the procedure [35]. A combination of neuraxial, regional and general anaesthesia is often employed to ensure the safest conditions for the patient and to optimise post-operative pain control management [36–38]. As there is a possibility for considerable blood loss during the case as well as prolonged recumbency, the anaesthetic team should be prepared for high-volume fluid shifts, and invasive intraarterial and central venous monitoring is often required. High-volume fluid shifts may result in pulmonary oedema and upper airway and facial swelling [37]. Liaison with intensive care specialist is recommended in anticipation of a period of intensive post-operative monitoring until the patient is stable enough to return to the general ward.

16.3.1 Positioning

The patient is usually positioned in the "floppy lateral" position (Fig. 16.1). In this position the patient is held with side supports at the sternum and thoracic region with the abdomen, flank and pelvis free for any approach. With the side supports

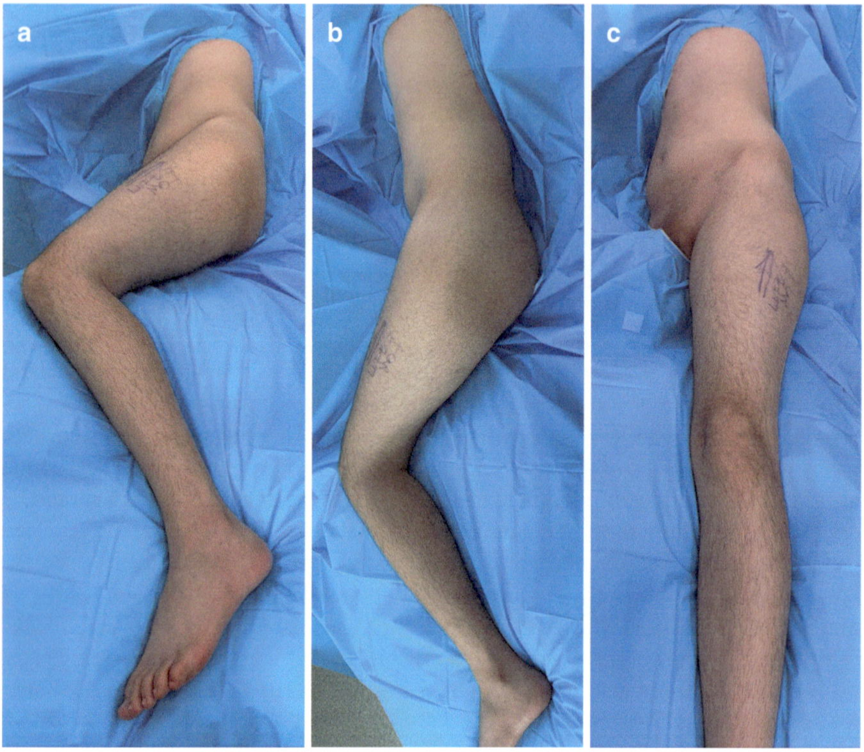

Fig. 16.1 The patient is held in the floppy lateral position with a sternal and mid thoracic rest. This allows good exposure of the abdomen and the entire hemipelvis and lower leg. This allows the patient to be held in (**a**) the lateral position, (**b**) rolled inward into a semi-prone position and (**c**) rolled outward into a semi-supine position. This allows an excellent approach to the pelvis from the front, the side and the back. Preparing the leg free also permits harvest of the ipsilateral fibula

securely positioned opposite the sternum and mid thorax, the patient may be rolled forward from the lateral position (Fig. 16.1a) to the semi-prone position to expose the posterior pelvis/buttock (Fig. 16.1b) and to the semi-supine position (Fig. 16.1c) to expose the anterior lower abdomen and pelvis as required [39]. Careful padding of the pressure points on the underside of the patient is mandatory because of the duration of the operation.

16.3.2 Surgical Considerations

Pelvic surgery is complex because of the close proximity of vital structures and viscera. The pelvic ring may be divided into four parts which bear special relevance when planning surgery (Fig. 16.2).

The ring consists of (I) the iliac wing (superior and inferior halves), (II) the peri-acetabulum, (III) the symphysis and pubic rami and (IV) the sacrum. This

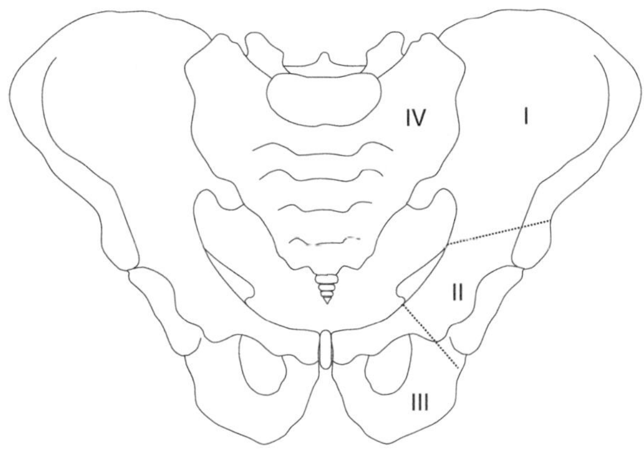

Fig. 16.2 The pelvis is divided into four zones (Type I, II, III, and IV). Tumours are classified according to where they are located (e.g. Type I tumour is in the ilium, Type II is periacetabular, Type III is ischio-pubic, and Type IV is sacral). Crossover of tumours from one zone to another is reflected in the nomenclature (e.g. Types I–IV are ilio-sacral tumours)

classification (Types I–IV) is a consensus nomenclature to allow surgeons expert in the field to discuss tumour locations, resections, reconstructions and outcomes [40].

16.3.2.1 Type I Tumours

Tumours of the iliac wing are classified as Type I tumours. The least complicated position is the superior half of the wing of the ilium. Here, the main structures to consider when planning surgery are the muscles on either side of the bone, namely, ilio-psoas and the abductors.

Resection of tumours of the superior part of the iliac wing may occur without disrupting the pelvic ring. Leg lengths are usually maintained, and the function of the hip usually remains normal unless there has been sacrifice of the gluteus medius.

Involvement of the inferior half of the iliac wing usually complicates the contents of the sciatic notch. Here the internal iliac vessels emerge as the superior and inferior gluteal vessels and the internal pudendal vessels. If an extraosseous extension of bone tumour or a soft tissue sarcoma obstructs the sciatic notch, then limb-sparing surgery may be difficult or impossible without sacrificing the sciatic nerve and the internal iliac vessels. Securing the sciatic notch is critical for limb-sparing surgery, and appreciation of this must occur early in the planning of surgical margins (Fig. 16.3).

Reconstruction of the iliac wing is usually unnecessary if the pelvic ring is not disrupted. If, however, disruption occurs, there are a number of reconstructive options available.

(a) No reconstruction – Leaving the defect as is will result in the two ends of the "broken" ring approximating each other. The side of the surgery will close like a book hinging on the symphysis pubis. Doing so, there are usually a limb length discrepancy and slight outward rotation of the ipsilateral leg [41, 42].

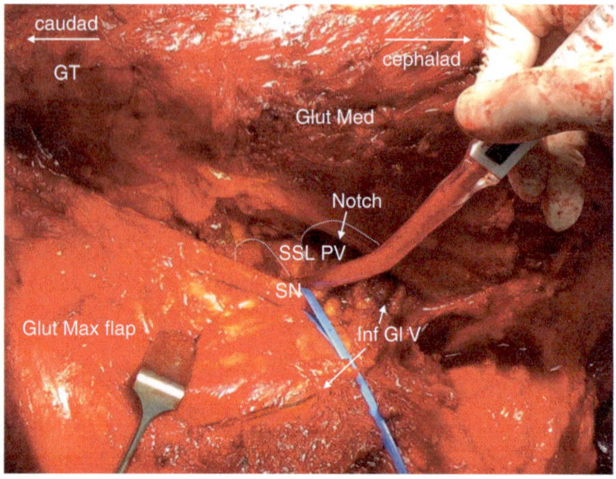

Fig. 16.3 Securing the notch is critical for safe surgery. Key anatomic landmarks from behind include the sacrospinous ligament (SSL), the pudendal vessels (PV), the sciatic nerve (SN) and the inferior gluteal vessels (Inf Gl V)

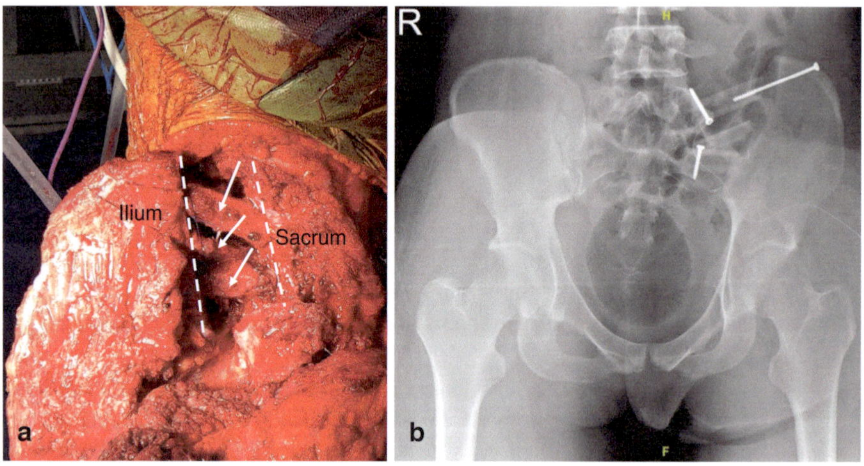

Fig. 16.4 (**a**) Posterior view of Type I–IV resection demonstrating the cut surfaces of the ilium and sacrum (dashed lines) and the three fibular grafts spanning the defect (arrows). (**b**) Plain anteroposterior radiograph demonstrating the reconstruction. Sacral cut performed just lateral to the sacral foramina

Patients tend to do very well after this type of surgery and are able to partially weight bear with walking aids about 3 months after surgery. With increasing comfort, patients may be graduated onto greater weight bearing as tolerated. It may be helpful to have a patient in a hip spica initially to stabilise the pelvis, thus making it more comfortable for the patient when mobilising.

(b) Biological reconstruction – The defect in the ilium may be spanned by vascularised or non-vascularised autogenous bone [43–47] (Fig. 16.4). The outcome of non-vascularised bone may be similar to vascularised grafts and, therefore, may be chosen because of a shorter, less complicated surgery (Fig. 16.4).

The defect may also be spanned using allograft bone [1, 48, 49]. The availability of large amounts of bone of different dimensions usually means that allograft bone is a satisfactory option. This can be considered when the gap top span is wide. Whether allograft bone survives longer than autograft bone or is as strong depends on variables such as whether the bone is fresh-frozen or irradiated. The latter is usually of less structural quality than fresh-frozen bone. However, the need to protect the graft and recipient from infection usually requires irradiation, and therefore, the risk of late fracture, dissolution or non-union exists.

(c) Bespoke prosthetic reconstructions of the pelvic wing – These are less commonly used because of the expense and complexity of manufacture. Their use in specialist centres usually reflects surgeon or institutional preferences [50–54]. Modern three-dimensional additive manufacturing has opened renewed interest in such bespoke implants because of the ability to address not only the shape but also the strength and the surface characteristics of the prosthesis. Although modern bespoke manufactured prostheses have enjoyed great attraction, they are not regarded as conventional because of costs and the lack of long-term data.

16.3.2.2 Type II Tumours

Tumours of the periacetabulum are referred to as Type II tumours. Tumours here usually involve the hip joint, and treatment almost always leads to sacrifice of that joint. The extent to which part of the hip joint can be spared in any Type II resection will depend on the nature of the tumour, its response to neoadjuvant therapy and whether the preserved part of periacetabular bone is actually worth preserving. Reconstructions are complex and associated with high intra- and post-operative risk [55].

Resections of the periacetabulum usually require dissection through the sciatic notch; therefore, it is critical that control of the contents of the sciatic notch is achieved and that achieving control retains good margins around the periacetabular tumour. The spine of the pelvis and the ischial tuberosity form the posterior column of the acetabulum. Wide resection of tumours therefore will usually include these two landmarks. It is important that the sacro-spinous and the sacro-tuberous ligaments are safely identified and divided prior to performing the osteotomies, as these structures may impede manipulation of the osteotomised fragment and prevent its extraction if the ligaments, which are very robust, remain intact.

If the hip joint is involved with tumour within the joint, then an extra-articular resection is required which includes the hip joint (unopened). To achieve this, the femoral osteotomy should follow the line of the femoral attachment of the capsule or at least at the subtrochanteric region or below.

Exposure of the periacetabulum is facilitated by a trochanteric osteotomy which will allow reflection of the abductors superiorly to demonstrate the underlying bone. If trochanteric osteotomy is possible, then reattachment at the end of the procedure will usually facilitate good abductor function and hip joint stability later.

Reconstructions after periacetabular resections may include joint reconstruction or non-joint reconstructing procedures.

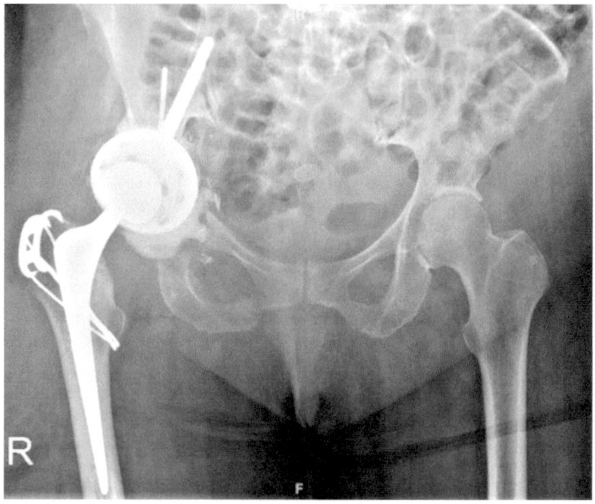

Fig. 16.5 Pedestal cup impacted into position using computer guidance to reconstruct a Type II resection

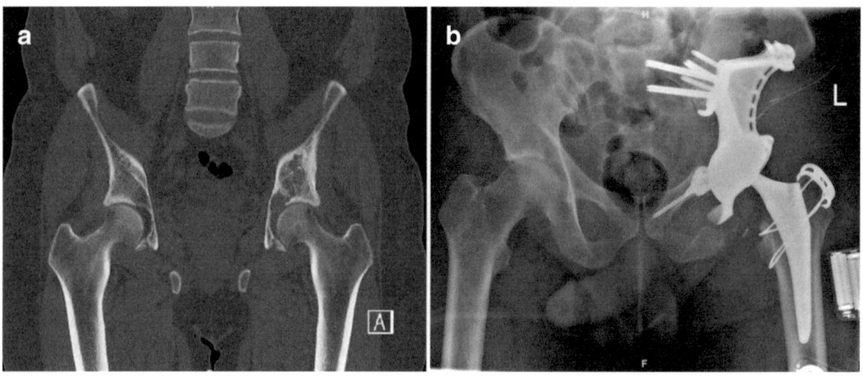

Fig. 16.6 (**a**) CT scan demonstrating left periacetabular chondrosarcoma. (**b**) Type I–II resection and reconstructed with bespoke 3D printed implant

Joint reconstructing procedures aim to re-establish the hip joint. This usually involves a prosthetic solution or an autograft/allograft prosthetic composite.

Prosthetic solutions include standard acetabular reconstructions, pedestal cup type reconstructions (Fig. 16.5) or bespoke pelvic prostheses (Fig. 16.6).

Biologic reconstructions alone are uncommon and are usually combined with prosthetic solutions. These include pelvic allografts or pelvic autografts (post-extracorporeal irradiation) (Fig. 16.7) in combination with standard hip prosthetic implants.

Non-joint reconstructing procedures include flail hip, ilio-femoral arthrodesis or ischio-femoral pseudarthrosis. Ilio-femoral arthrodesis is a reliable means of achieving stable weight-bearing ability after resection of the acetabulum. However, this procedure is always associated with a limb length deficiency, unless an intercalary graft is also used to build up the deficit of bone. Patients with ilio-femoral

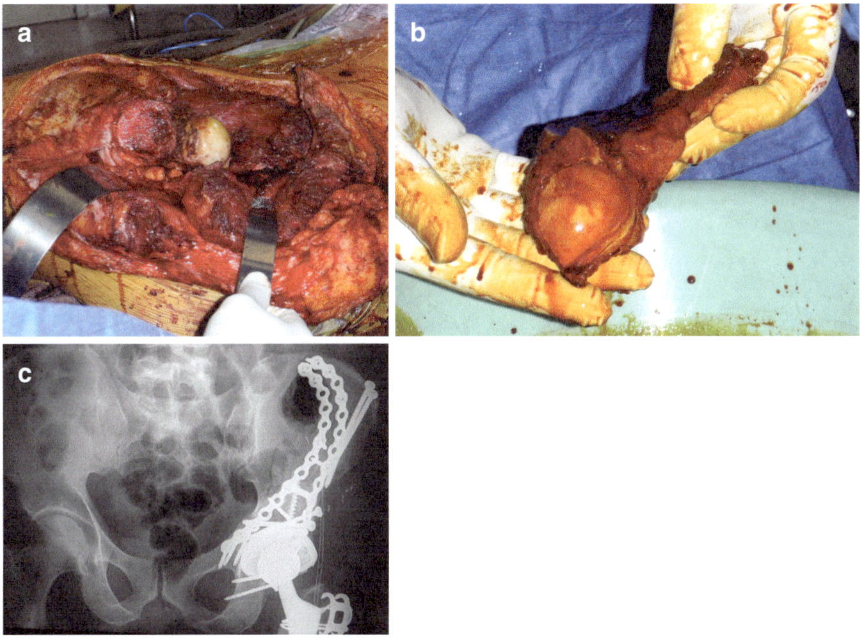

Fig. 16.7 (**a**) Type I–II resection. Note exposed femoral head and trochanteric osteotomy for exposure. (**b**) Segment of resected bone containing periacetabular chondrosarcoma. (**c**) Following extracorporeal irradiation, Type I–II reconstruction with pelvic plates, large interfragmentary screws and total hip replacement

pseudarthroses rely on increased activity and mobility of the ipsilateral knee, contralateral hip and lumbar regions to compensate for the loss of mobility through the arthrodesis.

Ischio-femoral pseudarthrosis (Fig. 16.8) is an excellent reconstructive solution for patients who have had periacetabular resections. The reconstruction itself is simple and essentially consists of lashing the proximal femur to the superior and inferior pubic ramus with cerclage cables and grafting around the pseudarthrosis with femoral head graft if possible. The limb hinges on the pubic symphysis allowing some movement to compensate for the stiffness of the pseudarthrosis. A jog of movement at the pseudarthrosis adds to the movement imparted at the pubic symphysis.

Type II reconstructions if successful provide the patient with a useful lower limb, and therefore, these reconstructions should be considered where feasible. However, the complications and risks associated with this type of reconstruction are significant [56], particularly when considering the use of novel bespoke prostheses. Careful consideration is required when discussing the pros and cons of such surgery with the patient to ensure that a fully informed decision is made and that post-operative expectations of patient and surgeon are matched. Because of these high risks, the patient must understand the potential for limb or life lost as a result of these complications.

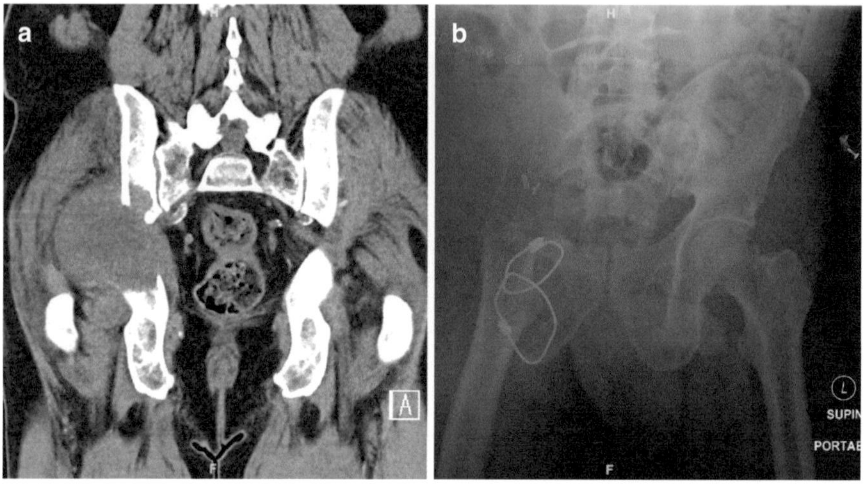

Fig. 16.8 (**a**) Coronal CT scan demonstrating large periacetabular sarcoma. (**b**) Type I-II-IV resection followed by ischio-femoral pseudarthrosis reinforced by two cables

16.3.2.3 Type III Tumours

Type III resections remove the bone from the symphysis pubis to the acetabular margin. Surgery in this area exposes the femoral and obturator neurovascular structures to injury. In addition, the bladder is at risk of tumours that are midline in the anterior pelvis. The urethra is also at risk as it passes under the pubic arch. Post-operatively, anterior pelvic resections may be complicated by large direct inguinal hernias that include bowel and bladder.

Bone reconstructions following Type II resections are uncommon. Weight bearing does not require a reconstruction of the bony pubis even if bilateral pubic rami resections (four-poster) are required.

Direct hernia of the lower anterior abdominal wall is common after unilateral or bilateral pubic rami resections. However, it is uncommon for such hernias to become complicated. Some patients may develop pressure symptoms related to bowel or bladder herniation. Reconstruction of the lower anterior abdominal wall is difficult and usually requires supplementary material such as synthetic mesh to provide sufficient strength to hold back the pressure of abdominal contents [57]. The main problem of such reconstructions is identifying suitable attachment points on the residual bone or soft tissue to act as a robust foundation for anchoring sutures. Soft tissue reconstructions with fascia or muscle flaps have also been tried with varying success.

16.3.2.4 Type IV Tumours

Type IV resections involve resections of the sacral body or alar. Sacral resections are employed either for the treatment of chordomas or where the lateral sacral alar is included as part of the margin when resecting Type I tumours.

Resections of the Sacral Alar.

Resections of the sacral alar usually occur lateral to the sacral foramina. The emerging nerve roots are the landmarks for the most medial extent of the resection. The nerve roots may be identified anteriorly as they emerge from the foraminae or from behind as the nerve roots are followed out laterally during the course of a sacral laminectomy. The use of computer-assisted techniques borrowed from spinal and joint replacement surgery now allows navigation of the line of the osteotomy, thus increasing the efficiency and safety of the procedure.

Sacrectomy for sacral chordoma is a challenging operation [58–60] particularly if it requires resections above the level of the S2–3 interval. At this level, decisions are required as to whether to spare at least one sacral nerve root, if possible, to provide a level of urinary and bowel continence [61]. Moreover, resections that are above the S2–3 interval stand to increase the stresses on the remaining sacral segments (S1, partial S2) because of the transmission of the body weight through this weakened part of the pelvic ring. The risk of stress fracture through the sacral remnant is high with such resections [62] and if present will lead to pain and deformity. Under such circumstances, modifications to rehabilitation and reconstruction with spinal instrumentation supplemented by allograft/autograft bone [60] should be considered.

Sacrectomy below the S2 has been well described and can usually occur without significant compromise of bowel or bladder dysfunction or injury to the lumbosacral plexus. Bone reconstruction is unnecessary. However, soft tissue reconstruction to close a soft tissue deficit may be required [58]. The use of pedicled myocutaneous rectus abdominis flaps has been successful at facilitating soft tissue defect closure of upper and lower sacral chordomas. This will depend on the extent of soft tissue involvement posteriorly or laterally to the sacrum by tumour extension. Bilateral gluteus maximus flaps may also be used in a keystone manner to close midline sacral lesions. Reconstruction allows the introduction of thicker tissue into the sacral defect which can help to reduce the occurrence or size of a rectocoele.

In some centres, sacrectomy other than for very low and small sacral tumours has been replaced by radiotherapy [63–65]. The results of proton or carbon ion beam radiotherapy have demonstrated equivalent local control of disease in certain circumstances that are equivalent to surgery. The advantage of this treatment is that it avoids the morbidity of surgery and is not associated with loss of bowel or bladder function as a direct result of radiotherapy and the soft tissue toxicity of radiotherapy is acceptable. A higher dose that is more targeted and therefore sparing to surrounding unaffected tissues is said to be better. The disadvantages of this type of radiotherapy are the cost and limited availability of this modality with only few centres around the world being able to deliver such specialised care.

A combined radiotherapy-surgery approach is being popularised because of preliminary retrospective results indicating better local control in sacral tumours treated preoperatively with radiotherapy.

Margins

Local control of disease is directly related to the quality of the surgical margin in the majority of cases. Sometimes, however, local recurrence may occur despite excellent surgical margins. This is most likely the local manifestation of a biologically aggressive tumour, just as systemic metastases are a manifestation of a high-grade tumour.

Achieving wide surgical margins can be a challenge when resecting bone and soft tissue sarcomas of the pelvis. Sacrifice of important bone, muscle, visceral or neurovascular structures may be required to achieve local control of disease with a curative intent. Neoadjuvant therapies (chemotherapy, radiotherapy) may afford additional control of local disease if surgical margins are anticipated to be less than wide. Should radiotherapy be recommended, then it is best to be delivered in the pre-operative setting when there is a target for the radiation and where a margin of sterilisation may be included around the tumour. This is despite the recognition that radiotherapy may cause induration to the mesentery and other soft tissues, as well as the possibility of anastomotic and wound healing complications.

Amputation

External hemipelvectomy (amputation) should be considered when tumours of the pelvis arise in situations which preclude the possibility of a functional limb. An inability to close a wound and achieve adequate oncologic margins, gross tumour contamination by inadvertent excision and tumour fungation are indications for external hemipelvectomy.

Sacrifice of the femoral vasculature, sciatic nerve or hip joint may occur as part of a pelvic resection. These are compatible with limb-sparing surgery if resection is limited to one of the vessels, nerve or joint but not two. Should two or more of these structures require sacrifice, then attempts at limb salvage surgery should be avoided, and surgery should proceed directly to amputation.

Amputations may be based on an anterior or posterior flap [66]. Anterior flap hemipelvectomies rely on a patent femoral artery system. A posterior flap hemipelvectomy relies on the buttock musculature which is based around the inferior gluteal vessels. In this regard, careful pre-operative staging imaging is critical to clarify the involvement of the internal and external iliac systems from which the inferior gluteal and femoral arteries arise, respectively. Occasionally, there may be insufficient soft tissue to close a hemipelvectomy. In this case, a free vascularised flap harvested from the amputated limb may provide a solution without further morbidity to the patient [67].

References

1. Aach M, Gebert C, Ahrens H, Dieckmann R, Gosheger G, Hardes J, et al. The primary stability of pelvic reconstruction after partial supraacetabular pelvic resection due to malignant tumours of the human pelvis: a biomechanical in vitro study. Med Eng Phys. 2013;35(12):1731–5.
2. Akiyama T, Saita K, Ogura K, Kawai A, Imanishi J, Yazawa Y, et al. The effect of an external hip joint stabiliser on gait function after surgery for tumours located around the circumference of the pelvis: analysis of seven cases of internal hemipelvectomy or proximal femur resection. Int Orthop. 2016;40(3):561–7.
3. Wilson RJ, Freeman TH Jr, Halpern JL, Schwartz HS, Holt GE. Surgical outcomes after limb-sparing resection and reconstruction for pelvic sarcoma: a systematic review. JBJS Rev. 2018;6(4):e10.

4. Ferguson JL, Turner SP. Bone Cancer: diagnosis and treatment principles. Am Fam Physician. 2018;98(4):205–13.
5. Morley N, Omar I. Imaging evaluation of musculoskeletal tumors. Cancer Treat Res. 2014;162:9–29.
6. Patel A, Davies AM, James SL. Imaging of extremity soft tissue masses: pitfalls in diagnosis. Br J Hosp Med (Lond). 2015;76(6):344–52.
7. Patel DB, Matcuk GR Jr. Imaging of soft tissue sarcomas. Chin Clin Oncol. 2018;7(4):35.
8. Wenaden AE, Szyszko TA, Saifuddin A. Imaging of periosteal reactions associated with focal lesions of bone. Clin Radiol. 2005;60(4):439–56.
9. Stramare R, Beltrame V, Gazzola M, Gerardi M, Scattolin G, Coran A, et al. Imaging of soft-tissue tumors. J Magn Reson Imaging. 2013;37(4):791–804.
10. Rajiah P, Ilaslan H, Sundaram M. Imaging of sarcomas of pelvic bones. Semin Ultrasound CT MR. 2011;32(5):433–41.
11. Arkun R, Argin M. Pitfalls in MR imaging of musculoskeletal tumors. Semin Musculoskelet Radiol. 2014;18(1):63–78.
12. Chan WP. Magnetic resonance imaging of soft-tissue tumors of the extremities: a practical approach. World J Radiol. 2013;5(12):455–9.
13. Subhawong TK, Wilky BA. Value added: functional MR imaging in management of bone and soft tissue sarcomas. Curr Opin Oncol. 2015;27(4):323–31.
14. van der Woude HJ, Bloem JL, Pope TL Jr. Magnetic resonance imaging of the musculoskeletal system. Part 9. Primary tumors. Clin Orthop Relat Res. 1998;347:272–86.
15. Andersen KF, Jensen KE, Loft A. PET/MR Imaging in Musculoskeletal Disorders. PET Clin. 2016;11(4):453–63.
16. Behzadi AH, Raza SI, Carrino JA, Kosmas C, Gholamrezanezhad A, Basques K, et al. Applications of PET/CT and PET/MR imaging in primary bone malignancies. PET Clin. 2018;13(4):623–34.
17. Guimaraes JB, Rigo L, Lewin F, Emerick A. The importance of PET/CT in the evaluation of patients with Ewing tumors. Radiol Bras. 2015;48(3):175–80.
18. Kandathil A, Subramaniam RM. PET/computed tomography and precision medicine: musculoskeletal sarcoma. PET Clin. 2017;12(4):475–88.
19. Partovi S, Chalian M, Fergus N, Kosmas C, Zipp L, Mansoori B, et al. Magnetic resonance/positron emission tomography (MR/PET) oncologic applications: bone and soft tissue sarcoma. Semin Roentgenol. 2014;49(4):345–52.
20. Zhang X, Guan Z. PET/CT in the diagnosis and prognosis of osteosarcoma. Front Biosci (Landmark Ed). 2018;23:2157–65.
21. Choong PF, Nizam I, Ngan SY, Schlict S, Powell G, Slavin J, et al. Thallium-201 scintigraphy--a predictor of tumour necrosis in soft tissue sarcoma following preoperative radiotherapy? Eur J Surg Oncol. 2003;29(10):908–15.
22. Jo I, Gould D, Schlicht S, Taubman K, Choong PF. Diagnostic accuracy of functional imaging modalities for chondrosarcoma: a systematic review and meta-analysis. J Bone Oncology. 2019;19:100262.
23. Jo O, Schlicht S, Slavin J, Di Bella C, Pang G, Powell G, et al. The role of Thallium-201 scintigraphy and Tc-99m pentavalent dimercaptosuccinic acid in diagnosis and grading of chondrosarcoma. Eur J Radiol. 2020;125:108846.
24. Wu G, Xie R, Li Y, Hou B, Morelli JN, Li X. Histogram analysis with computed tomography angiography for discriminating soft tissue sarcoma from benign soft tissue tumor. Medicine (Baltimore). 2020;99(2):e18742.
25. Miwa S, Taki J, Yamamoto N, Shirai T, Nishida H, Hayashi K, et al. A novel combined radiological method for evaluation of the response to chemotherapy for primary bone sarcoma. J Surg Oncol. 2012;106(3):273–9.
26. Adigun IA, Rahman GA, Ogundipe KO. Soft tissue sarcoma of the thigh: need for angiography in the developing countries. Ann Afr Med. 2010;9(1):39–43.
27. Shapeero LG, Vanel D. Imaging evaluation of the response of high-grade osteosarcoma and Ewing sarcoma to chemotherapy with emphasis on dynamic contrast-enhanced magnetic resonance imaging. Semin Musculoskelet Radiol. 2000;4(1):137–46.

28. Olieman AF, van Ginkel RJ, Hoekstra HJ, Mooyaart EL, Molenaar WM, Koops HS. Angiographic response of locally advanced soft-tissue sarcoma following hyperthermic isolated limb perfusion with tumor necrosis factor. Ann Surg Oncol. 1997;4(1):64–9.
29. Lang P, Vahlensieck M, Matthay KK, Johnston JO, Rosenau W, Gooding CA, et al. Monitoring neovascularity as an indicator to response to chemotherapy in osteogenic and Ewing sarcoma using magnetic resonance angiography. Med Pediatr Oncol. 1996;26(5):329–33.
30. Wang JH, Li MJ, Tang DX, Xu S, Mao JQ, Cai JB, et al. Neoadjuvant transcatheter arterial chemoembolization and systemic chemotherapy for treatment of clear cell sarcoma of the kidney in children. J Pediatr Surg. 2019;54(3):550–6.
31. Ni JY, Sun HL, Chen YT, Luo JH, Wang WD, Jiang XY, et al. Drug-eluting bead transarterial chemoembolization in the treatment for unresectable soft tissue sarcoma refractory to systemic chemotherapy: a preliminary evaluation of efficacy and safety. J Cancer Res Clin Oncol. 2018;144(1):157–63.
32. Hansch A, Neumann R, Gajda M, Marintchev I, Pfeil A, Mayer TE. Transarterial catheter embolization of a sarcoma for preoperative conditioning. Vasa. 2010;39(2):185–8.
33. Trieu J, Sinnathamby M, Di Bella C, Pianta M, Perera W, Slavin JL, et al. Biopsy and the diagnostic evaluation of musculoskeletal tumours: critical but often missed in the 21st century. ANZ J Surg. 2016;86(3):133–8.
34. Trieu J, Schlicht SM, Choong PF. Diagnosing musculoskeletal tumours: how accurate is CT-guided core needle biopsy? Eur J Surg Oncol. 2016;42(7):1049–56.
35. Molnar R, Emery G, Choong PF. Anaesthesia for hemipelvectomy--a series of 49 cases. Anaesth Intensive Care. 2007;35(4):536–43.
36. Grap SM, Fox E, Freeman M, Blackall GF, Dalal PG. Acute postoperative pain management after major limb amputation in a pediatric patient: a case report. J Perianesth Nurs. 2019;34(4):801–9.
37. Couto AG, Araujo B, Torres de Vasconcelos RA, Renni MJ, Da Fonseca CO, Cavalcanti IL. Survival rate and perioperative data of patients who have undergone hemipelvectomy: a retrospective case series. World J Surg Oncol. 2016;14(1):255.
38. Malawer MM, Buch R, Khurana JS, Garvey T, Rice L. Postoperative infusional continuous regional analgesia. A technique for relief of postoperative pain following major extremity surgery. Clin Orthop Relat Res. 1991;266:227–37.
39. Chretien PA, Sugarbaker PH. Surgical technique of hemipelvectomy in the lateral position. Surgery. 1981;90(5):900–9.
40. Shao QD, Yan X, Sun JY, Xu TM. Internal hemipelvectomy with reconstruction for primary pelvic neoplasm: a systematic review. ANZ J Surg. 2015;85(7–8):553–60.
41. Kollender Y, Shabat S, Bickels J, Flusser G, Isakov J, Neuman Y, et al. Internal hemipelvectomy for bone sarcomas in children and young adults: surgical considerations. Eur J Surg Oncol. 2000;26(4):398–404.
42. Jin T, Liu W, Xu H, Li Y, Hao L, Niu X. How does iliosacral bone tumor resection without reconstruction affect the ipsilateral hip joint? BMC Musculoskelet Disord. 2018;19(1):102.
43. Houdek MT, Rose PS, Bakri K, Wagner ER, Yaszemski MJ, Sim FH, et al. Outcomes and complications of reconstruction with use of free vascularized fibular graft for spinal and pelvic defects following resection of a malignant tumor. J Bone Joint Surg Am. 2017;99(13):e69.
44. Pieroh P, Spindler N, Langer S, Josten C, Bohme J. A double-barrelled fibula graft restoring pelvic stability after late posterior ring instability related to a surgical treated osteitis pubis: a case report. Arch Orthop Trauma Surg. 2016;136(1):47–53.
45. Ogura K, Sakuraba M, Miyamoto S, Fujiwara T, Chuman H, Kawai A. Pelvic ring reconstruction with a double-barreled free vascularized fibula graft after resection of malignant pelvic bone tumor. Arch Orthop Trauma Surg. 2015;135(5):619–25.
46. Akiyama T, Clark JC, Miki Y, Choong PF. The non-vascularised fibular graft: a simple and successful method of reconstruction of the pelvic ring after internal hemipelvectomy. J Bone Joint Surg Br. 2010;92(7):999–1005.
47. Sakuraba M, Kimata Y, Iida H, Beppu Y, Chuman H, Kawai A. Pelvic ring reconstruction with the double-barreled vascularized fibular free flap. Plast Reconstr Surg. 2005;116(5):1340–5.

48. Campanacci D, Chacon S, Mondanelli N, Beltrami G, Scoccianti G, Caff G, et al. Pelvic massive allograft reconstruction after bone tumour resection. Int Orthop. 2012;36(12):2529–36.
49. Langlais F, Lambotte JC, Thomazeau H. Long-term results of hemipelvis reconstruction with allografts. Clin Orthop Relat Res. 2001;388:178–86.
50. Wei R, Guo W, Yang R, Tang X, Yang Y, Ji T, et al. Reconstruction of the pelvic ring after total en bloc sacrectomy using a 3D-printed sacral endoprosthesis with re-establishment of spinopelvic stability: a retrospective comparative study. Bone Joint J. 2019;101-B(7):880–8.
51. Smolle MA, Andreou D, Tunn PU, Leithner A. Advances in tumour endoprostheses: a systematic review. EFORT Open Rev. 2019;4(7):445–59.
52. Gomez-Palomo JM, Estades-Rubio FJ, Meschian-Coretti S, Montanez-Heredia E, De Santos-de la Fuente FJ. Internal Hemipelvectomy and reconstruction assisted by 3D printing technology using premade intraoperative cutting and placement guides in a patient with pelvic sarcoma: a case report. JBJS Case Connect. 2019;9(4):e0060.
53. Fang C, Cai H, Kuong E, Chui E, Siu YC, Ji T, et al. Surgical applications of three-dimensional printing in the pelvis and acetabulum: from models and tools to implants. Unfallchirurg. 2019;122(4):278–85.
54. Angelini A, Trovarelli G, Berizzi A, Pala E, Breda A, Ruggieri P. Three-dimension-printed custom-made prosthetic reconstructions: from revision surgery to oncologic reconstructions. Int Orthop. 2019;43(1):123–32.
55. Choong PF. Reconstructive surgery following resection of primary and secondary tumours of the hip. J Orthop Surg. 2000;8(2):83–94.
56. Capanna R, van Horn JR, Guernelli N, Briccoli A, Ruggieri P, Biagini R, et al. Complications of pelvic resections. Arch Orthop Trauma Surg. 1987;106(2):71–7.
57. Reddy S, Bloom N. En bloc resection of extra-peritoneal soft tissue neoplasms incorporating a type III internal hemipelvectomy: a novel approach. World J Surg Oncol. 2012;10:222.
58. Reynolds JJ, Khundkar R, Boriani S, Williams R, Rhines LD, Kawahara N, et al. Soft Tissue and Bone Defect Management in Total Sacrectomy for Primary Sacral Tumors: A Systematic Review With Expert Recommendations. Spine (Phila Pa 1976). 2016;41 Suppl 20:S199-S204.
59. Kayani B, Hanna SA, Sewell MD, Saifuddin A, Molloy S, Briggs TW. A review of the surgical management of sacral chordoma. Eur J Surg Oncol. 2014;40(11):1412–20.
60. Bederman SS, Shah KN, Hassan JM, Hoang BH, Kiester PD, Bhatia NN. Surgical techniques for spinopelvic reconstruction following total sacrectomy: a systematic review. Eur Spine J. 2014;23(2):305–19.
61. Ji T, Guo W, Yang R, Tang X, Wang Y, Huang L. What are the conditional survival and functional outcomes after surgical treatment of 115 patients with sacral Chordoma? Clin Orthop Relat Res. 2017;475(3):620–30.
62. Clair B, Ordway NR, Damron T, Lavelle WF. Sacral insufficiency fracture after partial sacrectomy. Am J Orthop (Belle Mead NJ). 2014;43(11):E272–4.
63. Imai R, Kamada T, Araki N. Working Group for B, soft tissue S. carbon ion radiation therapy for Unresectable sacral Chordoma: an analysis of 188 cases. Int J Radiat Oncol Biol Phys. 2016;95(1):322–7.
64. Nishida Y, Kamada T, Imai R, Tsukushi S, Yamada Y, Sugiura H, et al. Clinical outcome of sacral chordoma with carbon ion radiotherapy compared with surgery. Int J Radiat Oncol Biol Phys. 2011;79(1):110–6.
65. Imai R, Kamada T, Tsuji H, Sugawara S, Serizawa I, Tsujii H, et al. Effect of carbon ion radiotherapy for sacral chordoma: results of phase I-II and phase II clinical trials. Int J Radiat Oncol Biol Phys. 2010;77(5):1470–6.
66. Kulaylat MN, Froix A, Karakousis CP. Blood supply of hemipelvectomy flaps: the anterior flap hemipelvectomy. Arch Surg. 2001;136(7):828–31.
67. Roulet S, Le Nail LR, Vaz G, Babinet A, Dumaine V, Sallot A, et al. Free fillet lower leg flap for coverage after hemipelvectomy or hip disarticulation. Orthop Traumatol Surg Res. 2019;105(1):47–54.

17 Surgical Management of Chest Wall Sarcomas

Naveed Z. Alam

The chest wall is composed of the bony skeleton of the thorax along with associated cartilaginous elements. The functions of the chest wall are broadly to protect the underlying vital structures and to provide a scaffold for the muscles of the thorax which are ultimately responsible for adequate ventilation.

17.1 Historical Note

The first reported resection of a chest wall tumour was in 1778 by Osias Aimar. He removed an osteosarcoma involving the fifth, sixth, and seventh ribs but took care not to enter the pleura. It was only after the advent of positive pressure ventilation with endotracheal tube intubation that surgeons were able to breach the pleural space without fear of losing their patient to the immediately resultant ipsilateral pneumothorax. Reports of resections became more frequent after Parham published his experience in 1899 [1].

The principles of chest wall reconstruction evolved in the theatre of war as surgeons gained experience in the management of chest trauma and stabilisation of flail segments. Much of the early work in reconstruction was performed at the Mayo Clinic by Clagett [2].

17.2 Primary Chest Wall Malignancies

Primary tumours of the chest wall are rare, and as such, much of the historical management was based on anecdotal evidence and the few case series that were reported. More recently, extrapolation from management of sarcomas at other sites has influenced and informed current strategies and guidelines.

N. Z. Alam (✉)
Department of Surgery, University of Melbourne, Melbourne, VIC, Australia

Department of Cardiothoracic Surgery, St. Vincent's Hospital, Melbourne, VIC, Australia

P. F. M. Choong (ed.), *Sarcoma*, https://doi.org/10.1007/978-981-15-9414-4_17

Table 17.1 Primary chest wall malignancies

Histotype
Chondrosarcoma
Osteosarcoma
Ewing's sarcoma (including Askin's)
Myeloma (including solitary plasmacytoma)
Lymphoma
Malignant fibrous histiocytoma
Leiomyosarcoma
Liposarcoma
Neurofibrosarcoma
Rhabdomyosarcoma
Haemangiosarcoma

Chest wall tumours span the breadth of the spectrum from benign lesions to exceedingly aggressive malignancies. They also encompass a wide variety of histologically distinct entities. The focus of this discussion will be on primary sarcomas of the chest wall (Table 17.1).

17.3 Clinical Presentation

About 60 percent of chest wall tumours are malignant, though primary chest wall malignancies represent less than 2% of thoracic neoplasms. The mean age of presentation for patients with a primary malignant tumour of the chest wall is 40 with a male-to-female ratio of 2:1 [3]. They present as slow-growing masses that are initially painless but do begin to cause pain with continued growth. Associated symptoms including weight loss, fever, and shortness of breath are not common.

17.3.1 Diagnosis

Palpable masses should be measured and classified as fixed or mobile and soft or hard. In addition to history and physical examination, imaging is critical. Old imaging, if available, can help to establish the pace of growth of a lesion. In the first instance, a CT scan should be performed to assess the extent of involvement of the various structures including the pleura, the mediastinum, and any potential pulmonary involvement. MRI is useful in precisely defining tissue planes and may sometimes give better spatial resolution than CT.

PET has been shown to be valuable in many malignancies. In sarcoma, it has been shown to be more accurate than CT alone in staging. It is also helpful in assessing early responses to therapy and in restaging after completion of neoadjuvant therapy [4]. PET is also superior to CT alone in assessing lymph node involvement.

In most situations, a percutaneous biopsy should be performed, particularly if malignancy is suspected. A potential exception is for small tumours (< 2 cm) which can be treated with excisional biopsies provided they are performed with clear margins. The location of any biopsy should be planned to enable excision of the biopsy tract at the time of the planned resection of the mass.

17.3.2 Treatment

The mainstay of treatment for sarcomas of the chest wall is surgical resection. Surgery alone, however, has mixed results. The overall 5-year survival is approximately 65%. High-grade tumours fare worse than low-grade ones with 5-year survivals of 50% vs 90%, respectively. Metastases develop in 50% of patients with high-grade tumours and only 10% of low-grade ones [5]. In addition to the grade of the tumour, the most important prognostic factor seems to be adequacy of resection, but it is unclear what that means precisely.

The original recommendation for 4-cm resection margins was based on a series of 90 patients which suggested that those with margins of less than 2 cm had worse 5-year disease-free survival than those with margins greater than 4 cm [6]. Current guidelines call for oncologically appropriate margins [7]. This somewhat ambiguous term takes into consideration that margins often have to be determined by the proximity to vital major structures (nerves, vessels) such that a clear margin with minimal functional impairment may result in a superior outcome for the patient. In general, a 1-cm margin in soft tissue is thought to be adequate.

Specific subtypes of tumours should be treated differently, and this underscores the vital role that multidisciplinary care provides in this complex oncological setting. A recent randomised trial demonstrated that neoadjuvant epirubicin and ifosfamide improved survival of patients affected by five high-risk soft tissue sarcoma histologies of the trunk and extremities, including undifferentiated pleomorphic sarcoma, myxoid liposarcoma, synovial sarcoma, malignant peripheral nerve sheath tumours, and leiomyosarcoma [8]. The use of neoadjuvant radiotherapy also has merit in certain tumour types with concerning features, particularly if the potential for tumour shrinkage can decrease the morbidity of the planned resection.

Certain tumour types are not amenable to surgery as the primary treatment modality. Ewing's sarcomas present in younger patients and are treated with systemic therapy as the primary treatment with localised therapy (usually surgery but occasionally radiation) used as the adjuvant therapy.

17.3.3 Preoperative Evaluation

Chest wall resections are major surgical procedures, and patients need to have their underlying cardiopulmonary reserve assessed to enable appropriate risk stratification. Often fitness for one lung ventilation is required. Underlying chest wall mechanics are disrupted, at least in the near term, which can result in significant perioperative morbidity, particularly with regard to splinting and retention of pulmonary secretions. A well-thought-out analgesic plan for the perioperative and postoperative period is critical. The use of epidurals, fascial blocks, and paravertebral or extrapleural catheters should be considered.

17.4 Principles of Surgery

17.4.1 Resection

Apart from the grade of the tumour, clear and adequate resection margins are the most important prognostic factor in sarcoma surgery. As discussed above, the early recommendations in chest wall sarcomas were for 4-cm margins, but the current guidelines emphasise oncologically appropriate margins. Early recommendations also suggested that normal ribs above and below should be resected, but those recommendations need to be placed in the larger context of the specific patient's situation. For example, having a 4 cm and an uninvolved rib of clear caudal margin to the tumour at the expense of function may not be that significant if there is only scope to have 0.5 cm of clear margin cephalad to the tumour. It must be noted that the extent of the resection should not be limited by the size of the resulting defect, as most defects can be reconstructed. If the treating clinicians are uncertain of their ability to repair resulting defects, patients should be referred to specialist centres with extensive chest wall reconstructive experience.

The skin incision (if the underlying soft tissue is not involved) should be made in an elliptical fashion encompassing the biopsy tract. If the skin or deeper tissues are involved, then adequate margins need to be taken with planned soft tissue flap coverage if primary repair is not possible. Muscles overlying the tumour should be excised en bloc with the mass up to a depth where there is a plane without tumour involvement.

Our practice is to resect the intercostal muscle below the lowest involved rib. If the intercostal muscle is involved, then part of the rib below (or above) should be removed with a margin of at least 1 cm radial to the tumour. If the tumours are high grade, then wider excision of the ribs laterally is preferred because of the risk of subperiosteal or intramedullary spread.

If underlying viscera is involved, this should similarly be resected as required. Lung parenchyma should be wedged en bloc with the chest wall segment, if involvement is suspected, along with a generous cuff of the parietal pleura. If the posterior table of the sternum or manubrium are breached, consideration should be given to thymectomy along with removal of the anterior mediastinal and/or pericardial fat. In these instances, care must be taken to avoid injuring the phrenic nerves.

If major vessels have partial thickness involvement or close margins, partial thickness resections with side-biting clamps and primary repair can be performed. If the lumen of the vessel (e.g. SVC) is too narrowed for primary repair, then patch repairs with native or bovine pericardium can be used. In rare cases, Dacron or PTFE grafts can be interpositioned for larger vascular defects.

17.4.2 Reconstruction

The goals of chest wall reconstruction are shown in Table 17.2. Not all chest wall defects need reconstruction. The size and location of the defect will dictate whether a reconstruction needs to be performed and with which materials. Some authors suggest that defects smaller than 5 cm in the chest wall can be managed with only soft tissue coverage. Certainly, in the posterior chest wall, under the scapulae, larger defects are acceptable. However, in our experience, in the anterior and lateral chest wall, any defect larger than 4 cm, or involving resection of two or more ribs, is often served well with at least a mesh repair to prevent lung herniation and maintain chest wall dynamic integrity.

17.4.3 Choice of Material

A large number of options are available for reconstruction of the chest wall. They vary in terms of their inherent material components, rigidity, resistance to infection, and ability to be customised for specific applications. A non-exhaustive list is provided in Table 17.3. Decisions regarding the use of rigid or semirigid reconstructive materials are often dictated by both patient-specific characteristics and surgeon or institutional preference.

Table 17.2 Goals of chest wall reconstruction

Goals
Protection of underlying viscera (heart, great vessels)
Restoration of rigidity to facilitate ventilation
Support for arm and shoulder movement
Prevention of lung herniation
Prevention of trapping of the scapula
Good cosmetic result

Table 17.3 Choice of materials for reconstruction of rib cage

Reconstruction	Material	Rigidity
Autografts	Rib	Rigid
	Myocutaneous flaps	Nonrigid
Synthetic mesh	Polypropylene	Semirigid
	PTFE	Semirigid
	Nylon	Semirigid
	Polyglactin	Semirigid
	Methyl methacrylate (MMA)	Rigid
Bioprosthetics	Bovine pericardium	Nonrigid
	Porcine dermis	Nonrigid
Osteosynthesis systems	Stratos (titanium)	Rigid
	MatrixRIB (titanium)	Rigid

Table 17.4 Selected series of prosthetic chest wall reconstructions adopted from [9]

Series Author	No. of recons	Material used	Complications (%)	Prosthesis removal (%)	Mortality (%)
Deschamps [10]	197	Mesh alone	46.2	2.5	4.1
Lardinois [11]	26	MMA	23	7.7	0
Walsh [12]	33	Mesh alone and MMA	24	6.1	0
Mansour [13]	93	Various	24	n/a	7
Weyant [14]	209	Mesh alone and MMA	33	4.3	3.8
Daigeler [15]	62	Mesh alone	42	6.5	5.4
Kachroo [16]	42	Mesh alone and MMA	16	4.8	0

Results of chest wall resections show substantial postoperative complications. A list of published case series is shown in Table 17.4.

17.4.4 Tips/Tricks

Reconstruction in certain anatomic areas can be challenging. However, potential pitfalls can be avoided with experience and planning.

For the largest potential resections, particularly if there is potential for full-thickness resections, multidisciplinary input should be sought. Plastic surgeons should be involved early in the preoperative planning process so that they can assess what myocutaneous options they have for repairing the soft tissue defects. Their choices will gravitate to the natural workhorses of chest wall reconstruction, latissimus dorsi, and pectoralis major, if these pedicles are available and viable. In their absence, other options are available, including rectus abdominis and free tissue transfer.

Small defects (two ribs) can be repaired with a simple mesh closure between the ribs. This prevents lung herniation and can be sutured in place tightly enough to contribute to chest wall rigidity.

In the posterior chest wall, larger defects (up to 8 cm) under the scapulae can be left without repair; however, if the defect involves the fifth or sixth ribs, then at a minimum, a semirigid repair with a synthetic mesh will remove the chance of the tip of the scapula being trapped at the site of the defect.

In the upper anterior and lateral chest wall, large defects can be repaired effectively with an MMA sandwich. A piece of synthetic mesh is chosen that is larger than the defect which is then placed within the defect. The contour of the opening is then marked with a pen. MMA is then mixed on the back table and painted on to the mesh, with a second layer of mesh added above the MMA to form a sandwich. The

MMA can be painted as a single block or in bands as *neo-ribs*. It is important to leave at least a centimetre cuff from the edge of the MMA to the edge of the native chest wall so that there is no friction between these rigid elements which could result in pain or a clicking sensation postoperatively. The MMA sandwich can be contoured on the patient's hip or ASIS or on a kidney basin to approximate the contour of the chest wall. Once it becomes rigid, it is sewn into the chest with interrupted permanent sutures that are placed around the adjacent ribs and deeply into the surrounding tissues (see Fig. 17.1).

Osteosynthetic systems can also be used, often in conjunction with synthetic mesh. The two most common systems use titanium and are the MatrixRIB and the Stratos system. The potential advantage of titanium over other rigid prostheses, such as stainless steel or ceramics, is its greater tensile strength and resistance to infection. The disadvantages are related to cost and perhaps some limitations in the ability to customise for certain applications. There have also been reports of high proportions of late failure of the prostheses mandating removal [17].

When the lower ribs are resected, particularly in the anterior chest wall, part of the diaphragm is often sacrificed. Standard principles of diaphragmatic resection are applicable, with circumferential rather than radial resections preferred to preserve the phrenic innervation. If the abdomen is entered, primary repair of the peritoneum is performed. If the costal margin is sacrificed, then an abdominal augmentation procedure can be employed. This involves closing the diaphragm either primarily or with a PTFE patch and then attaching it to the lowest remaining rib.

A similar technique can be used in the posterior and lateral chest if the floating ribs (11 and 12) are resected. This can aid in preventing incisional hernias.

For tumours involving the sternum, reconstruction needs to be tailored to the extent of the resection. If only part of the sternum is resected and the heads of the clavicles and superior manubrium remain intact, then an MMA sandwich as described above is effective in protecting the viscera and preserving chest wall rigidity. If the heads of the clavicles are resected along with the manubrium, then restoration of the integrity of the clavicular axis is mandated to maintain optimal shoulder and arm function. This can be accomplished by plates or titanium prostheses. Our preferred reconstruction, however, involves harvesting a length of rib, long enough to bridge the gap between the resected ends of the clavicle, and attaching the ends with steel cables that are clamped flush. This cabling system is used primary in sternotomy closures following cardiac surgery. An MMA sandwich is then used to close the defect between the neo-clavicle and the body of the sternum (see Fig. 17.2).

17.4.5 As in all thoracic surgery, controlling the pleural space(s) is mandatory in the perioperative period. Chest drains need to be placed, and discussion with

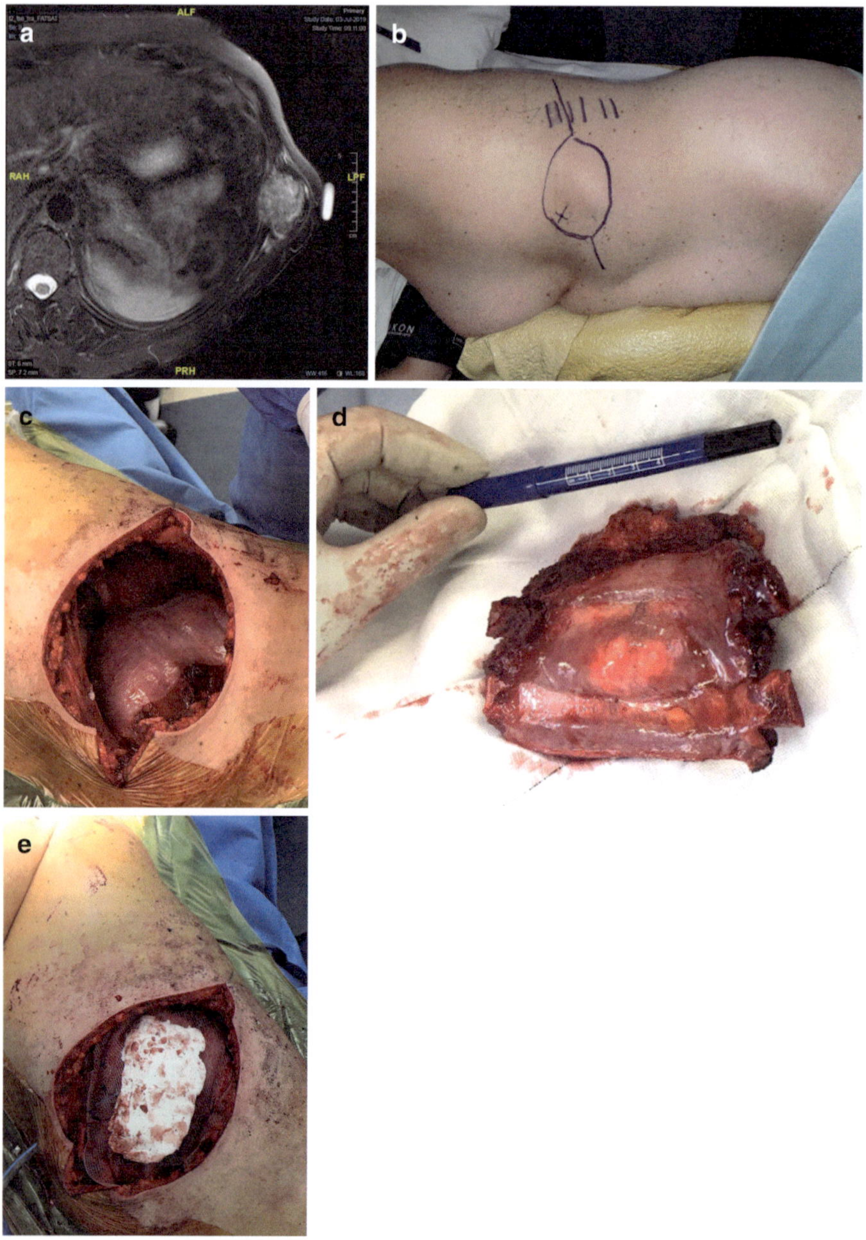

Fig. 17.1 (**a**) MRI of lateral chest wall fibromyxoid sarcoma. (**b**) Biopsy site marked with X. (**c**) En bloc resection of two ribs, intercostal muscles above and below, and peripheral diaphragm. (**d**) Specimen with cuff of the diaphragm. (**e**) Reconstruction with MMA sandwich. The diaphragm was primarily repaired and sutured to lower ribs

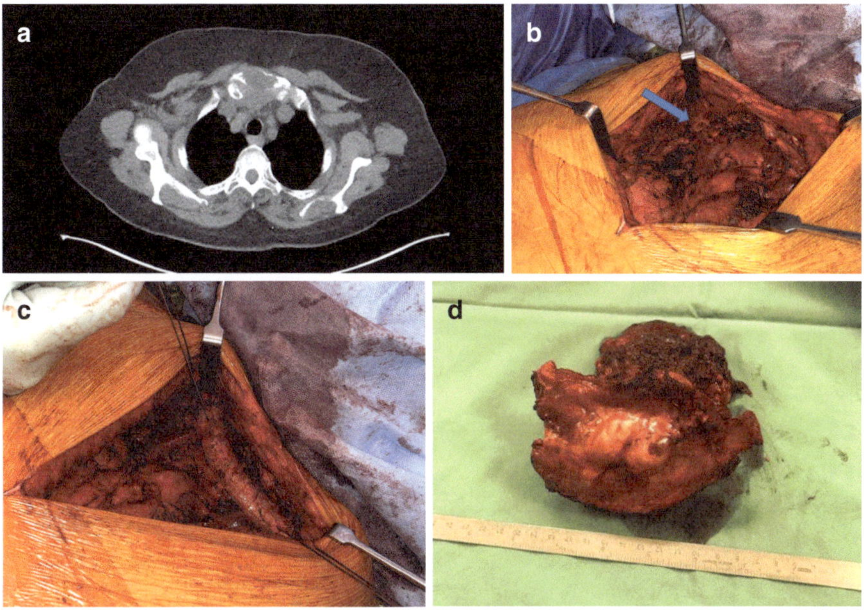

Fig. 17.2 (**a**) Manubrial-based osteosarcoma involving clavicular heads. (**b**) Specimen resected. Arrow points to cut edge of the right clavicle. (**c**) Right fourth rib harvested through the same incision and secured to clavicular heads with steel cables. (**d**) Resected manubrium and clavicular heads

the plastic surgeons beforehand may be helpful so as to avoid injuring any tissue that may be required in the soft tissue reconstructive phase.

17.5 Future Directions

While there will no doubt be new medicines in the treatment of chest wall sarcomas, potentially with new immunotherapy agents, and new radiotherapy techniques to help with close margins or tumour shrinkage, the mainstay of sarcoma therapy will likely be surgery for the foreseeable future.

Resection techniques will likely not change dramatically, though the use of real-time imaging may play some role. The main gains in the future will likely be in the reconstruction of defects in the chest wall. The most predictable of these developments is the use of three-dimensional printing to fashion customised prostheses. In fact, it is somewhat disingenuous to call this a future direction. A number of reports of 3D printed prostheses with various materials have already been implanted in patients [18–20].

The main problems with this method currently are the costs and the time required to produce the prostheses. These hurdles will surely be overcome. Even more interesting will be the development of prostheses that are composed of variable materials such as resins, polymers, metals, and degradable biomaterials that can be made quickly and accurately [21]. Furthermore, there may be development of 3D printed bioscaffolds that afford the patient's own cells the opportunity to colonise and proliferate [22].

Animal models already exist for absorbable meshes, demineralised bone matrix, and bone marrow stromal cells [23]. And perhaps the ultimate goal will be the bioengineering of vascularised osseomyocutaneous chest wall grafts grown from the patient's own stem cells [24].

17.6 Summary

Chest wall sarcomas are a rare but often surgically curable disease. A multidisciplinary approach is critical at several points in the care pathway. Pre-therapeutic planning with medical and radiation oncologists will aid in the selection of appropriate neoadjuvant treatment strategies. Preoperative consultation with resection and reconstruction in mind may often require different surgical craft groups as well, as well as the input of anaesthesiology. Clear surgical margins are of paramount importance, and the degree of resection should not be compromised for fear of the reconstruction. Centres with significant experience can manage very complex reconstructions with minimal morbidity.

References

1. Hedblom CA. Open pneumothorax in its relation to the extirpation of tumors of the bony chest wall. Arch Surg. 1922;4(3):588–97.
2. Pascuzzi CA, Dahlia DC, Clagget OT. Primary tumors of the ribs and sternum. Surg Gynecol Obstet. 1957;104:390.
3. Graeber GM, Jones DR, Pairolero PC. Primary Neoplasms. In: Pearson FG, Cooper JD, editors. Thoracic Surgery. Philadelphia: Churchill Livingstone; 2005. Chapter 53.
4. Piperkova E, Mikhaeil M, Mousavi A, et al. Impact of PET and CT in PET/CT studies for staging and evaluating treatment response in bone and soft tissue sarcomas. Clin Nucl Med. 2009;34(3):146–50.
5. Gordon MS, Hajdu SI, Bains MS, et al. Soft tissue sarcomas of the chest wall. Results of surgical resection. J Thorac Cardiovasc Surg. 1991;101(5):843–54.
6. King RM, Pairolero PC, Trastek VF, et al. Primary chest wall tumors: factors affecting survival. Ann Thorac Surg. 1986;41:597–601.
7. NCCN Guidelines Version 2. Soft tissue sarcoma; 2019. https://www.nccn.org/professionals/physician_gls/PDF/sarcoma.pdf
8. Gronchi A, Ferrari S, Quagliuolo V, et al. Neoadjuvant chemotherapy in high-risk soft tissue sarcomas: a randomised clinical trial from the Italian sarcoma group (ISG), the Spanish sarcoma group (GEIS), the French sarcoma group (FSG) and the polish sarcoma group (PSG). Lancet Oncol. 2017;18(6):812–22.

9. Khullar OV, Fernandez FG. Prosthetic reconstruction of the Chest Wall. Thorac Surg Clin. 2017;27(2):201–8.
10. Deschamps C, Tirnaksiz BM, Darbandi R, et al. Early and long-term results of prosthetic chest wall reconstruction. J Thorac Cardiovasc Surg. 1999;117(3):588–91. [discussion: 591–2
11. Lardinois D, Muller M, Furrer M, et al. Functional assessment of chest wall integrity after methylmethacrylate reconstruction. Ann Thorac Surg. 2000;69(3):919–23.
12. Walsh GL, Davis BM, Swisher SG, et al. A single-institutional, multidisciplinary approach to primary sarcomas involving the chest wall requiring full-thickness resections. J Thorac Cardiovasc Surg. 2001;121(1):48–60.
13. Mansour KA, Thourani VH, Losken A, et al. Chest wall resections and reconstruction: a 25-year experience. Ann Thorac Surg. 2002;73(6):1720–5. [discussion: 1725–6]
14. Weyant MJ, Bains MS, Venkatraman E, et al. Results of chest wall resection and reconstruction with and without rigid prosthesis. Ann Thorac Surg. 2006;81(1):279–85.
15. Daigeler A, Druecke D, Hakimi M, et al. Reconstruction of the thoracic wall-long-term follow-up including pulmonary function tests. Langenbeck's Arch Surg. 2009;394(4):705–15.
16. Kachroo P, Pak PS, Sandha HS, Lee C, Elashoff D, Nelson SD, Chmielowski B, Selch MT, Cameron RB, Holmes EC, Eilber FC, Lee JM. Single-institution, multidisciplinary experience with surgical resection of primary chest wall sarcomas. J Thorac Oncol. 2012;7(3):552–8.
17. Berthet JP, Gomez Caro A, Solovei L, et al. Titanium implant failure after chest wall osteosynthesis. Ann Thorac Surg. 2015;99(6):1945–52.
18. Turna A, Kavakli K, Sapmaz E, et al. Reconstruction with a patient-specific titanium implant after a wide anterior chest wall resection. Interact Cardiovasc Thorac Surg. 2014;18:234–6.
19. Wang L, Huang L, Li X, et al. Three-dimensional printing PEEK implant: a novel choice for the reconstruction of Chest Wall defect. Ann Thorac Surg. 2019;107(3):921–8.
20. Moradiellos J, Amor S, Córdoba M, et al. Functional Chest Wall reconstruction with a biomechanical three-dimensionally printed implant. Ann Thorac Surg. 2017;103(4):e389–91.
21. Ng CS. Recent and future developments in Chest Wall reconstruction. Semin Thorac Cardiovasc Surg. 2015;27(2):234–9.
22. Michalski MH, Ross JS. The shape of things to come: 3D printing in medicine. J Am Med Assoc. 2014;312:2213–4.
23. Tang H, Xu Z, Qin X, et al. Chest wall reconstruction in a canine model using polydioxanone mesh, demineralized bone matrix and bone marrow stromal cells. Biomaterials. 2009;30(19):3224–33.
24. Sandler G, Hayes-Jordan A. Chest wall reconstruction after tumor resection. Semin Pediatr Surg. 2018;27(3):200–6.

18 Surgical Management of Pulmonary Metastases from Sarcoma

Gavin Wright

18.1 Introduction

Sarcomas, despite being a disparate group of malignant diseases, share a common propensity to metastasise to the lungs, regardless of origin of the primary. This risk correlates with location, size, grade and histological subtype [1]. Often this is the only clinical evidence of disease in patients after appropriate complete resection of their primary sarcoma. They may appear at the time of local recurrence in an incompletely resected or inappropriately treated primary sarcoma.

Approximately 20% of patients with resected sarcoma will develop isolated pulmonary metastatic disease at some point in the course of their disease [2]. There appear to be particular subtypes of sarcoma with higher pulmonary metastatic rates, such as tenosynovial sarcoma, spindle cell sarcoma from extremities and extra-skeletal osteosarcoma [3, 4]. As a more general rule, high-grade sarcomas make up 90% of pulmonary metastatic disease and low-grade sarcomas only 10%. The observation that pulmonary metastatic disease is common, and often isolated, is a strong impetus to target that disease aggressively.

Since the introduction of safe methods of anaesthesia and resection of pulmonary tissue, pulmonary metastasectomy for colorectal and other malignancies, including sarcoma, have become an increasingly popular therapy. The hope is that the burden of disease will be reduced, time to further progression will be prolonged and direct invasive complications and further "tertiary" spread will be prevented. Systemic agents may be considered relatively ineffective or held in reserve, whilst surgical control is possible, and finally, some patients may be considered cured of

G. Wright (✉)
Department of Surgery, University of Melbourne, Melbourne, VIC, Australia

Department of Cardiothoracic Surgery, St. Vincent's Hospital, Melbourne, VIC, Australia

Lung Oncology Service, Peter MacCallum Cancer Centre, Melbourne, VIC, Australia
e-mail: gavin.wright@svha.org.au

P. F. M. Choong (ed.), *Sarcoma*, https://doi.org/10.1007/978-981-15-9414-4_18

Table 18.1 Criteria for prognostication of metastasectomy from the International Registry of Lung Metastases [5]

Prognostic factor			Prognostic group	Median survival (months)
DFI[a] > 3 years	Solitary	Complete resection		
TRUE	TRUE	TRUE	1	61
TRUE	FALSE	TRUE	2	34
FALSE	TRUE	TRUE		
FALSE	FALSE	TRUE	3	24
ANY	ANY	FALSE	4	14

[a]*DFI* Disease free interval between primary resection and metastasectomy
Prognosis worsens significantly with increasing group number

their metastatic disease in that they die of unrelated causes or achieve incredibly long disease-free intervals.

The complex interplay between patient selection and class effect of an intervention is rarely as evident as in the mainstream practice of pulmonary metastasectomy. Using the much cited but somewhat anachronistic criteria from the International Registry of Lung Metastases [5] (Table 18.1), a surgeon could choose only to operate on patients with a solitary lung metastasis from a primary malignancy that was resected more than 3 years ago. With modern peri-operative care, minimally invasive techniques and optimal lung parenchymal preservation, that surgeon would be expected to have exceptional results in terms of low mortality, good early return to normal activity and prolonged disease-free and overall survival. However, if there are therapeutic benefits of metastasectomy beyond the selection of "winners", that same surgeon is doing a disservice to the patients who present with two metastases, or present with their solitary metastasis just 2.5 years after original diagnosis. Conversely a surgeon who attempts to resect all lung metastases in all patients without discrimination may impose greater harms than any expected benefits on that patient population. This raises the question of whether there is a state of oligometastatic disease for which intervention is beneficial that can be distinguished from a more generalised state of systemic disease for which surgical intervention is futile and harmful.

18.2 The Oligometastatic Disease Concept

The concept of oligometastatic disease is that between the states of loco-regional malignancy and widespread metastatic malignancy, there exists a state of limited systemic metastatic disease for which local ablative therapy could be curative [6]. The definition of oligometastatic disease is elusive. It is easy to identify the extremes – solitary, single organ involvement is definitely an indication; widespread innumerable lesions are definitely not. But what of six metastases in one organ? What of a single metastasis in each of two disparate organs? Where is the blurred line between the two putative metastatic states? Is it probabilistic or stochastic events that result in failure of disease control? Does removing four metastases necessarily bring poorer results than removing three? What about the inherent biology of the particular patient's malignancy and their individual host response?

The above conundrums drive clinicians to define their own therapeutic guidelines, arbitrary as they must be, without high-quality evidence. Being the largest and most promulgated series, the International Registry of Lung Metastases (IRLM) provides the basis for most clinical guidelines. These are particularly relevant for sarcoma as 2173 of the 5206 cases reported were for sarcoma. However, IRLM predated the introduction of ^{18}FDG-PET scanning and wide-scale use of minimally invasive and complex sublobar resection techniques. There have also been advances in therapeutic agents for some sub-groups of sarcoma in the decades since the IRLM was published.

The other problem with definition of an oligometastatic disease state in sarcoma is the extreme heterogeneity of disease under the sarcoma umbrella. Well-differentiated soft tissue sarcoma, osteosarcoma and Ewing's tumours are not all likely to respond to the same surgery as a class effect. An elderly patient with significant comorbidity clearly has much less to gain (and greater potential for harm) than a fit 40-year-old. Therefore, some groupings must be looked at individually within any guidelines.

Historical experience of the natural history of these diseases and their response to pulmonary metastasectomy are the only evidence we have. For example, a 15-year experience of soft tissue sarcoma at Memorial Sloan Kettering Cancer Center at the turn of the century yielded 719 cases of pulmonary metastatic disease from over 3000 cases [7]. As there was a consistent therapeutic protocol to resect this disease from the lungs, we can get some insight into the expected outcomes. The entire metastatic group 3-year survival rate was 25%, with a median survival of 15 months, from time of detection of pulmonary metastases. At one extreme, those with completely resected disease had a 3-year survival rate of 46%, with a median survival of 33 months, but those with no resection had a median survival of only 11 months.

There is a point when treating teams decide there is too much disease to justify intervention, even in such a centre. This defines their local institutional definition of oligometastatic disease, but is also a self-fulfilling prognosticator. The ideal use of pulmonary metastasectomy would result in improved survival of the entire population by not imposing harms on futile cases, but reaping the benefits of intervention in all other cases. The authors were able to define groups for which pulmonary metastasectomy yielded disappointing results, namely, liposarcoma, peripheral nerve sheath tumour and patients over 50.

Given the ubiquitous finding of complete resection as the most important factor for prolonged survival, the concept of oligometastatic disease is not just defined by a number or a size of a lesion. Special patterns of disease are either particularly amenable to resection or particularly adverse. Some patterns correlate with aggressive or indolent tumour biology. The following have been gleaned from the author's direct and secondary experience over the last two decades:

- The "contaminated" lobe.
- Bilateral mirror image involvement.

- Direct invasion of adjacent structures.
- The “kissing metastasis” vs pleural spread.
- Endobronchial disease.
- “The Sky by Night” appearance.

The contaminated lobe is the finding of multiple metastases in the distribution of a single pulmonary artery branch. This may manifest itself in the basal segments of a lower lobe, or the lingula, for example. These are relatively easy to take anatomically and eradicate the known disease in that lobe or segment, but also include any disease below the sensitivity of imaging detection. Thus, numerically unfavourable disease may in fact be successfully controlled with minimal loss of lung.

Bilateral disease as a prognosticator has conflicting evidence. The plethora of small case series from single institutions makes it difficult to distinguish the numerical from the bilaterality prognosticator, given that by definition, there must be two or more lesions. In the larger series, it appears that there is no difference between 2 and 3 metastases in a single lung or divided between two lungs [5, 8–10]. Mirror image metastases, especially affecting the upper or lower lobes, may in fact be prognostically better than a metastasis in each lobe of one lung.

A solitary metastasis that directly invades an adjacent structure, such as aorta, azygos, vertebra, oesophagus, diaphragm or rib is another special case that warrants aggressive intervention. Prolonged disease-free survival is seen with en bloc resection of aortic wall, diaphragm and ribs and is far more favourable than droplet or kissing metastasis of the pleural cavity. For involvement of head or neck of ribs, dislocation of the rib from its transverse process or even limited resection of adjacent vertebral body can achieve local control. More extensive involvement of the vertebral body is difficult to justify resection in the metastatic setting. Multi-level posterior rod stabilisation and anterior expandable cage insertion is usually a major 12-hour undertaking with the risks of paraplegia, chronic implant infection and chronic pain.

The “kissing metastasis” is an entity seen where a subpleural metastasis invades through the surface of the visceral pleura of the lung and rubs against either diaphragmatic, mediastinal or parietal pleura. The mechanism for this, as opposed to widespread droplet metastases, or trans-coelomic spread is unclear. However, it appears to confer much better prognosis than multiple or remote pleural metastases and is worth resecting radically en passant. It is usually not detectable preoperatively in any case, as the kissing metastasis appears fused with the lung metastasis of origin.

Endobronchial disease is a feature of some metastatic sarcoma, particularly epithelioid sarcoma. The latter may even mimic the behaviour of a non-small cell lung cancer, with spread to draining lymph nodes. Lung-sparing resectional surgery can be undertaken where appropriate, such as sleeve lobectomy or segmentectomy, as long as good surgical margins are achievable. Failing this, endobronchial therapies such as laser, stenting and brachytherapy can result in good palliation and prolongation of survival.

The CT appearance of "The Sky at Night" is a clearly unfavourable phenotype. Multiple small lesions, randomly distributed throughout the lungs, are not only suggestive of biologically aggressive disease that can thrive in different micro-environments; it is technically near-impossible to embark on a radical metastasectomy whilst preserving adequate lung function for quality survival. Conversely, scattered, but peripherally based metastases can be completely resected bilaterally ("pruning" of the lung), with the prospect of prolonged disease-free survival. Thus, the surgeon must consider the pattern of disease as much as the number and location of metastases.

18.3 Assessment for Surgery

The typical patient presenting with metastatic sarcoma is significantly different to the far more common patient requiring resection of non-small cell lung cancer. Not only is the median age much younger (55 years cf. 69 years; author's data), but they have much lower rates and dosage of tobacco exposure, therefore relatively free of chronic obstructive pulmonary and atherosclerotic vascular disease.

Spirometry and carbon monoxide diffusing capacity are commonly tested prior to lung resection, but, in the asymptomatic non-smoker under 60 years having pulmonary metastasectomy, is a cost without benefit. Patients requiring more than lobectomy and repeat surgery and higher-risk patients should have appropriate physiological testing such as echocardiography, cardio-pulmonary exercise testing or angiography if indicated by symptoms, known comorbidity or cardiovascular risk factors. Death is a very rare occurrence for metastasectomy in specialist centres, but care must be taken not to inflict significant respiratory disability in a previously well-functioning individual.

The main aim of assessment is related to tumour factors. Despite upstaging rates of less than 5% [11], fluorodeoxyglucose (^{18}FDG)-positron emission tomography (PET) scan has long been a standard of care prior to consideration of metastasectomy. This is particularly important to rule out local relapse at the primary site. Such disease should be completely resected with curative intent prior to pulmonary metastasectomy. PET scans can also identify unusual sites of extra-pulmonary metastases, such as mediastinal fat, mesentery, tongue, and peripheral muscle, that may be missed with a conventional CT scan. In general, these would rule out pulmonary metastasectomy.

PET scans have poor positive predictive value for extra-thoracic disease in tumours that do not avidly uptake ^{18}FDG. Therefore, magnetic resonance imaging of the primary tumour site may be required to rule out concomitant local relapse. SPECT bone scans should be used if there are any undiagnosed skeletal symptoms in such patients. These are also useful in patients with myxoid or round cell liposarcomas as they have an additional predilection for bony metastases [12].

18.4 Surgical Oncology Principles

Thoracic surgeons dealing with pulmonary metastases have to negotiate the conflict between preservation of maximal lung parenchyma and fulfilling the requirement for good radial margins around a sarcoma. Whilst the wide margins mandated for primary resection are not required in the lung, any close or involved margin will likely result in local recurrence and predicts for poor survival as an independent risk factor [5].

Metastases to the lung are blood-borne and therefore can be subject to the fluid mechanics of the pulmonary vasculature as well as their tropism for the lung micro-environment. Therefore, for small multiple lesions within a single vessel delta, it may make oncological sense to perform an anatomical segmental, multi-segmental or lobar resection, rather than attempting a non-anatomic wedge resection. This would ensure that any undetected disease in that distribution would be removed along with the macroscopic disease.

For lung cancer, the accepted rule of wedge resection is to achieve a radial margin of at least the diameter of the tumour. For sarcoma metastases, this is not so vital, as they grow radially from a pulmonary vessel base, whereas lung cancer is a bronchiolo-alveolar and bronchial-based disease, which can more widely spread microscopically, either directly (lepidic growth) or as spread through alveolar spaces. Therefore, a margin of 5 mm after removal of the conventional triple row of staples (equating to at least 10 mm in total) is the minimum adequate margin for an intra-parenchymal metastasis. Visceral pleural margins are often measured in fractions of a millimetre for subpleural deposits, but as the next structure is the pleural cavity, it is either completely resected, or there will be pleural contamination no matter what the surgeon does. Therefore, there is no advantage in taking additional parietal pleura unless there is direct invasion or a kissing metastasis.

Lung-sparing techniques allow for good margins whilst achieving the thoracic surgeon's other aim of preservation of lung function. These include bronchoplastic or sleeve resections at the lobar, segmental or, rarely, the carinal level. The specifics of sleeve resection will be discussed in the conduct of surgery section. Anatomic sublobar resections can allow resection of larger deep lesions, or geographic resections of impalpable deep lesions whilst sparing substantial portions of the involved lobe. A description of anatomically straightforward sublobar resections will be presented in the conduct of surgery section and listed in Table 18.2.

Navigational bronchoscopy can be used to mark small or impalpable lesions with either methylene blue for direct visualisation, indocyanine green (ICG) for near-infrared imaging or radio-opaque material for cone beam CT localisation in hybrid operating theatres. These techniques extend the reach of minimally invasive techniques, where palpation of small lesions can be difficult or, in the case of robotic surgery, impossible.

Table 18.2 A list of standard anatomical segmental resections for resection of deep, impalpable or multiple lesions in a single geographic region of lung

Resection name	Segments removed[a]	Segmental loss
Apico-anterior Bisegmentectomy	LUL or RUL anterior and apical segments (S1 & S3)	2
Lingulectomy	Lingula (S4-S5)	2
Superior Trisegmentectomy	LUL superior division (S1-S3)	3
Superior Segmentectomy	LLL or RLL apical segment (S6)	1
Apex-sparing lower lobectomy	LLL or RLL basal segments (S7-S10)	4

[a]Segment nomenclature: Apical (1), Posterior (2), Anterior (3), RML or Lingula (4–5), Superior (6), RLL Medial basal (7), Anterior basal (8), Lateral basal (9), Posterior basal (10)

From the notional 19 segments in normal lungs, an estimate can be made of post-operative lung volume

LUL left upper lobe, *RUL* right upper lobe, *LLL* left lower lobe, *RLL* right lower lobe

18.5 Conduct of Surgery

18.5.1 Access

The "gold standard" access for lung resection has long been one or other variation of the thoracotomy. These variations include the posterolateral thoracotomy, which involves the division of latissimus dorsi and trapezius muscles. The rib below the entry space (usually the sixth rib) is either divided posteriorly, shingled with 1 cm excised posteriorly or simply allowed to fracture. The costo-vertebral ligament may or may not be lysed to facilitate rib-spreading.

Muscle-sparing variations include those that enter the same space by mobilising the trapezius and latissimus muscles and retracting them in the posterior auscultatory triangle. An anterior muscle-sparing thoracotomy can be achieved by making an incision from the inferior border of the scapula anteriorly. The latissimus, pectoral and serratus anterior muscles are mobilised and split or retracted, and the fourth or fifth interspace is entered. Whilst muscles are spared, all of these procedures involve rib-spreading, the major cause of short- and long-term morbidity for simple lung resections.

Bilateral lesions have traditionally been accessed by sternotomy, or, less commonly, clamshell incisions. Sternotomy is less painful than thoracotomy, but may result in significant medium- to long-term morbidity from superficial or deep sternal wound infection, sternal dehiscence or instability. This is a particular risk for patients with diabetes, obesity or chronic obstructive pulmonary disease. It also has the disadvantage of poor access to lower lobe, particularly left lower lobe, without compromising cardiac function by pressure of the surgeon's hands or retractors. Clamshell incisions give superior access but are also quite morbid, with division of the sternum and internal thoracic vessels transversely and the intercostal neuralgia of bilateral thoracotomies at a single sitting.

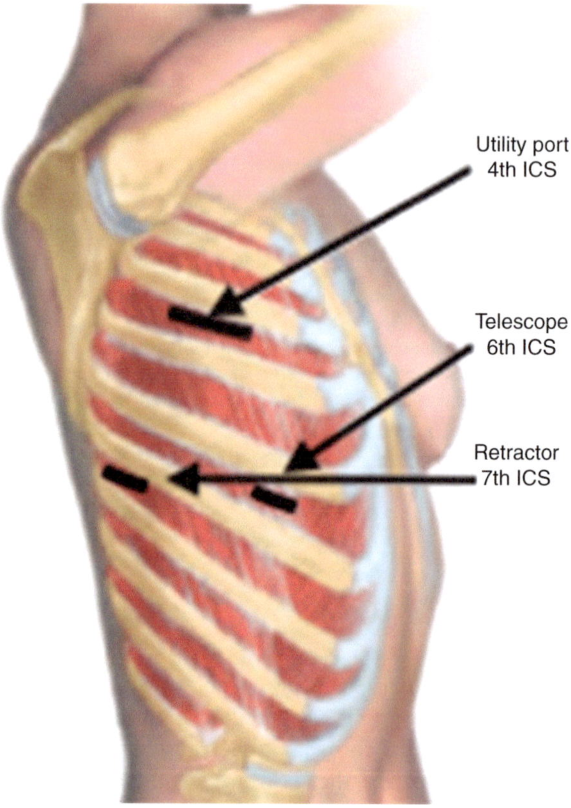

Fig. 18.1 Port placement for a standard three-port thoracoscopic (VATS) technique

Video-assisted thoracic surgery (VATS) or thoracoscopic surgery has considerably minimised the morbidity of access to the lungs for metastasectomy. This is especially the case for bilateral disease, which can be comfortably dealt with in staged resections separated by as little as a week. There are now many variations of VATS, including port number and placement, robotic-assisted techniques and uniportal techniques.

The standard VATS procedure for wedge resection is arguably the three-port technique (Fig. 18.1). This allows multiple angles to visualise and manipulate the lung, the ability to "bring the lung to the finger" for palpation of deeper nodules, and multiple angles for best stapler application.

For simple subpleural nodules, or if an anatomic resection is mandated, a two-port VATS is quite useful, with two angles for both visualisation and stapling. Uniportal VATS techniques can be employed by enlarging the axillary utility incision and placing a wound protector sleeve. Palpation of the lung is more limited, however.

Uniportal VATS also has some advantages in the setting of simple resection of a subpleural, easily identified lesion, or for cases where an anatomic segmental or lobar resection is required. Visualisation is more akin to the thoracotomy view, which leads to less disorientation for the less expert VATS surgeon; however palpation and localisation is far more difficult than multi-port VATS. Despite the displeasing aesthetics of placing the intercostal catheter through the access incision and therefore more awkward closure, there are possibly fewer superficial wound problems and neuralgia than normally associated with the same catheter placed in a two-port or three-port telescope port. The main advantages of uniportal surgery are the ease of teaching the technique and its low cost compared to all other minimally invasive techniques. It is therefore well suited to low-income countries and emerging economies.

Other than for anatomic segmental or lobar resections, robotic surgery is not the ideal approach for metastasectomy. It requires four intercostal ports and a subcostal port, is expensive (in capital and disposable expenditure) for a simple wedge metastasectomy and adds considerable theatre time to what should be a quick procedure for staff and the patient. The only value for an institution is to improve setup skills and efficiency for technical and nursing staff and to amortise the large capital cost of the robot across more cases. However, deeper lesions requiring segmental resections after preoperative localisation with ICG lend themselves well to the robotic approach, especially for posterior and lateral basal segments of the lower lobe.

18.5.2 Wedge Metastasectomy

Once access to the lung is achieved by any means above, consideration turns to how a surgical margin will be achieved whilst minimising loss of lung parenchyma and avoiding prolonged air leakage from the cut surface.

By far the most useful and widespread technique is a stapled wedge metastasectomy. Commercial staplers usually provide three rows of staggered staple lines on either side of a proposed lung incision and simultaneously divide the tissue with an integrated blade. Other than severely emphysematous lungs, this results in an airtight, haemostatic seal of the cut lung surface. Stapling of particularly thick tissue can result in air leaks from nearby fracturing of visceral pleura or the cutting out of a portion of staples. This can be minimised by compressing the tissue for longer and by intermittently and slowly advancing the stapler firing to allow further compression of the progressing staple line. For severely emphysematous lungs, a thicker tissue staple cartridge with a reinforcing sheet of absorbable material is recommended to prevent staples cutting out or missing lung tissue altogether by stapling "air".

For very small peripheral surface lesions, pinpoint diathermy is useful to preserve lung, especially if multiple wedge metastasectomies or additional anatomic segmental or lobar resections are required. This focussed diathermy ablation is usually sufficient to weld the very peripheral bronchioles and vessels, and the apposition of these wounds against parietal pleura is usually sufficient to prevent prolonged air leaks.

Laser incisions are even more haemostatic and airtight than pinpoint diathermy, but increases the capital expenditure and disposable costs. For very peripheral lesions, it is particularly effective. It is also technically effective for deeper lesions where lung-sparing is critical, but its drawback is the difficulty in achieving reliable oncological margins without techniques such as suture fixation of the lesion, which potentially results in trans-coelomic spread or disruption of tumour.

18.5.3 Anatomic Sublobar Resections

One way of avoiding lobectomy for deep lesions is to determine what anatomic segment is affected by tumour and divide the relevant bronchial, venous and arterial supply.

The simplest segmentectomy is the lingulectomy. The fissure is more often complete, and even if it isn't, access to the interlobar pulmonary artery is usually straightforward. The superior pulmonary vein usually has very obvious lingular and upper division tributaries. Once the singular vessels are divided, the upper lobe bronchus can be clear of the segmental node and the singular branch isolated for stapler division. A notional "neo-fissure" is created along the approximation of the inter-segmental plane, taking care to secure good oncologic margins.

By exclusion, the next most useful and straightforward sublobar resection is the left upper lobe superior trisegmentectomy (or divisionectomy). This is otherwise known as a lingula-sparing left upper lobectomy. Basically, the lingular structures are preserved, meaning the truncus anterior, and any posterior pulmonary arteries are divided after dividing the superior division tributary of the superior pulmonary vein. Once the superior division bronchus has been cleared and divided, the neo-fissure is staple-divided exactly as for lingulectomy.

Lower lobe superior segmentectomies of either lung are usually straightforward, especially if there is a good fissure, or at least good access to the interlobar pulmonary artery. The superior segmental tributary of the inferior pulmonary vein (V6) and the superior segmental pulmonary artery (A6) are divided then, after removing the segmental node, the superior segmental bronchus (B6) is divided. The neo-fissure is then estimated, taking care to secure good oncologic margins.

Once again, by exclusion, it is possible to perform apex-sparing lower lobectomies by dividing all structures except the superior segmental artery, bronchus and vein. The neo-fissure is then estimated as for a superior segmentectomy. The resulting superior segment is the largest segment of the lower lobe and very useful for filling the pleural space and preserving lung function.

Other more unusual segmental or bisegmental resections are possible with increasingly detailed knowledge of pulmonary vascular anatomy and its variations. Apico-anterior bisegmentectomy of either upper lobe is possible by dividing the truncus anterior and then chasing the upper lobe vein deep into the hilum to preserve the posterior tributary. By exclusion, a posterior segmentectomy on the right is also possible. In the lower lobe, a superior segmentectomy can be extended to an apico-posterior bisegmentectomy, or by exclusion, antero-medial or postero-lateral bisegmentectomies can be achieved by dividing the relevant terminal pulmonary artery branches beyond the lingular or middle lobe branches on the left or right, respectively.

18.5.4 Bronchoplastic Resections

Pneumonectomy should be avoided at almost any cost when the indication is metastasectomy. The mortality is significantly higher than all other lung resections; the reduction in quality of life is obvious even in fit patients. Future interventions other than stereotactic radiation may be prohibitive. Meticulous anatomic surgery may allow a lobectomy or (right side) bilobectomy to be performed in many cases. This may require a hand cut and sewn anastomosis for a close bronchial margin, or resection of a lobe and an adjacent segment across a fissure to achieve an en bloc resection.

If a bronchial margin cannot be secured without division of the origin of a main bronchus, then every endeavour should be made to perform some form of bronchoplastic resection. The simplest is the sleeve bronchoplasty, where the sleeve of bronchus that the involved segment, lobe or lung arises from is removed en bloc with the intended lung resection. The two open ends of bronchus proximally and distally are then carefully re-anastomosed, taking care not to strip too much of the peri-bronchial tissue during preparation. A running suture is quite acceptable as long as any size discrepancy is accommodated. The other favoured method is to perform a running anastomosis of the membranous portion, which can be cut to leave it slightly longer than the bronchial cartilage. The membrane is cinched on the larger bronchus and small bites taken on the smaller bronchus. Individual simple or figure-of-eight sutures can then be placed under vision and held. Cardiac snuggers are useful to bring the bronchial ends together and distribute tension evenly whilst each suture is tied. This technique is favoured over continuous suture if there is obvious tension in the anastomosis.

The most common and straightforward sleeve bronchoplasty is the right upper lobe with attached right main bronchus. The bronchus intermedius or even the lower lobe or lower lobe basal segments can be anastomosed as high as the ostium of the main bronchus if necessary (Fig. 18.2a, b). For more than just right upper lobe

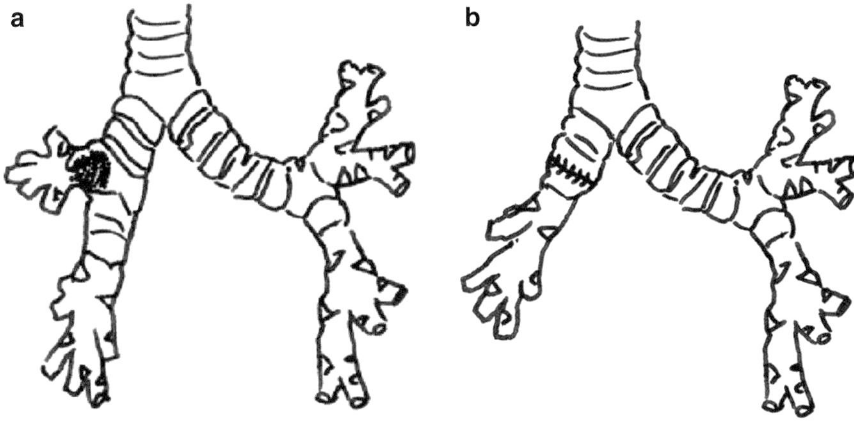

Fig. 18.2 The prototype sleeve bronchoplastic resection of the right upper lobe and right main bronchus is required for tumours involving the origin of the right upper lobe (**a**). After removal of the specimen, the bronchus intermedius is anatomised to the residual right main bronchus or carina (**b**)

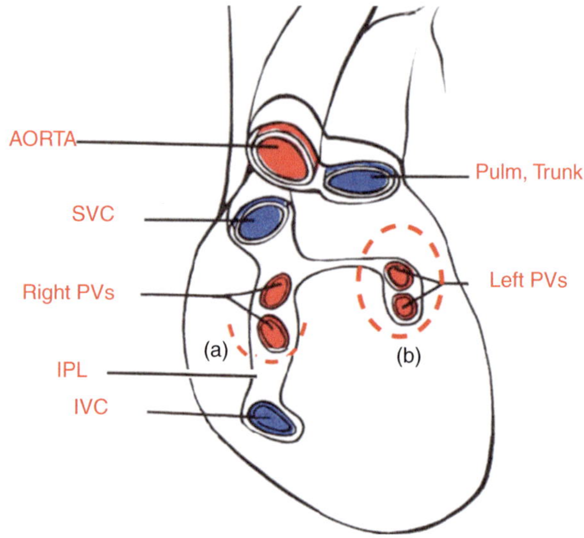

Fig. 18.3 The hilum can be mobilised to facilitate bronchial re-anastomosis after sleeve resection. A pericardial U-release (**a**) and the more extensive O-release (**b**) are depicted by dashed red line. These allow the pulmonary veins (PVs) and peri-bronchial tissues to move comfortably towards the carina. *SVC* superior vena cava, *IVC* inferior vena cava, *IPL* inferior pulmonary ligament

sleeve resection, a pericardial release will be required to allow the vascular hilum to move towards the carina. This is achieved by either curved incision of the pericardium below the inferior pulmonary vein (U-release) or circumcision of pericardium all the way around the pulmonary veins (O-release). These provide several centimetres of advancement of the bronchus towards the carina (Fig. 18.3a, b).

Sleeve resections can also be applied to segmental resections, especially the superior segment of the left lower lobe. On the right side, the position of the middle lobe bronchus may not allow a sleeve superior segmentectomy; therefore a "cruciate" sleeve resection is indicated, whereby the right middle lobe and superior segment bronchi are resected en bloc with a continuous sleeve of bronchus from the bronchus intermedius to the right lower lobe basal bronchus. This results in the loss of three segments, compared to five segments for a complete right lower lobectomy or seven segments for a right middle and lower bilobectomy (Fig. 18.4).

Variations of bronchoplastic techniques include the wedge bronchoplasty and the hinge bronchoplasty. The wedge bronchoplasty is indicated when a hand cut margin of the origin of a lobar bronchus cannot be closed without risking a stricture. A V-excision is made in the lateral sides of the bronchus starting either side of the resection defect. The bronchus can now be closed axially rather than transversely. This will result in some angulation, but it is usually of no functional consequence.

The hinge bronchoplasty is particularly useful on the left side when a hand cut bronchial margin of the secondary carina results in a large bronchial defect medially. The left lower lobe can be rotated inferiorly and medially with the previously inferior lingular bronchial margin being anastomosed to the medial wall of the left main bronchus. Careful suture placement is required to prevent accidental closure or stricturing of the lingular bronchial ostium. An analogous hinge bronchoplasty can be performed on the right if a right middle and lower bilobectomy requires en bloc resection of the right main bronchus opposite the right upper lobe ostium. The

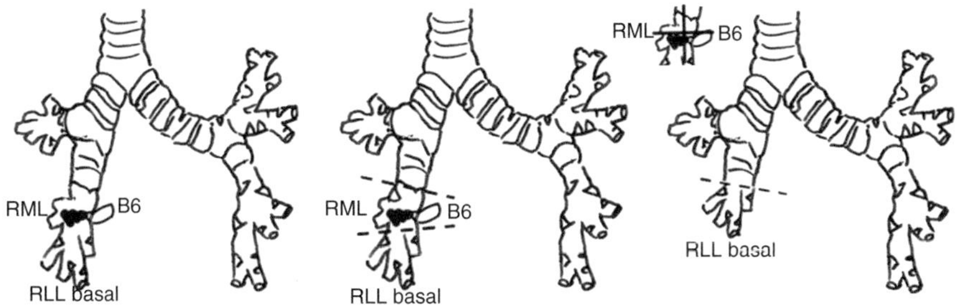

Fig. 18.4 Cruciate sleeve resection is employed for tumours involving the origin of either the right middle lobe bronchus or the superior segment bronchus of the right lower lobe. Both the middle lobe and the superior segment are sacrificed along with the attached bronchus intermedius and lower lobe bronchus, culminating in a cross-shaped resection specimen, hence the name (inset). The lower lobe basal bronchus is then re-anastomosed into the residual bronchus intermedius

previously inferior side of the right upper lobe bronchus is swung inferiorly and medially to anastomosed to the medial wall of the main bronchus. The result is a very functional residual lung (Fig. 18.5a, b). Finally, hinge bronchoplasty is also useful for an extended right lower lobectomy with angled hand cut resection of the posterolateral bronchus intermedius opposite the right middle lobe ostium. This may be required for encroachment of a tumour slightly superior to the superior segment bronchus take-off, but only involving a small area of bronchus intermedius. Once again, the middle lobe bronchus is swung on its remaining attachment, this time superiorly and posteriorly.

18.6 Complications of Surgery

As mentioned previously, the average patient having sarcoma metastasectomy is usually free of significant comorbidity. However, there is a cohort of patients in their sixth and seventh decades in whom unexpected non-technical complications are possible. Prolonged air leak or subcutaneous emphysema despite a functioning intercostal catheter are the most common technical complications of any lung resection. Subcutaneous emphysema, whilst dramatic in appearance, is usually benign and self-limiting. There appears to be a higher incidence of this in the VATS era, but this may just be because it is the most obvious reason for prolonged hospital stay beyond 1 or 2 days. This may need intervention for patient comfort and to reduce alarm amongst nursing staff and visiting relatives. The author has found that re-opening the VATS utility port down to the emphysematous plane and applying a VAC dressing (KCI, TX) connected to continuous wall suction is highly effective and can usually prevent a return to the operating room. Prolonged air leak beyond 7 days should trigger the question of whether a thoracoscopic exploration should be undertaken on the next available operating list. Sometimes these are due to unfavourable adhesions resulting in inadequate drainage, or fracturing of peri-staple

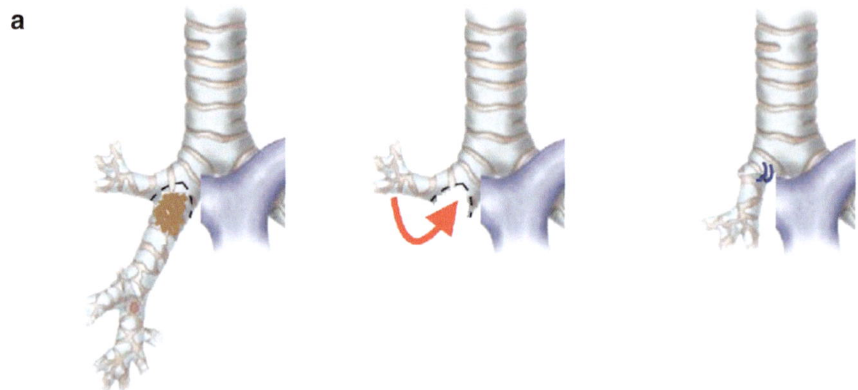

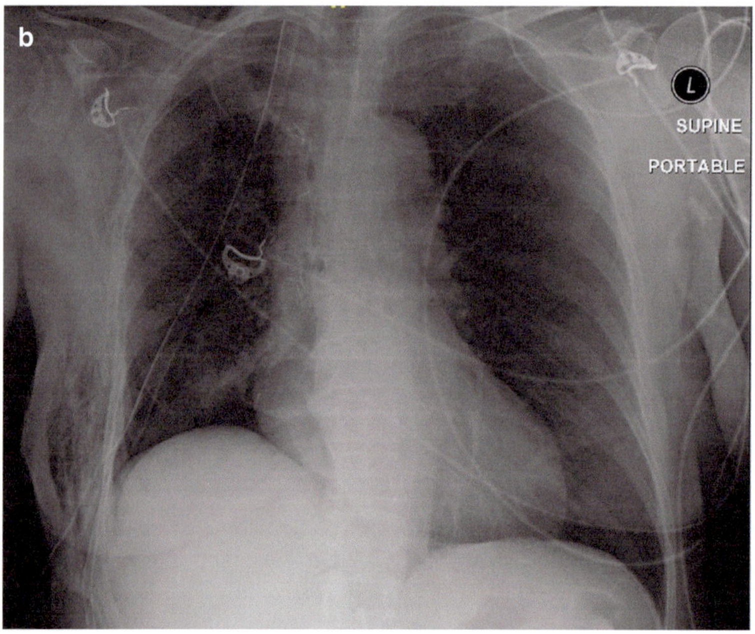

Fig. 18.5 Hinge bronchoplasty of the right upper lobe may be indicated during bilobectomy if the tumour involves the medial wall of the main bronchus opposite the right upper lobe ostium. The right upper lobe is swung inferiorly and medially to anastomose onto the end of the main bronchus to create a valuable functioning neo-lung (**a**). A post-operative chest X-ray demonstrates the re-positioned lobe almost filling the pleural cavity (**b**)

lung. In most cases re-draining and starting over will eliminate the problem. This is preferred over waiting until an empyema develops.

Bleeding is an unusual complication of wedge metastasectomy, although a port site can continually ooze and form a clotted haemothorax. This should be cleared operatively. For lobar and sublobar anatomic resections, the source of bleeding comes from the hilar vessels themselves and from the bronchial and other small arteries supplying the lymph nodes and bronchi. The hilar vessels are more likely to be an intra-operative problem. Bronchial and nodal vessel bleeding are the most likely to result in return to the operating room. Preventative measures include liberal use of clips and energy such as ultrasonic shears or "smart" bipolar diathermy. This will also prevent prolonged lymphatic ooze.

Anastomotic complications are exceedingly rare for lobar stumps, but are a specific risk for pneumonectomy and sleeve resections. The tension required to close a main bronchial stump actually puts it at greater risk of dehiscence than a sleeve anastomosis at the same site, which allows the bronchial lumina to maintain their natural shape. For right-sided pneumonectomy, a flap reinforcement is strongly advised. The simplest form is to mobilise the pericardial fat pad, which will reach most anastomotic locations. Reversed pleural or pericardial pedicled flaps are another alternative. The intercostal muscle of the thoracic access space can also be mobilised as a pedicled flap, but this will increase the chest wall morbidity from somatic and neuropathic pain.

As with all major surgery in the presence of advanced malignancy, the risk of pulmonary embolus is elevated, and therefore all patients should be placed on prophylactic low molecular weight heparins (LMWH) unless there is a specific contraindication. The addition of sequential calf compression devices or thromboembolic stockings should be in accordance with institutional policy. These adjuncts may be required in lieu of LMWH if there is a known contraindication to that drug class.

When patients have been exposed to chemotherapeutic agents prior to surgery, consideration must be given to the possibility of pneumonitis or cardiac injury. Marrow suppression may result in poor haemopoietic response to blood loss; therefore the threshold for consideration of blood transfusion may be lowered if there has been significant blood loss intra-operatively or post-operatively.

References

1. Mariani L, Miceli R, Kattan MW, Brennan MF, Colecchia M, Fiore M, et al. Validation and adaptation of a nomogram for predicting the survival of patients with extremity soft tissue sarcoma using a three-grade system. Cancer. 2005;103:402–8.
2. Gadd MA, Casper ES, Woodruff JM, McCormack PM, Brennan MF. Development and treatment of pulmonary metastases in adult patients with extremity soft tissue sarcoma. Ann Surg. 1993;218:705–12.
3. Lewis JJ, Brennan MF. Soft tissue sarcomas. Curr Probl Surg. 1996;33:817–72.
4. Vezeridis MP, Moore R, Karakousis CP. Metastatic patterns in soft-tissue sarcomas. Arch Surg. 1983;118:915–8.
5. Pastorino U, Buyse M, Friedel G, Ginsberg RJ, Girard P, Goldstraw P, et al. Long-term results of lung metastasectomy: prognostic analyses based on 5206 cases. J Thorac Cardiovasc Surg. 1997;113:37–49.
6. Kaneda H, Communications YSCT. Oligometastases: defined by prognosis and evaluated by cure: Clin Lung Cancer; 2015.
7. Billingsley KG, Burt ME, Jara E, Ginsberg RJ, Woodruff JM, Leung DH, et al. Pulmonary metastases from soft tissue sarcoma: analysis of patterns of diseases and postmetastasis survival. Ann. Surg. 1999;229:602–10–discussion610–2.

8. Cheung F, Alam N, Wright G. Pulmonary metastasectomy: analysis of survival and prognostic factors in 243 patients. ANZ J Surg. John Wiley & Sons, Ltd (10.1111); 2018;88:1316–21.
9. Migliore M, Jakovic R, Hensens A, Klepetko W. Extending surgery for pulmonary Metastasectomy what are the limits? J Thorac Oncol. 2010;5:S155–60.
10. Dear RF, Kelly PJ, Wright GM, Stalley P, McCaughan BC, Tattersall MHN. Pulmonary metastasectomy for bone and soft tissue sarcoma in Australia: 114 patients from 1978 to 2008. Asia Pac J Clin Oncol. 2012;8:292–302.
11. Roberge D, Vakilian S, Alabed YZ, Turcotte RE, Freeman CR, Hickeson M. FDG PET/CT in initial staging of adult soft-tissue sarcoma. Sarcoma. 2012;2012:960194.
12. Moreau L-C, Turcotte R, Ferguson P, Wunder J, Clarkson P, Masri B, et al. Myxoid\round cell Liposarcoma (MRCLS) revisited: an analysis of 418 primarily managed cases. Ann Surg Oncol. 5 ed. Springer-Verlag; 2011. 19:1081–8.

Management of Retroperitoneal Sarcomas

19

Michelle J. Wilkinson, Jennifer Downs, and David E. Gyorki

Retroperitoneal sarcomas (RPS) represent approximately 10–20% of all soft tissue sarcomas. The anatomical location and relationship to important structures pose unique complexities in the management of these patients. These often giant tumours have been described in literature dating back to 1761, but it is only in the last few decades that the understanding and treatment of these tumours has begun to consolidate and advance [1].

19.1 Epidemiology and Staging

As described earlier, soft tissue sarcoma staging is based on tumour size, location (superficial versus deep) and grade, and this is modified from the classical TNM because lymph node metastases are rare. Given that retroperitoneal sarcoma is all deep by definition and most are greater than 10 cms in diameter, the staging system has previously been a poor prognostic discriminator. In this regard, the AJCC eighth Edition now has a specific staging system for sarcomas located in the retroperitoneum which is strongly influenced by tumour grade due to it being a significant prognostic factor [2]. The first three stages (I, II, IIIA) are stratified by increasing the grade and size, whilst stages IIIB and IV reflect local nodal and distant involvement, respectively.

M. J. Wilkinson · J. Downs · D. E. Gyorki (✉)
Division of Cancer Surgery, Peter MacCallum Cancer Centre, Melbourne, VIC, Australia

Division of Surgical Oncology, Peter MacCallum Cancer Centre, Melbourne, VIC, Australia
e-mail: michelle.wilkinson@petermac.org; jennifer.downs@petermac.org; david.gyorki@petermac.org

P. F. M. Choong (ed.), *Sarcoma*, https://doi.org/10.1007/978-981-15-9414-4_19

19.2 Histologic Subtypes

19.2.1 Liposarcomas

The most common sarcoma subtype arising in the retroperitoneum is liposarcoma (LPS). These tumours arise from perinephric and retroperitoneal adipocytes on either the right or left side of the retroperitoneum. As they grow, they displace the viscera medially, progressively displacing them into the contralateral abdomen.

As shown in the largest Australian and UK reviews of retroperitoneal sarcomas, one-third of LPS are homogeneous well-differentiated tumours. Approximately two-thirds are more aggressive heterogeneous tumours containing dedifferentiated components [3–5]. The extent and grade of differentiation predict tumour behaviour. After complete resection, patients with WDLPS have a local recurrence (LR) risk of approximately 20% and distant metastasis (DM) of 1%. By contrast, patients with grade 3 DDLPS have a risk of LR of 30% and DM of 40–50% [6]. This high risk of local recurrence even for low-grade tumours dictates optimal management as discussed later.

19.2.2 Leiomyosarcomas

Leiomyosarcomas develop from smooth muscle cells. In the retroperitoneum, they often arise from large blood vessels such as the gonadal vein, renal vein or inferior vena cava and have the potential for intra- or extra-luminal growth. These tumours have a high propensity for distant spread, with approximately 50% developing distant metastases at 5 years [6].

19.2.3 Other Histologies

Other histological subtypes that occur in the retroperitoneum include undifferentiated pleomorphic sarcoma (UPS), solitary fibrous tumour, synovial sarcoma and extraskeletal Ewing sarcoma.

19.3 Patient Presentation

Patients most commonly present with either a palpable abdominal mass or a lesion discovered incidentally on imaging for other indications. RPS are rarely symptomatic and can be very large at presentation. They typically arise insidiously and progress undetected whilst they expand from the retroperitoneum into the spacious abdominal cavity. Furthermore, unlike other intra-abdominal cancers, these tumours rarely cause pain, anorexia, weight loss, lethargy or symptoms from invasion of adjacent viscera. Symptoms (usually early satiety, nausea and vomiting) only tend to arise when tumours are large, causing compression of the adjacent viscera. The median size of these tumours at presentation is 12–14 cm but ranges between 2 and 42 cm [3].

Distinguishing between the different RPS histological types, epithelial tumours (e.g. lymphoma, germ cell tumour) and benign aetiology such as lipoma, angiomyolipoma and leiomyoma is important as they can require different oncological approaches and surgical strategies.

19.4 Diagnostic Pathway

When an RPS is suspected, it is important to establish the diagnosis, accurately stage the patient and assess fitness for surgery. This is achieved through a combination of clinical assessment, imaging and core needle biopsy (CNB). Early referral of patients to a specialist sarcoma centre is recommended as it is associated with improved outcomes [7].

19.4.1 Imaging

Due to the rarity of these tumours, the radiology and clinical team involved in the patients' care at presentation may not have experience of the imaging appearances. Failure to recognise an RPS on imaging can lead to inappropriate management in non-specialist centres [8]. The minimum imaging requirement and most useful primary investigation is a computerised tomography (CT) scan with intravenous contrast of the thorax, abdomen and pelvis. CT enables accurate assessment of the extent of the tumour, visceral involvement, establishes if solitary or multifocal and the presence of any metastatic disease.

Other imaging modalities which may be required include magnetic resonance imaging (MRI), positron emission tomography/CT (PET/CT) and others such as formal vascular assessment depending on tumour location and the suspected histological subtype.

The utility of MRI imaging in RPS is limited but is particularly valuable in patients with pelvic disease and in tumours with indeterminate bone (especially the sciatic notch and vertebral foramina) or muscle involvement on CT. It can also be used as an alternative to contrast CT in those with allergies to iodinated contrast agents or during pregnancy.

FDG-PET/CT provides important supplementary information beyond simple cross-sectional imaging. Functional imaging provides information on the grade of tumour, as Glut-1 expression and glucose metabolism have been shown to correlate with tumour grade [9]. Identifying the areas of maximal glucose uptake can be useful to ensure that preoperative CNB targets the areas of greatest uptake and therefore highest grade. In retroperitoneal liposarcomas, a PET/CT SUV_{max} of 4.5 has been shown to be highly predictive of Fédération Nationale des Centres de Lutte Contre le Cancer (FNCLCC) grade 3 tumours and an SUV_{max} >4.5 can be used as a prognostic factor for recurrence-free survival and overall survival before obtaining the histopathology [10].

19.4.2 Core Needle Biopsy

Tumours within the retroperitoneum can cause diagnostic dilemmas. It has been shown that the correct diagnosis of an RPS based on imaging alone is challenging [11]. Therefore, CNB is needed to definitively establish the diagnosis, aid clinical decision-making and help guide surgical strategy [12].

In retroperitoneal lesions, the four main reasons to obtain a core needle biopsy are:

1. To establish the diagnosis of RPS and exclude other malignant processes, e.g. lymphoma or benigXn lesions (lipoma, schwannoma) and secondary metastatic lesions.
2. To identify chemosensitive pathology such as Ewing sarcoma, synovial sarcoma or GISTs in which neoadjuvant treatment may be indicated to downsize the lesion, reduce its biological activity and potentially facilitate organ-preserving surgery and better oncological outcomes.
3. To identify the presence of a dedifferentiated component within a WD/DDLPS, as a solid component within a LPS may just represent a solid component of WDLPS.
4. To plan the optimal extent of surgery specific to tumour histology (see below).

CNB should be performed under imaging guidance using a retroperitoneal approach targeting the highest-grade component of the tumour. Potential post-procedure risks of CNB are bleeding, rectus sheath haematoma, tumour rupture, sampling error and delay in treatment; however, in experienced centres, these risks are low. There is a very low risk of tumour seeding with CNB which is further reduced with the use of a coaxial needle. These risks are significantly outweighed by the benefits of an accurate preoperative diagnosis [13].

The use of open biopsy is limited to the rare case where CNB is non-diagnostic. However, where PET/CT is used to guide biopsy localisation, the inability to accurately confirm a diagnosis on CNB is very rare.

19.4.3 The Transatlantic Retroperitoneal Sarcoma Working Group

The combination of RPS being both rare (with further division into multiple histological subtypes) and complex has led to the development of an international multicentre collaboration – the Transatlantic Retroperitoneal Sarcoma Working Group (TARPSWG) – in 2013. The aim of this group is to combine knowledge and experience from high-volume sarcoma specialist centres, to critically evaluate the current evidence and to establish consensus regarding various aspects of patient management with the overall aim of improving oncological outcomes in this difficult disease. They secondarily have set up a prospective registry. In line with this, the TARPSWG collaboration has published consensus statements regarding the management of primary retroperitoneal sarcoma [14], recurrent RPS [15] and metastatic RPS [16].

In an era of increased movement towards individualised patient care, the ability to predict prognosis following surgery for RPS is essential. This enables therapeutic strategies to be tailored to individual patient and facilitates adequate patient counselling. The outcomes of patients who have undergone resection for RPS can be predicted using tools such as nomograms [17]. One such useful tool for prediction of both overall survival and disease-free survival is Sarculator (www.sarculator.com). This can be used for both primary and recurrent RPS and also has a predictor for extremity soft tissue sarcoma.

19.5 Management

The primary curative-intent modality of treatment for patients with RPS is surgery, and the best chance of cure is at the time of primary presentation.

19.5.1 Multidisciplinary Team

In accordance with the Trans-Atlantic RPS working group, RPS is a, complex malignancy and is best managed in specialist centres [14]. The patient's history, imaging and histology should be reviewed and discussed at a sarcoma-specific multidisciplinary meeting (MDM) with a surgeon trained in RPS resection. The clinical approach and extent of surgical resection is tailored to the individual patient and tumour characteristics. The factors that must be considered are:

1. The patient's wishes, performance status, past medical history and previous abdominal surgery.
2. The tumour's location and involvement of critical and noncritical abdominal structures.
3. The tumour's histology and grade.
4. Is it unifocal or multifocal disease?
5. Is it a primary diagnosis or recurrent disease?

19.5.2 When Is a Retroperitoneal Sarcoma Deemed Unresectable?

Retroperitoneal sarcomas are typically large tumours, but very few of them are unresectable. Curative-intent surgery necessitates a complete en bloc resection of the tumour. Patients with tumours that involve the superior mesenteric artery/root of the mesentery, coeliac trunk, portal vein, bilateral renal vessels and extension into the spinal canal or into the vertebral bodies are considered unresectable.

19.6 Preoperative Assessment

If the decision at the MDM is to proceed with surgery, whether for primary or recurrent disease, patients require assessment by the anaesthetic team for surgical fitness. RPS resections are often prolonged procedures with multivisceral resection and significant risk of blood loss and fluid shifts. Preoperative review allows for assessment of baseline, optimisation of co-morbidities and treatment of modifiable risk factors. Unit-specific protocols should be in place for this at specialist centres. A minimum review includes a detailed medical, surgical and anaesthetic history, current medications, baseline blood tests, cardiac assessment and standardised functional testing such as cardiopulmonary exercise testing (CPET) or walk test, e.g. 6-min walk or shuttle walk test.

Prehabilitation is useful in RPS patients. Surgery places significant demands on patients, both physically and psychologically. Prehabilitation offers the possibility of improving their ability to meet these demands. This includes a physiological assessment of surgical patients and targeted programmes to alter modifiable risk factors such as anaemia, poor nutrition and impaired lung function. The aim is to optimise patients for surgery and enhance their recovery by reducing postoperative complications. Small studies have shown that interventions such as single counselling sessions or supervised exercise programmes have halved postoperative complications in patients undergoing major abdominal surgery [18].

However, the benefit of delaying surgery to modify risk factors should be weighed up against the risk of progression of disease, and decisions should be made on a case-by-case basis with multidisciplinary input.

19.7 The Surgical Strategy

Excision of RPS with clear margins is the best chance for cure. Surgical resection of RPS is complex and requires the surgeon to have extensive anatomical knowledge and technical skills in the resection and reconstruction of the retroperitoneum including the autonomic and somatic nerves, lymphatics, paravertebral vessels and retroperitoneal and abdominal viscera to successfully manage these patients. Single-organ/single-site expertise is not sufficient to minimise the risk of morbidity and mortality and provide the best possible oncological outcomes [6, 19]. The primary surgeon may need to bring together a team with diverse surgical expertise, e.g. involvement of vascular surgery, to achieve optimal outcomes.

The main surgical consideration is balancing the extent of the surgery required for oncological clearance against potential morbidity. The anatomical constraints of the retroperitoneum often restrict the ability to achieve wide resection margins.

Decision-making around the extent of surgery relies on an understanding of the diverse tumour biology based on histologic subtypes. Patients with LMS have a 5-year local recurrence (LR) rate <10%, a distant metastasis (DM) rate of 50% and an OS of around 55% [6]. These patients can be treated with resection of the tumour mass alone with preservation of adjacent organs unless there is clear invasion evident on imaging. By contrast, patients with LPS have an LR rate of 20–40%. In this histology, organ invasion can be difficult to predict based on imaging alone [20], and therefore, a multivisceral resection including adjacent organs in particular the kidney and colon should be considered. This allows complete clearance of the ipsilateral retroperitoneal fat.

The resection described below is designed for liposarcoma (LPS), the most common RPS (Fig. 19.1). A compartmentectomy aims to achieve complete tumour

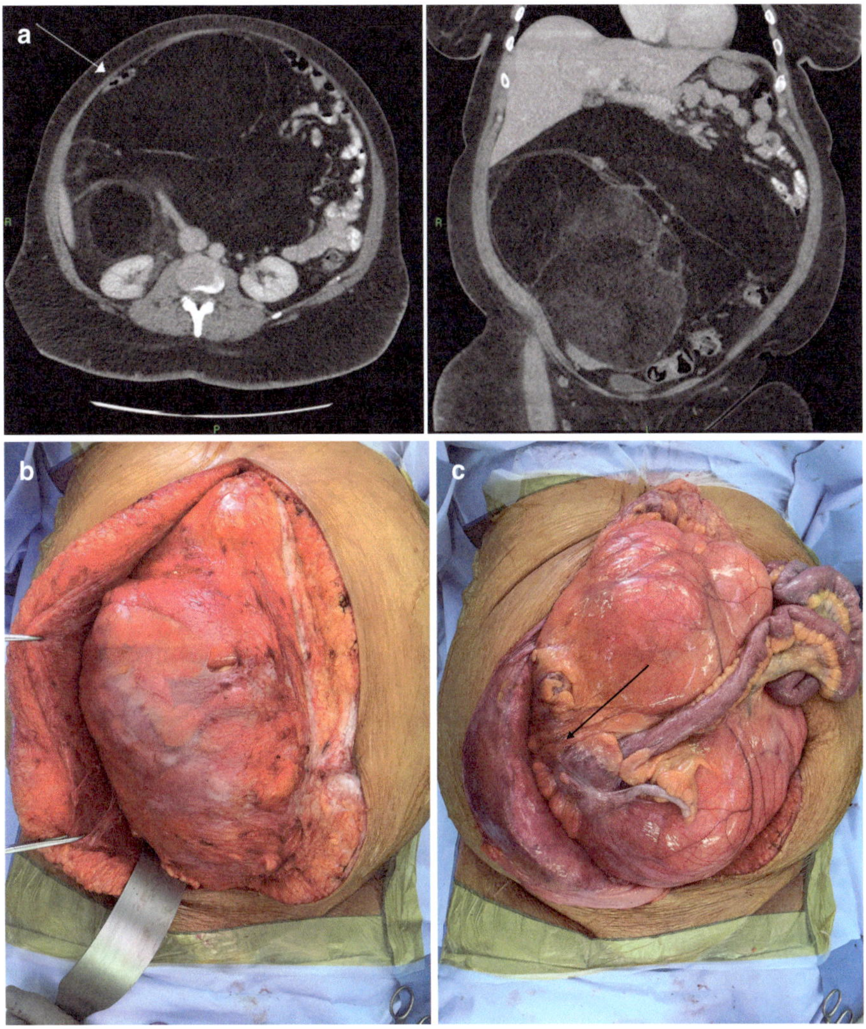

Fig. 19.1 Large right retroperitoneal liposarcoma in a 56-year-old female patient who underwent en bloc multivisceral resection with extended right hemicolectomy and right nephrectomy and remains free of disease after 3 years of follow-up: (**a**) CT shows large lipomatous mass encasing the right kidney posteriorly and the right colon anteriorly (arrow), displacing the uninvolved viscera to the left. (**b**) Initial extraperitoneal dissection dissecting tumour off the lateral abdominal wall preserving peritoneal margin. (**c**) Subsequent transperitoneal approach demonstrating involvement of the right colon (arrow). (**d**) Resected specimen demonstrating en bloc multivisceral specimen containing extended right hemicolectomy and right nephrectomy (not seen). (**e**) Surgical footprint demonstrating IVC with right renal vein stump (arrow) as well as skeletonised posterior abdominal wall with fascia retained on tumour surface as deep margin

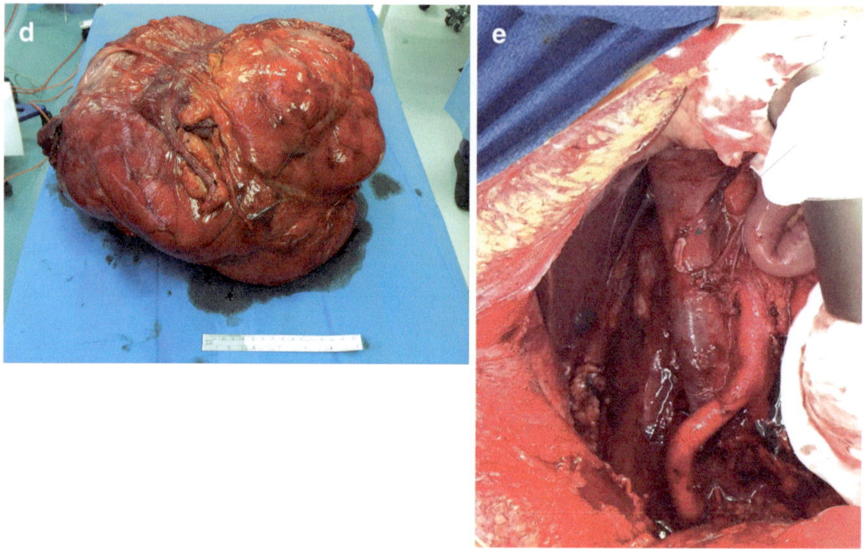

Fig. 19.1 (continued)

resection whilst minimising the chance of positive microscopic margins. This is achieved by removing the RPS en bloc with its contiguous noncritical surrounding viscera (even when not preoperative imaging does not identify overt tumour infiltration) and clearing the ipsilateral retroperitoneal fat. When considering resection of critical neurovascular structures, the surgeon must assess the risks and benefits of achieving local control versus potential long-term morbidity.

Resection of an LPS commonly involves either a right nephrectomy and colectomy or left nephrectomy and colectomy. For left-sided tumours, a distal pancreatectomy and splenectomy may also be required. Right-sided tumours may require partial duodenal resection, but the liver is rarely involved. In accordance with the 'Milan approach', the RPS resection has been described as a six-stage procedure [19]:

1. Midline laparotomy and careful dissection into the retroperitoneal space, with assessment of tumour resectability (Fig. 19.1b).
2. Division of the gastrocolic ligament and transverse colon (plus distal ileum if on the right side) and assessment of the duodenum/head of the pancreas (right side) or body/tail of the pancreas and spleen (left side).
3. Mobilisation of duodenum/head of the pancreas (right side) or body/tail of the pancreas and spleen and duodenojejunal junction (left side). Partial duodenal resection or pancreaticoduodenectomy is uncommon (<5%) (right side). However, distal pancreatectomy and splenectomy are more common (up to 50%) in left-sided retroperitoneal sarcomas or if adherent to or invaded by tumour.
4. Major vascular dissection of the inferior vena cava (IVC) or aorta as appropriate, with ligation and division of ipsilateral renal vessels and other collaterals, and dissection of the tumour from the iliac system (Fig. 19.1e).

5. Peritonectomy and resection of the psoas fascia in the pelvis (plus rectal resection if on the left side) after preservation of the femoral nerve (unless directly invaded). Femoral cutaneous branch and the genitofemoral and ilioinguinal nerves are expendable and may need to be resected, as these lie between the tumour and the psoas fascia.
6. With psoas invasion by tumour, the origin of the psoas is resected from the spine whilst sparing the roots of the femoral nerve (L2, L3, L4) and possibly the ilio-hypogastric nerve. Mobilising the costo-diaphragmatic fold facilitates removal of the specimen.

Whilst subcapsular hepatic dissection or partial hepatectomy for right-sided tumours are infrequently required, mobilisation of the right lobe of the liver is recommended. Gastric procedures such as sleeve or proximal gastrectomy are infrequent for left-sided tumours. Vascular resections including iliac vessels and IVC (right side) are infrequently required (4%).

Patients require intensive anaesthetic support throughout the procedure with invasive monitoring and goal-directed fluid management. These operations are often prolonged with the potential for significant blood loss and fluid shifts putting patients at risk of hypothermia, hypovolaemia, acidosis and coagulopathy. Therefore, intraoperative and postoperative management of these patients should be directed by experienced staff, and standardised approaches should be implemented where possible (warming techniques, fluid management, transfusion requirements, anticoagulants, analgesia and postoperative care).

Prior series have shown a rate of return to theatre for all causes of 10% [21]. The commonest cause of early return to theatre is for bleeding. Delayed return may be due to overt or suspected anastomotic leak, infected haematoma or collection. The post-procedure mortality rate is approximately 3%. The commonest causes of death are multisystem organ failure, often secondary to sepsis, cardiac failure, myocardial infarction and pulmonary embolus [4, 5, 22]. Postoperative complications that should be consented for include bleeding and return to theatre, infection (collections, overwhelming post-splenectomy infection or lower respiratory tract infection), bowel ischaemia, pulmonary embolus or deep vein thrombosis, pleural effusions, anastomotic leak, pancreatic leak, ileus, delayed wound healing, dehiscence and wound infection.

19.8 Prognosis

The local control rates for RPS are worse than for extremity sarcomas. This is due to both non-modifiable tumour factors, such as histology, grade and anatomical location, and modifiable factors, e.g. tumour resection margins. It is therefore paramount that the treatment of these tumours is focused on achieving complete resection margins to optimise patient outcomes.

Patients with primary tumours who undergo complete macroscopic resection have an overall local recurrence rate of 38–40%. The risk of recurrence does not plateau over time. At 5 years, local recurrence-free survival is 50–55%, and overall survival is 68–70% (Gyorki JSO, Strauss BJS 2010 TA group plus Ferrario et al). Survival is also related to tumour grade, and when the outcomes are analysed by tumour grade, the 5-year overall survival in low-grade lesions (G1) increases to 82–92%, for intermediate (G2) 54–77%, compared to 43–48% 5-year survival in patients with high-grade (G3) tumours [23, 24].

The poorest outcomes are often seen in retroperitoneal leiomyosarcoma involving the inferior vena cava where the 5-year survival rate is between 35 and 65% with a disease-free survival of only 25–30% [25, 26].

19.8.1 Neoadjuvant and Adjuvant Therapies

There is no high-level evidence to date that the use of neoadjuvant therapies for RPS improves local control rates or overall survival. However, it is very difficult to perform prospective randomised trials for RPS due to the rarity of the disease and the variation in tumour size, grade and histological subtype.

19.8.1.1 Radiotherapy

Given the importance of local control in a majority of RPS subtypes, radiation therapy (RT) has been an important component in the multimodal treatment of this disease. There has been great debate over the use of RT in either the adjuvant or the neoadjuvant setting, based on lessons learned from extremity sarcomas [27]. The neoadjuvant approach is preferred as the tumour is readily identifiable and displaces radiosensitive structures out of the radiation fields, allowing delivery of adequate radiation dose to the tumour, with low toxicity and without significantly increased perioperative morbidity or mortality.

In analysis of the Peter MacCallum Cancer Centre patients, the use of neoadjuvant radiotherapy was associated with lower rates of local recurrence [3]. Historically extended compartmental resection in LPS was not routinely practiced, and therefore the influence of RT may have been overestimated.

The first prospective randomised controlled trial designed to evaluate the efficacy of neoadjuvant radiotherapy on RPS (ACOSOG Z9031) was closed prematurely in 2004 due to low accrual rates, concerns over treatment toxicity and delays in surgery. More recently, the STRASS trial, an EORTC international randomised controlled trial assessing oncologic outcomes in patients undergoing neoadjuvant RT followed by surgery versus those undergoing upfront surgery alone, has completed accrual. This was reported in 2019 and failed to demonstrate a benefit of preoperative RT for RPS at 3 years. However, in the exploratory analysis, preoperative RT showed benefit for the LPS subgroup with 3-year abdominal recurrence-free survival of 71.6% (61.3–79.6%) and 60.4% (49.8–69.5%) in the radiotherapy plus surgery group versus surgery groups (HR = 0.64, 95%CI 0.40–1.01, $p = 0.049$). It will be interesting to see if this trend continues and becomes more significant at the 5- and 10-year time points.

19.8.1.2 Chemotherapy

The strongest indication for neoadjuvant therapy is in RPS with chemotherapy (synovial sarcoma, leiomyosarcoma). Neoadjuvant therapy may downsize these tumours, enable resection with negative margins and improve patient outcomes. Furthermore, neoadjuvant chemotherapy allows an in vivo assessment of chemosensitivity by allowing assessment of pathological response.

To date, there have not been any studies of neoadjuvant chemotherapy in patients with RPS. Following on from the STRASS trial, a multicentre randomised EORTC clinical trial is currently investigating whether neoadjuvant chemotherapy, as an adjunct to curative-intent surgery, improves the prognosis of high-risk DDLPS (dedifferentiated Liposarcoma) and LMS (Leiomyosarcoma) patients as measured by disease-free survival.

The use of adjuvant chemotherapy, external beam radiotherapy and brachytherapy has no clinical study-proven value in the treatment of RPS.

19.8.2 Follow-Up

There is no evidence to guide follow-up for patients following definitive surgical resection of RPS. Clinical evaluation accompanied by appropriate imaging every 4–6 months for the first 5 years is recommended with annual follow-up thereafter. The optimal imaging modality for follow-up is CT chest/abdomen/pelvis, covering both local recurrence and likely sites of distant metastasis. In young patients, especially females of child-bearing age, MRI of the abdomen and pelvis with CXR may be considered to reduce radiation exposure.

19.9 Management of Recurrent Disease

The commonest type of relapse in completely treated RPS is local recurrence. This may be single site or multifocal and can be slow growing or rapidly progressive. Recurrent disease is often detected on radiological surveillance whilst the patient is asymptomatic.

In patients with recurrent disease, the most important factors to consider are:

1. To exclude the presence of distant metastatic disease.
2. Time interval from previous resection and tumour growth rate.
3. Is it resectable?
4. Is the patient symptomatic?

Unfortunately, 20% of patients present with synchronous local recurrence and metastatic disease. Resectability is less likely in recurrent disease compared to primary presentation, but if it is resectable, this correlates with a median overall survival of 60 months compared to 20 months in unresectable recurrence [28]. The speed of tumour growth is also predictor of disease-specific survival in recurrent disease with a tumour growth rate of >0.9 cm/month having a median DSS of 21 months compared to 100 months if growth was <0.9 cm/month [29].

Even after a complete resection of recurrent disease, there is still a 10% risk of systemic recurrence and an ongoing risk of further local recurrence. After each recurrence, the time interval between recurrences shortens, and the operative morbidity increases. However, if complete surgical resection is possible, then the role of surgery for recurrent RPS is with curative intent and in most cases is still the best treatment option. However, the optimal timing of surgery is critically important.

The decision to operate on patients with locally recurrent RPS depends on multiple factors, not resectability alone. These include the patient's symptoms, fitness for surgery, number of previous resections and timing of recurrence interval, tumour growth and presence of multifocal disease. There is no high-level evidence to help guide this often difficult decision-making process, and therefore expert review is required. The options should be clearly explained to the patient as shared decision-making and multidisciplinary input are vital. Overall, these patients are challenging to manage, and the risks and benefits or surgery must be carefully reviewed on a case-by-case basis. Early surgery may not provide optimal outcomes, and a period of watchful waiting is often advisable [30].

In patients with unresectable disease or in whom surgery is unlikely to provide benefit, the options of treatment are surveillance, trial of chemotherapy, radiotherapy or in rare symptomatic cases palliative debulking.

Palliative debulking should be reserved for patients with symptomatic disease. There is no role for an incomplete resection for patients with asymptomatic recurrence. For symptomatic patients, the risks and benefits need to be considered as symptoms tend to recur rapidly and patients are at high risk of postoperative complications.

19.10 Management of Metastatic Disease

In RPS, the commonest cause of death is local recurrence leading to cachexia and bowel obstruction. The commonest sites of systemic metastatic disease are the lung and liver. Metastatic disease may also present as intra-abdominal multifocal peritoneal sarcomatosis.

Whilst surgery may be considered for patients, it is important to acknowledge that the probability of cure in metastatic RPS is low. Although there are some long-term survivors after metastectomy, this is likely a reflection of patient selection. Those considered for metastectomy are often those with more favourable disease biology.

Patients shown to have the greatest benefit from metastectomy are:

1. Those with a good performance status.
2. Those who have a prolonged time between primary resection and distant disease (greater than 12 months).

3. Low-volume metastases in whom complete disease eradication is possible.

For systemic oligometastatic disease, local therapies can be considered in appropriate patients such as resection, microwave or radiofrequency ablation and stereotactic radiotherapy. Less invasive modalities should be used where possible as they have the benefit of fewer side effects and less disruption to any ongoing systemic treatment. They can be used alone or in combination with surgery to attempt complete disease clearance [16].

The majority of patients with metastatic RPS will require palliative treatment and have a median survival of 12 months. Systemic therapy, with an anthracycline-based regimen, is the commonest form of first-line treatment but may also be used in those for consideration of resection to evaluate tumour biology. Radiotherapy may be used for symptomatic relief especially in those with pain, spinal cord compression or breathlessness.

References

1. Tseng WW, Wang SC, Eichler CM, Warren RS, Nakakura EK. Complete and safe resection of challenging retroperitoneal tumors: anticipation of multi-organ and major vascular resection and use of adjunct procedures. World J Surg Oncol. 2011;9:143.
2. Fisher SB, Chiang YJ, Feig BW, Cormier JN, Hunt KK, Torres KE, et al. An evaluation of the eighth edition of the American joint committee on Cancer (AJCC) staging system for retroperitoneal sarcomas using the National Cancer Data Base (NCDB): does size matter? Am J Clin Oncol. 2019;42(2):160–5.
3. Snow HA, Hitchen TX, Head J, Herschtal A, Bae S, Chander S, et al. Treatment of patients with primary retroperitoneal sarcoma: predictors of outcome from an Australian specialist sarcoma Centre. ANZ J Surg. 2018;88(11):1151–7.
4. Strauss DC, Hayes AJ, Thway K, Moskovic EC, Fisher C, Thomas JM. Surgical management of primary retroperitoneal sarcoma. Br J Surg. 2010;97(5):698–706.
5. Smith HG, Panchalingam D, Hannay JA, Smith MJ, Thomas JM, Hayes AJ, et al. Outcome following resection of retroperitoneal sarcoma. Br J Surg. 2015;102(13):1698–709.
6. Gronchi A, Strauss DC, Miceli R, Bonvalot S, Swallow CJ, Hohenberger P, et al. Variability in patterns of recurrence after resection of primary retroperitoneal sarcoma (RPS): a report on 1007 patients from the multi-institutional collaborative RPS working group. Ann Surg. 2016;263(5):1002–9.
7. Bonvalot S, Rivoire M, Castaing M, Stoeckle E, Le Cesne A, Blay JY, et al. Primary retroperitoneal sarcomas: a multivariate analysis of surgical factors associated with local control. J Clin Oncol. 2009;27(1):31–7.
8. Messiou C, Morosi C. Imaging in retroperitoneal soft tissue sarcoma. J Surg Oncol. 2018;117(1):25–32.
9. Tateishi U, Yamaguchi U, Seki K, Terauchi T, Arai Y, Hasegawa T. Glut-1 expression and enhanced glucose metabolism are associated with tumour grade in bone and soft tissue sarcomas: a prospective evaluation by [18F]fluorodeoxyglucose positron emission tomography. Eur J Nucl Med Mol Imaging. 2006;33(6):683–91.
10. Rhu J, Hyun SH, Lee KH, Jo SJ, Lee KW, Park JB, et al. Maximum standardized uptake value on (18)F-fluorodeoxyglucose positron emission tomography/computed tomography improves outcome prediction in retroperitoneal liposarcoma. Sci Rep. 2019;9(1):6605.
11. Morosi C, Stacchiotti S, Marchiano A, Bianchi A, Radaelli S, Sanfilippo R, et al. Correlation between radiological assessment and histopathological diagnosis in retroperitoneal tumors:

analysis of 291 consecutive patients at a tertiary reference sarcoma center. Eur J Surg Oncol. 2014;40(12):1662–70.
12. Gyorki DE, Choong PFM, Slavin J, Henderson MA. Importance of preoperative diagnosis for management of patients with suspected retroperitoneal sarcoma. ANZ J Surg. 2018;88(4):274–7.
13. Wilkinson MJ, Martin JL, Khan AA, Hayes AJ, Thomas JM, Strauss DC. Percutaneous core needle biopsy in retroperitoneal sarcomas does not influence local recurrence or overall survival. Ann Surg Oncol. 2015;22(3):853–8.
14. Trans-Atlantic RPSWG. Management of primary retroperitoneal sarcoma (RPS) in the adult: a consensus approach from the Trans-Atlantic RPS working group. Ann Surg Oncol. 2015;22(1):256–63.
15. Trans-Atlantic RPSWG. Management of Recurrent Retroperitoneal Sarcoma (RPS) in the adult: a consensus approach from the Trans-Atlantic RPS working group. Ann Surg Oncol. 2016;23(11):3531–40.
16. Trans-Atlantic Retroperitoneal Sarcoma Working G. Management of metastatic retroperitoneal sarcoma: a consensus approach from the Trans-Atlantic retroperitoneal sarcoma working group (TARPSWG). Ann Oncol. 2018;29(4):857–71.
17. Tattersall HL, Callegaro D, Ford SJ, Gronchi A. Staging, nomograms and other predictive tools in retroperitoneal soft tissue sarcoma. Chin Clin Oncol. 2018;7(4):36.
18. Barakat HM, Shahin Y, Khan JA, McCollum PT, Chetter IC. Preoperative supervised exercise improves outcomes after elective abdominal aortic aneurysm repair: a randomized controlled trial. Ann Surg. 2016;264(1):47–53.
19. Almond LM, Gronchi A, Strauss D, Jafri M, Ford S, Desai A. Neoadjuvant and adjuvant strategies in retroperitoneal sarcoma. Eur J Surg Oncol. 2018;44(5):571–9.
20. Fairweather M, Wang J, Jo VY, Baldini EH, Bertagnolli MM, Raut CP. Surgical Management of Primary Retroperitoneal Sarcomas: rationale for selective organ resection. Ann Surg Oncol. 2018;25(1):98–106.
21. Bonvalot S, Gaignard E, Stoeckle E, Meeus P, Decanter G, Carrere S, et al. Survival benefit of the surgical Management of Retroperitoneal Sarcoma in a reference center: a Nationwide study of the French sarcoma group from the NetSarc database. Ann Surg Oncol. 2019;26(7):2286–93.
22. MacNeill AJ, Gronchi A, Miceli R, Bonvalot S, Swallow CJ, Hohenberger P, et al. Postoperative morbidity after radical resection of primary retroperitoneal sarcoma: a report from the transatlantic RPS working group. Ann Surg. 2018;267(5):959–64.
23. Ferrario T, Karakousis CP. Retroperitoneal sarcomas: grade and survival. Arch Surg. 2003;138(3):248–51.
24. Abdelfatah E, Guzzetta AA, Nagarajan N, Wolfgang CL, Pawlik TM, Choti MA, et al. Long-term outcomes in treatment of retroperitoneal sarcomas: a 15 year single-institution evaluation of prognostic features. J Surg Oncol. 2016;114(1):56–64.
25. Teixeira FJR Jr, do Couto Netto SD, Perina ALF, Torricelli FCM, Ragazzo Teixeira L, Zerati AE, et al. Leiomyosarcoma of the inferior vena cava: survival rate following radical resection. Oncol Lett. 2017;14(4):3909–16.
26. Blair AB, Reames BN, Singh J, Gani F, Overton HN, Beaulieu RJ, et al. Resection of retroperitoneal sarcoma en-bloc with inferior vena cava: 20 year outcomes of a single institution. J Surg Oncol. 2018;118(1):127–37.
27. Dumitra S, Gronchi A. The diagnosis and Management of Retroperitoneal Sarcoma. Oncology (Williston Park). 2018;32(9):464–9.
28. Gyorki DE, Brennan MF. Management of recurrent retroperitoneal sarcoma. J Surg Oncol. 2014;109(1):53–9.
29. Park JO, Qin LX, Prete FP, Antonescu C, Brennan MF, Singer S. Predicting outcome by growth rate of locally recurrent retroperitoneal liposarcoma: the one centimeter per month rule. Ann Surg. 2009;250(6):977–82.
30. Ikoma N, Roland CL, Torres KE, Chiang YJ, Wang WL, Somaiah N, et al. Salvage surgery for recurrent retroperitoneal well-differentiated Liposarcoma: early reoperation may not provide benefit. Ann Surg Oncol. 2018;25(8):2193–200.

Soft Tissue Reconstructions After Sarcoma Resection

20

Eldon Mah, Sophie Ricketts, Michael Lo, Satomi Koide, and Sarah Lonie

20.1 Challenges of Sarcoma Reconstruction

Sarcoma reconstruction is a challenging area of plastic surgery that demands careful defect assessment, critical considerations of all options and balanced approach to maximise patient's recovery. The purpose of this chapter is to define the difficulties surgeon face in sarcoma reconstructions and to provide a structured framework that would stimulate problem-solving process and assist in choosing the most appropriate reconstructive solutions.

The challenges in sarcoma reconstruction are directly attributed to the following:

- Site of the disease
- Size of the defect
- Neoadjuvant radiotherapy
- Functional loss consequent to the resection

Soft tissue sarcoma can occur at any site; thus reconstructive requirement changes according to the defect anatomy, presence of critical structures, functional needs and resultant contour deformity. While general principle applies everywhere, each anatomical region requires some special considerations. These are discussed in detail in this chapter.

Due to the malignancy and local aggressiveness of many of these tumours, surgical resection frequently demands wide margins and involve multiple tissue compositions such as muscles, nerves and vessels. Some of the larger defects push the limits of reconstructions, while others with multiple complex reconstructive needs challenges a surgeon's thought process and maturity. A 'one flap fits all' approach

E. Mah (✉) · S. Ricketts · M. Lo · S. Koide · S. Lonie
Department of Plastic and Reconstructive Surgery, St. Vincent's Hospital, Melbourne, VIC, Australia

P. F. M. Choong (ed.), *Sarcoma*, https://doi.org/10.1007/978-981-15-9414-4_20

simply does not work in sarcoma reconstruction. Rather, the focus should be on principles backed by a large armamentarium of reconstructive options.

Radiotherapy frequently plays an integral part of soft tissue sarcoma management. Its role in regional disease control has been well documented. While many centres debate the timing of radiotherapy, neoadjuvant radiotherapy is the preference at our institution. This approach has an immediate impact on the condition of the defects, only making the role of a plastic surgeon more crucial in these circumstances. Radiotherapy has both acute and long-term impact on these wounds that appropriate choice of reconstruction not only is critical in early wound healing phase but also long term in minimising tissue fibrosis, atrophy and necrosis.

The functional deficit resulting from the resection can be significant but often overlooked in the process of achieving cancer clearance and primary wound healing. Considerations in functional restoration is much more than selecting the latest reported technique; it is having a thorough understanding of the biomechanics that would prevent additional morbidity in flap selection with the aim of maximising the global functional improvement.

While much of this book focuses on the best oncological treatment possible, the role of the plastic and reconstructive surgeon is to maximise the quality of life of ones' cancer survival. The reconstructive team at St Vincent's Hospital believe that the success of sarcoma reconstruction lies with the following principles:

- Honest and precise communication between treating teams.
- Clear reconstructive goals and principles.
- Consideration of a wide selection of reconstructive options.
- Flexibility in adapting to each defect/patient needs.
- Balanced approach to minimise overall morbidity.

20.2 Goals and Principles of Reconstruction

Every sarcoma defect is unique. When faced with a complex three-dimensional defect with multiple factors to consider and range of treatment options to choose from, it is important to reflect on the goals and principles of reconstruction in order to gain clarity on how to approach the problem.

Goals of Sarcoma Reconstruction

- Primary wound healing.
- Functional restoration.
- Minimise overall morbidity.
- Optimise cosmesis.

Principles of Sarcoma Reconstruction

- Repair with well-vascularised healthy tissue.
- Aim for dermis to dermis closure.
- Obliterate dead space.
- Replace like with like.
- Consider all functional repairs options.
- Choose donor flap with least morbidity.
- Early correction of aesthetic concerns.

Wound healing is the primary role of a reconstructive surgeon in surgical management of sarcoma. It is a crucial component of a patient's recovery and should be the minimum requirement in any sarcoma reconstruction. Resections frequently create defects that are large, deep and with exposed critical structures such as major vessels, nerves and/or exposed reparative devices such as plate and screws or vascular reconstructions. Neoadjuvant or adjuvant radiotherapy only adds to the difficulties. The ability to cover difficult wounds is one of the primary influences in achieving limb salvage surgeries. It allows surgical resection of more complex tumours and can significantly change patients' quality of life.

In achieving primary wound healing in the shortest time possible, several principles of reconstruction need to be considered in choosing the best option. For most of the defects encountered at our institution, the size of the defect and addition of neoadjuvant radiotherapy demands the introduction of a vascularised healthy tissue into the defect with the use of a flap. Flap selection process (discussed later in this chapter) depends on assessment of the defect size, depth and structures involved, matched with available donor tissue.

It is important in the flap selection to consider how to obliterate the dead space. Dead space is a common problem post-resection of a large deep defect. It leads to the formation of seroma that prevents adequate flap inset and integration, causes discomfort and can harbour infection. If not prevented early or treated early, an infected rigid chronic seroma after surrounding fibrosis has set in is a difficult problem to manage.

Our preference in the flap selection is to aim for skin-to-skin closure of the defect, i.e. choosing a cutaneous component of the flap and avoid skin graft on muscle. This allows early wound healing time, dermal vascular integration and less wound healing complication. The long-term benefits include ease in future revisional surgery, improved aesthetics and reduced regional fibrosis. Even when there is no skin resection in tumour resection, adding a small island of skin in the flap repair improves wound healing in addition to the benefits listed.

One key, increasingly relevant goal is to restore functional loss or minimise functional deficit. Not all defects require functional restoration, but it should be part of every decision process. The approach is to list all functional deficits, e.g. from superficial sensory nerve loss to large compartmentectomy. Prioritise the need to repair them, and repair as much as possible. One other major advancement in our approach has been maximising the functional restoration potential with any flap we use. For example, an ALT flap to the sole of the foot should include the flap sensory nerve in order to sensitise the flap.

One last principle related to functional restoration is not to create more. A reconstruction surgeon needs to know the 'price to pay' with any surgical option and weigh it against the potential gain. This is not always an easy decision and an area much in need of future research. A global improvement in patient's functional state is the ultimate goal.

20.3 Wound Assessment and Flap Selection

All defects are different, and no reconstruction is exactly the same. The foundation of our decision-making process involves three main areas of considerations, each interact with another until the most balanced solution is reached. The three areas of considerations are (Fig. 20.1):

1. Defect characteristic.
   Defect size, depth, structures resected, structures preserved, recipient vessel quality, and critical structures that may need to be covered.
2. Functional deficit.
   Estimation of the actual and potential functional loss. What can be repaired and does it need to be repaired? Can we improve the deficit?
3. Flap selection.
   Choice of flap and its availability is match to the defect. What are the donor morbidities? What flap modification can be achieved to improve outcome?

The flow chart (Fig. 20.2) indicates broadly our decision process guided by the above mentioned principles. It is important to stress that this chart is NOT a flap selection protocol or algorithm. It also does not taken into account the exact flap

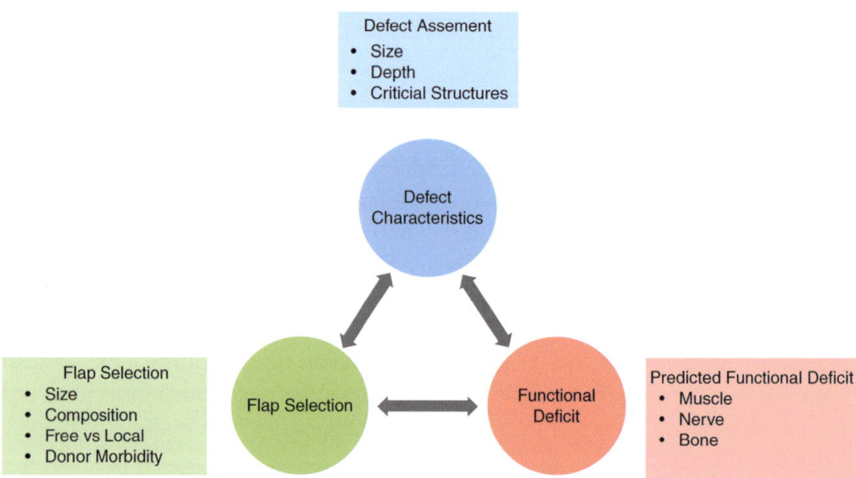

Fig. 20.1 Principles when considerations for flap selection

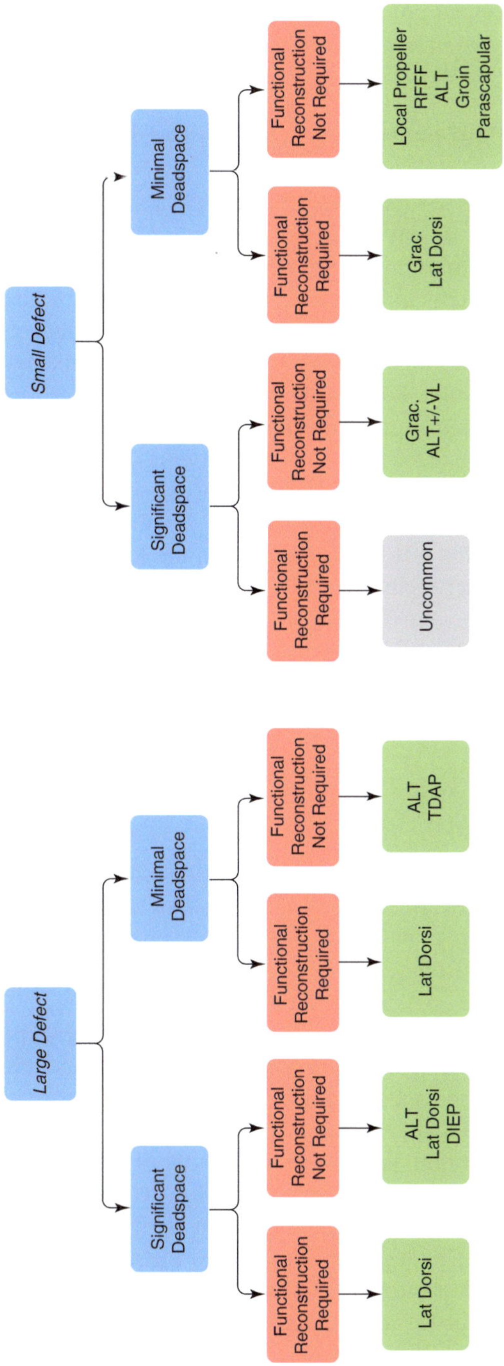

Fig. 20.2 Algorithm for selecting specific flaps for reconstructing soft tissue defects

design and modification which is different in each case. The chart simply summarises our usual thought process and choice of reconstruction as a reference for those who are interested in sarcoma reconstruction.

20.4 Regional Reconstruction: Lower Limb

A shift from amputation to limb salvage surgery [1] assisted by the advent of external beam radiotherapy in soft tissue sarcoma treatment [2–5] has necessitated a more sophisticated approach to limb reconstruction.

General principles apply in assessment of any given lower limb defect. Once an assessment of size and depth of the defect is made, one must then give special consideration to critical structures requiring coverage, as well as the functional requirements of the reconstruction. For defects that necessitate reconstruction with motor innervated muscle flaps to restore function, further careful planning is necessary with consideration given to location of recipient vessels in relation to the location of donor nerves, as well as accurate tensioning of the muscle flap for appropriate excursion.

Tradition has been for soft tissue coverage in the lower limb where remaining muscles are able to hypertrophy to carry out the function of those resected. The use of motor innervated free muscle flaps as part of our armamentarium in soft tissue sarcoma reconstruction [6–10] has shown great potential in achieving superior functional reconstructive outcomes without significant additional morbidity.

Unique considerations pertaining to regional defects of the lower limb are summarised below:

1. Thigh.
   (a) Anterior thigh

   Current reports on muscle reconstruction after quadriceps muscle sacrifice [7, 11] suggest free functioning latissimus dorsi muscle to be most useful in cases where three or more heads of the quadriceps group are sacrificed and impairment from resection of fewer heads to be only modest [12, 13].

   (b) Medial thigh

   The medial thigh comprises the adductor muscle group and vital structures of femoral artery and vein and femoral nerve. It is rare to see sacrifice of the adductors necessitating a functional reconstruction. More commonly we see skin and partial adductor muscle group sacrifice with exposure of the femoral vessels with or without vessel sacrifice requiring vascular reconstruction. In these scenarios, it is critical to offer a robust coverage and where possible a ‘double-layer’ closure of muscle/fascia over the vessels with direct skin-to-skin closure superficially. Common solutions include sartorius muscle turn over with pedicled ipsilateral ALT flap, pedicled recuts abdominus myocutaneous flap or free contralateral fasciocutaneous ALT flap.

   (c) Posterior thigh

Primary considerations in the posterior thigh are the hamstring muscle group (laterally biceps femoris and medially semimembranosus and semitendinosus muscles) and the sciatic nerve. Functional reconstruction of the hamstring muscles is generally considered with sacrifice of all four heads. The latissimus dorsi-free functioning muscle flap, including the skin, is most commonly used with its accompanying thoracodorsal nerve being coapted to an appropriate proximal motor branch of the sciatic nerve. This motor branch is identified with a hand-held nerve stimulator to distinguish it from purely sensory branches. Identification of this donor nerve must be done concurrent with the resection in order to ensure motor nerve axons suitable to innervate the muscle flap.

2. Leg
   (a) Anterolateral leg/foot

   Skin coverage is the key requirement of most defects in the anterolateral leg and foot. These areas frequently require free flap coverage due to a paucity of local options. More extensive resections will require consideration of resultant foot drop which is as a consequence of muscle and/or peroneal nerve resection. Complete anterior compartment resection (tibialis anterior, extensor digitorum longus and extensor hallucis longus) may be reconstructed with a free functioning myocutaneous gracilis muscle flap. Lateral compartment resection infrequently requires functional reconstruction.

   (b) Posterior leg

   The requirement for functional reconstruction of the posterior leg is less frequent due to the presence of both deep and superficial compartments with both soleus and gastrocnemius muscles making up the superficial compartment. If it is necessary to sacrifice both soleus and gastrocnemius muscles, a latissimus dorsi functioning muscle flap is preferred as a smaller muscle is unlikely to generate sufficient power.

3. Nerve

   Tumour resection often involves muscle groups in addition to any nerve sacrifice, so overall functional deficit needs to be considered, not just the morbidity of losing the nerve in isolation.

   Sciatic nerve (as well as peroneal or tibial nerve) sacrifice has previously been cited as an indication for amputation predominantly due to the loss of sensation [14]. Fuchs, however, reported on the outcomes of ten patients with limb salvage in the setting of sciatic nerve sacrifice with patients able to perform more than 70% of their daily activities with little or no difficulty [15]. Others have concurred with these findings [16]. Studies also report a greater level of disability after lower limb amputation than reconstruction in the setting of nerve sacrifice [17].

   Sensory loss of the skin of the sole of the foot should be considered as the one area of sensory loss worth reconstruction where possible.

   Sciatic nerve sacrifice is often in the setting of entire posterior thigh compartmentectomy, and therefore functional muscle reconstruction would be our preference (functional latissimus dorsi flap). More distal sensory nerves such as the sural nerve can be utilised as conduits for free nerve grafting of sciatic nerve gaps.

Peroneal nerve sacrifice and resultant foot drop may be in the setting of an intact anterior muscle compartment, in which case nerve transfer from the intact posterior compartment would be our preference. Other options would be tendon transfer as is usual for foot drop reconstruction.

20.4.1 Upper Limb

The shift to limb sparing surgery has been discussed earlier. Sarcoma of the upper limb faces some unique challenges largely due to the complex, functionally critical muscular and neurovascular structures that are in the resection. The role of reconstruction of upper limb has a large emphasis on functional restoration, and careful assessment of the resected structures and the residual function needs to be considered when reconstructive options are considered.

The application of general principles still applies in any defect, and a wide range of reconstructive options are available for coverage of the defect and reconstruction of the lost function [11, 18–25].

1. Arm

Elbow function. When sarcomas on the flexor or extensor surface of the arms are excised, the two most common flaps that are used to restore and reconstruct their functions are gracilis muscle and latissimus dorsi muscle. Latissimus dorsi flap can be transferred as a pedicle flap while maintaining its blood supply from the thoracodorsal vessels. The nerve supply can either remain as the thoracodorsal nerve or can be re-coaptated to the recipient nerve in the arm. The advantage of re-coaptation to the recipient nerve is the minimal requirement of patient training to initiate the action; however, the disadvantage is that the coaptation will be performed to an irradiated recipient nerve. Both gracilis muscle and latissimus dorsi can also act as a space filler, and the myofasciocutaneous flaps are excellent for skin recruitment and aesthetics of the defect.

2. Forearm and hand

Wrist/finger function. Resection of sarcoma from the forearm will often involve resection of muscle, tendons and neurovascular structures. Degree of functional deficit will depend on the location of the sarcoma, type of tumour and patient's body habitus and age.

In the reconstruction of the sarcoma of the forearm or hands, dead space becomes less of an issue, and functional reconstruction is often the most important factor to consider.

A variety of reconstructive techniques are available, and the surgeon will need to assess the defect and deficient function to determine the most suitable reconstructive technique. When flexor tendons in the forearm are resected, some tendons do not need reconstruction. In some where there are remaining functioning tendons, tenorrhaphy can be performed to allow the tendons to function as a bulk mover, or a vascularised or non-vascularised tendon graft can be used in conjunction with a fasciocutaneous flap. If a large portion of tendon-muscular unit is missing, it can be reconstructed with a gracilis or latissimus dorsi flap depending on the size of defect and requirement of pedicle and nerve length.

In a setting where nerve is resected together with the tumour, depending on the location of the nerve and the function it serves, several reconstructive options are available. Tendon transfers can be performed when a suitable tendon is available and if the functional recovery of the transfer is superior compared to other reconstructive options. For example, if the radial nerve needs reconstruction, tendon can be a simple and reliable reconstruction for the patient. If the nerve is a sensory nerve or if the nerve defect is close to the motor unit (point of muscle innervation), the nerve defect may be managed with cable nerve grafts. The alternative option will be nerve transfer or functional reconstruction with an innovated muscle flap. Again, each detail needs to be assessed by an experienced surgeon and the reconstructive decision made. In cases where tendon graft, tendon transfer, nerve graft and nerve transfer are performed, the defect will most always need a fasciocutaneous free flap to reconstruct the skin defect.

20.5 Common Flaps

Common flaps are listed below. This is certainly not the full list of flaps utilised at our institution but a list of common choices that allows to achieve our goal of reconstruction. It is important to have a wide range of flap options and be flexible and detailed in flap design in order to address the needs of the defect and the patient.

- Propeller styled perforator flap.
- Gracilis flap.
- Anterolateral thigh flap (ALT).
- Latissimus dorsi flap.
- Rectus abdominis flap.
- Parascapular flap.

20.6 Propeller Flap or Regional Fasciocutaneous Perforator Flaps

The concept of 'propeller flap' was defined in 1991 by Hyakusoku and others as a local fasciocutaneous flap skeletonised and completely islanded on a single perforating vessel and transposed or rotated 180° like a propeller into the defect [26–28].

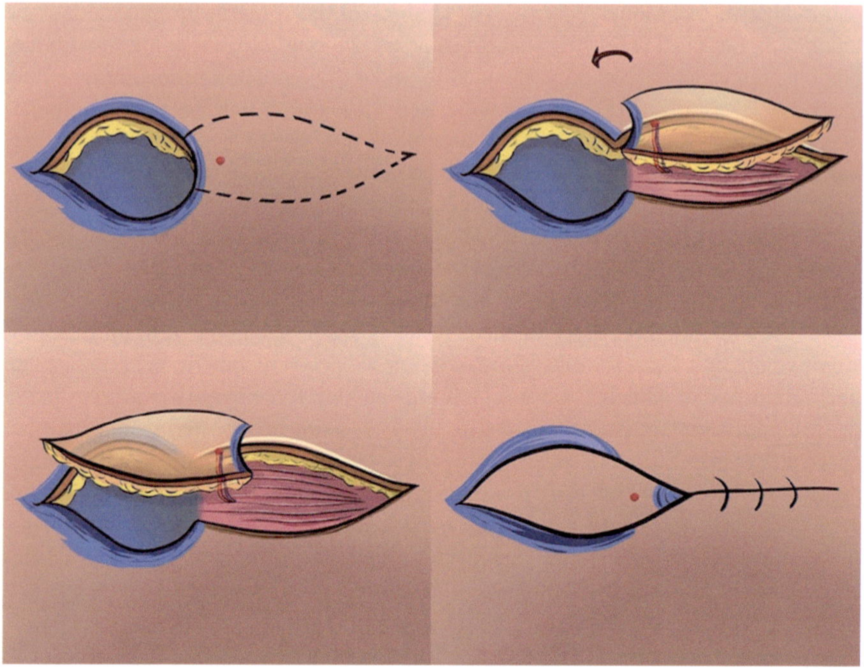

Fig. 20.3 Propeller flap reconstruction

20.6.1 Application in Sarcoma Reconstruction

Propeller flap design (Fig. 20.3) is suited for superficial defects that are small to moderately sized [26]. It is particularly useful in cases that have received neo-adjuvant radiotherapy by transposing a piece of well-vascularised non-irradiated adjacent skin into the irradiated defect and allowing dermis to dermis closure. It achieves several reconstructive principles by replacing like for like, promote healing with a vascularised tissue and minimise donor morbidity [29–33].

20.6.2 Latissimus Dorsi Flap

20.6.2.1 History

The latissimus dorsi flap is commonly used for reconstructive surgery owing to its long reliable pedicle and possibility to raise large area of muscle, myocutaneous or osteomyocutaneous pedicle or flaps. The latissimus dorsi was first described by Tansini in 1906 for coverage of an extensive mastectomy defect.

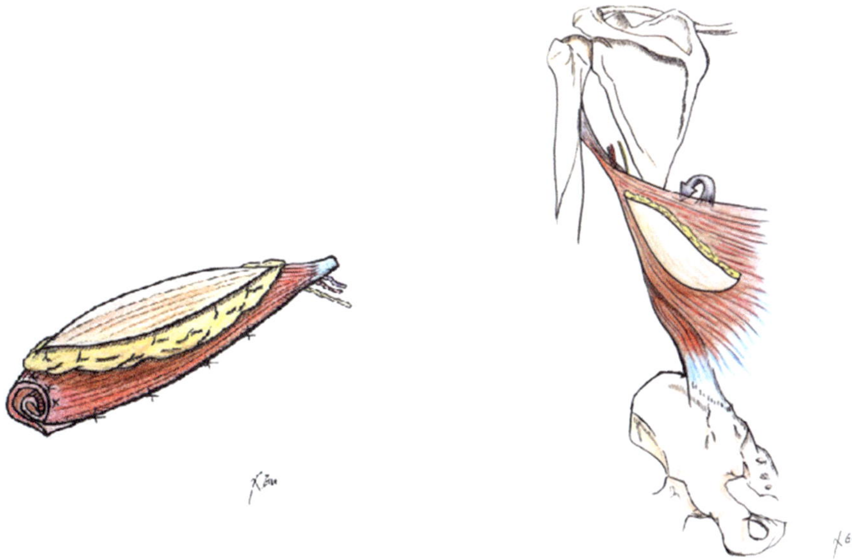

Fig. 20.4 The innovative role of latissimus dorsi free and rotational flaps for soft tissue reconstructions

20.6.3 Application in Sarcoma Reconstruction

Latissimus dorsi flap is a versatile workhorse flap in sarcoma reconstruction attributed to the size of the flap, the reach of the flap and the functional reconstruction capabilities [34, 35] (Fig. 20.4).

20.6.3.1 Free Flap

It is ideal for large defects and defects with large dead space. The size of skin paddle is limited by the tissue laxity to allow direct closure. Direct skin closure of the donor site is always preferable since skin graft on the back often results in prolonged healing and bad scarring. When in-setting a large latissimus dorsi flap, it is worth remembering that the most distal muscle and skin are often not well perfused; therefore it would be best to avoid using that portion of the flap to cover critical structures such as metal plates or vessels.

20.6.3.2 Local Flap

With the dominant vascular pedicle at one end of the flap (tendinous insertion), this allows the flap to have a great reach to defects on the anterior chest wall, shoulder and posterior arm. To minimise donor morbidity or reduce the bulk of the flap, the skin paddle can be designed over the anterior border by taking only the anterior 1/4 to 1/3 of muscle to ensure perfusion to the skin paddle.

20.6.3.3 Functional Reconstruction

One of few expendable muscle flaps, it is also the most commonly used flap for free functional muscle transfer at our institution. Harvested with the motor nerve to latissimus dorsi, it is used for anterior or posterior thigh partial or total compartmentectomy. To gain maximal power and excursion, it is our practice to align the muscle fibres of the flap by rolling it into a tubular structure (Fig. 20.4).

As a pedicle flap, it can also be utilised as a functional muscle transfer for biceps or triceps muscle defects.

20.6.4 Gracilis Flap

20.6.4.1 History

The use of the gracilis muscle in reconstructive surgery was first described in 1952. In 1990, O'Brien was the first to describe gracilis for functional free muscle transfer [36].

20.6.4.2 Application in Sarcoma Reconstruction

The gracilis can be used as a muscle or myocutaneous flap. The reliable anatomy allows safe harvest and donor morbidity is minimal [37–40].

1. Functional muscle transfer

   The anatomy of the flap makes it ideal choice of flap for functional reconstruction. The vascular pedicle and motor nerve are closely related to each other, and tendinous part allows secure insertion, commonly utilised for functional reconstruction of biceps, triceps defects or anterior compartment of lower leg.
2. Local flap

   Commonly used as a secondary flap to reduce dead space for defects around proximal thigh or perineal region.

   It is used on occasion as tendon transfer to replace vastus medialis.

For medical thigh defects where primary closure is considered, gracilis flap is frequently used.

20.6.5 Parascapular/Scapular Flaps

20.6.5.1 History

Manchot first described the perforators from the circumflex scapular artery emerging from the triangular space similar to spokes of a wheel [41]. Nassif et al. from France, in 1982 made use of the vertical branch of the superficial circumflex scapula and described the parascapular flap [42].

20.6.5.2 Application in Sarcoma Reconstruction

Parascapular flap is a fasciocutaneous flap that is well suited for a superficial defect of some thickness. It can be raised as local flap or free flap with very little donor morbidity [43, 44].

20.6.5.3 Local Flap

It is ideal for upper posterior trunk defects, posterior shoulder defects and proximal deltoid defects. This can be designed as a propeller flap or transpositional flap. The pedicle is sandwiched by dense fascia and needs to be released adequately to allow twisting of the flap.

20.6.5.4 Free Flap

It is also a good alternative fasciocutaneous flap that is thicker in composition than a radial forearm flap or groin flap but can often be thinner than ALT flap in some individuals. It also avoids re-positioning if the patient is in prone/lateral position. The reach of the pedicle however is shorter, so it is best to have selected the recipient vessel prior to harvesting this flap.

20.6.6 Anterolateral Thigh Flap

20.6.6.1 History

The anterolateral thigh (ALT) flap, first described by Song et al. in 1984, has become a workhorse flap for local and distant reconstruction [45].

20.6.6.2 Application in Sarcoma Reconstruction

The ALT is one of the most commonly used flaps. It is a large versatile flap that can be 'custom'-made to fit variety of defects to allow primary wound healing, obliteration of dead space and functional restoration and has minimal donor morbidity [46–49].

20.6.6.3 Free Flap

This is often the flap of choice for large superficial defect. The long pedicle allows better reach to recipient vessels, and the fascia enables additional closure of critical structures such as the plates, vessels or bone. Multiple tissue composition can be included with this flap on the same pedicle to meet the reconstructive need. Some examples are:

- Taking the sensory nerve with the skin paddle to reconstruct areas where protective sensation is important, e.g. sole of the foot.
- Taking larger amount of skin and subcutaneous fat, de-epithelised and used to obliterate dead space.
- Taking the fascia lata for tendon reconstruction.
- Using the descending branch of lateral circumflex femoral vessels to restore vascular supply as part of a flow through design.

20.6.6.4 Pedicle Flap

The long pedicle makes this flap ideal for regional defects. Common uses of a pedicle ALT flap are:

- Harvesting large sheath of fascia lata in lower abdominal wall reconstruction, adding further strength to mesh repair.
- Proximal 1/3 medial thigh defects.
- Defects over the hip/lower buttock.

References

1. Rosenberg SA, Tepper J, Glatstein E, Costa J, Baker A, Brennan M, et al. The treatment of soft-tissue sarcomas of the extremities: prospective randomized evaluations of (1) limb-sparing surgery plus radiation therapy compared with amputation and (2) the role of adjuvant chemotherapy. Ann Surg. 1982;196(3):305–15.
2. Jebsen NL, Trovik CS, Bauer HC, Rydholm A, Monge OR, Hall KS, et al. Radiotherapy to improve local control regardless of surgical margin and malignancy grade in extremity and trunk wall soft tissue sarcoma: a Scandinavian sarcoma group study. Int J Radiat Oncol Biol Phys. 2008;71(4):1196–203.
3. Lindberg RD, Martin RG, Romsdahl MM, Barkley HT Jr. Conservative surgery and postoperative radiotherapy in 300 adults with soft-tissue sarcomas. Cancer. 1981;47(10):2391–7.
4. Suit HD, Mankin HJ, Wood WC, Proppe KH. Preoperative, intraoperative, and postoperative radiation in the treatment of primary soft tissue sarcoma. Cancer. 1985;55(11):2659–67.
5. Yang JC, Chang AE, Baker AR, Sindelar WF, Danforth DN, Topalian SL, et al. Randomized prospective study of the benefit of adjuvant radiation therapy in the treatment of soft tissue sarcomas of the extremity. J Clin Oncol. 1998;16(1):197–203.
6. Doi K. Obstetric and traumatic pediatric palsy. In: Peimer C, editor. Surgery of the hand and upper extremity. 1st ed. New York: McGraw-Hill; 1996.
7. Doi K, Sakai K, Ihara K, Abe Y, Kawai S, Kurafuji Y. Reinnervated free muscle transplantation for extremity reconstruction. Plast Reconstr Surg. 1993;91(5):872–83.
8. Doi K, Sakai K, Kuwata N, Ihara K, Kawai S. Double free-muscle transfer to restore prehension following complete brachial plexus avulsion. J Hand Surg Am. 1995;20(3):408–14.
9. Ihara K, Shigetomi M, Kawai S, Doi K, Yamamoto M. Functioning muscle transplantation after wide excision of sarcomas in the extremity. Clin Orthop Relat Res. 1999;358:140–8.
10. Manktelow RT, Zuker RM, McKee NH. Functioning free muscle transplantation. J Hand Surg Am. 1984.;9A;9(1):32–9.
11. Muramatsu K, Ihara K, Taguchi T. Selection of myocutaneous flaps for reconstruction following oncologic resection of sarcoma. Ann Plast Surg. 2010;64(3):307–10.
12. Doi K, Kuwata N, Kawakami F, Hattori Y, Otsuka K, Ihara K. Limb-sparing surgery with reinnervated free-muscle transfer following radical excision of soft-tissue sarcoma in the extremity. Plast Reconstr Surg. 1999;104(6):1679–87.
13. Muramatsu K, Ihara K, Miyoshi T, Yoshida K, Hashimoto T, Taguchi T. Transfer of latissimus dorsi muscle for the functional reconstruction of quadriceps femoris muscle following oncological resection of sarcoma in the thigh. J Plast Reconstr Aesthet Surg. 2011;64(8):1068–74.
14. Williard WC, Hajdu SI, Casper ES, Brennan MF. Comparison of amputation with limb-sparing operations for adult soft tissue sarcoma of the extremity. Ann Surg. 1992;215(3):269–75.
15. Fuchs B, Davis AM, Wunder JS, Bell RS, Masri BA, Isler M, et al. Sciatic nerve resection in the thigh: a functional evaluation. Clin Orthop Relat Res. 2001;382:34–41.
16. Brooks AD, Gold JS, Graham D, Boland P, Lewis JJ, Brennan MF, et al. Resection of the sciatic, peroneal, or tibial nerves: assessment of functional status. Ann Surg Oncol. 2002;9(1):41–7.
17. Davis AM, Devlin M, Griffin AM, Wunder JS, Bell RS. Functional outcome in amputation versus limb sparing of patients with lower extremity sarcoma: a matched case-control study. Arch Phys Med Rehabil. 1999;80(6):615–8.
18. Hoy E, Granick M, Benevenia J, Patterson F, Datiashvili R, Bille B. Reconstruction of musculoskeletal defects following oncologic resection in 76 patients. Ann Plast Surg. 2006;57(2):190–4.
19. Megerle K, Sauerbier M. Reconstructive treatment of soft tissue sarcoma of the upper extremity. J Hand Surg Am. 2011;36(7):1241–7.
20. Mirous MP, Coulet B, Chammas M, Cupissol D, Lazerges C. Extensive limb-sparing surgery with reconstruction for sarcoma of the hand and wrist. Orthop Traumatol Surg Res. 2016;102(4):467–72.

21. Morii T, Mochizuki K, Takushima A, Okazaki M, Satomi K. Soft tissue reconstruction using vascularized tissue transplantation following resection of musculoskeletal sarcoma: evaluation of oncologic and functional outcomes in 55 cases. Ann Plast Surg. 2009;62(3):252–7.
22. Muramatsu K, Ihara K, Doi K, Hashimoto T, Taguchi T. Sarcoma in the forearm and hand: clinical outcomes and microsurgical reconstruction for limb salvage. Ann Plast Surg. 2009;62(1):28–33.
23. Slump J, Hofer SOP, Ferguson PC, Wunder JS, Griffin AM, Hoekstra HJ, et al. Flap choice does not affect complication rates or functional outcomes following extremity soft tissue sarcoma reconstruction. J Plast Reconstr Aesthet Surg. 2018;71(7):989–96.
24. Talbot SG, Mehrara BJ, Disa JJ, Wong AK, Pusic A, Cordeiro PG, et al. Soft-tissue coverage of the hand following sarcoma resection. Plast Reconstr Surg. 2008;121(2):534–43.
25. Wong JC, Abraham JA. Upper extremity considerations for oncologic surgery. Orthop Clin North Am. 2014;45(4):541–64.
26. D'Arpa S, Toia F, Pirrello R, Moschella F, Cordova A. Propeller flaps: a review of indications, technique, and results. Biomed Res Int. 2014;2014:986829.
27. Hallock GG. The propeller flap version of the adductor muscle perforator flap for coverage of ischial or trochanteric pressure sores. Ann Plast Surg. 2006;56(5):540–2.
28. Hyakusoku H, Yamamoto T, Fumiiri M. The propeller flap method. Br J Plast Surg. 1991;44(1):53–4.
29. D'Arpa S, Cordova A, Pignatti M, Moschella F. Freestyle pedicled perforator flaps: safety, prevention of complications, and management based on 85 consecutive cases. Plast Reconstr Surg. 2011;128(4):892–906.
30. Lecours C, Saint-Cyr M, Wong C, Bernier C, Mailhot E, Tardif M, et al. Freestyle pedicle perforator flaps: clinical results and vascular anatomy. Plast Reconstr Surg. 2010;126(5):1589–603.
31. Lonie S, Grinsell D, Mah E. Propeller flap reconstruction of irradiated sarcoma defects: a comparison(). J Plast Reconstr Aesthet Surg. 2019;72(2):181–7.
32. Saint-Cyr M, Wong C, Schaverien M, Mojallal A, Rohrich RJ. The perforasome theory: vascular anatomy and clinical implications. Plast Reconstr Surg. 2009;124(5):1529–44.
33. Taylor GI. The angiosomes of the body and their supply to perforator flaps. Clin Plast Surg. 2003;30(3):331–42. v
34. Germann G, Ohlbauer M. Latissimus Dorsi Flap. In: Wei F, Mardini S, editors. Flaps and reconstructive surgery. Philadelphia, PA: Saunders; 2009. p. 287–319.
35. Mathes S, Nahai F. Latissimus dorsi Flap. In: Mathes S, Nahai F, editors. Reconstructive surgery: principles, anatomy and technique. 1st ed. New York: Churchill Livingstone; 1997. p. 565.
36. O'Brien BM, Pederson WC, Khazanchi RK, Morrison WA, MacLeod AM, Kumar V. Results of management of facial palsy with microvascular free-muscle transfer. Plast Reconstr Surg. 1990;86(1):12–22; discussion 3-4
37. Chuang D. Gracilis flap. In: Wei F, Mardini S, editors. Flaps and reconstructive surgery. Philadelphia, PA: Saunders; 2009. p. 396–408.
38. Harii K, Ohmori K, Sekiguchi J. The free musculocutaneous flap. Plast Reconstr Surg. 1976;57(3):294–303.
39. Pickrell KL, Broadbent TR, Masters FW, Metzger JT. Construction of a rectal sphincter and restoration of anal continence by transplanting the gracilis muscle; a report of four cases in children. Ann Surg. 1952;135(6):853–62.
40. Yousif NJ, Matloub HS, Kolachalam R, Grunert BK, Sanger JR. The transverse gracilis musculocutaneous flap. Ann Plast Surg. 1992;29(6):482–90.
41. Manchot C. The cutaneous arteries of the human body. New York1983.
42. Nassif TM, Vidal L, Bovet JL, Baudet J. The parascapular flap: a new cutaneous microsurgical free flap. Plast Reconstr Surg. 1982;69(4):591–600.
43. Andrades P, Hallock GG. Circumflex scapular artery perforator flap. In: Blondeel P, Morris S, Hallock GG, Neligan P, editors. Perforator flaps: anatomy, technique and clinical applications. St. Louis: Quality Medical Publishing; 2006. p. 561–77.

44. dos Santos LF. The vascular anatomy and dissection of the free scapular flap. Plast Reconstr Surg. 1984;73(4):599–604.
45. Song YG, Chen GZ, Song YL. The free thigh flap: a new free flap concept based on the septocutaneous artery. Br J Plast Surg. 1984;37(2):149–59.
46. Koshima I, Fukuda H, Soeda S. Free combined anterolateral thigh flap and vascularized iliac bone graft with double vascular pedicle. J Reconstr Microsurg. 1989;5(1):55–61.
47. Koshima I, Fukuda H, Yamamoto H, Moriguchi T, Soeda S, Ohta S. Free anterolateral thigh flaps for reconstruction of head and neck defects. Plast Reconstr Surg. 1993;92(3):421–8. discussion 9-30
48. Mardini S, Lin C, Wiei F. Lateral circumflex femoral artery-vastus lateralis perforator flap. In: Blondeel P, Morris S, Hallock GG, Neligan P, editors. Perforator flaps: anatomy, technique and clinical applications. St. Louis: Quality Medical Publishing; 2006. p. 617–33.
49. Wei FC, Jain V, Celik N, Chen HC, Chuang DC, Lin CH. Have we found an ideal soft-tissue flap? An experience with 672 anterolateral thigh flaps. Plast Reconstr Surg. 2002;109(7):2219–26; discussion 27-30

Management of Metastatic Sarcoma

21

Sarat Chander, Catherine Ngan, and Peter F. M. Choong

One of the challenges of managing bone and soft tissue sarcomas is their propensity for hematogenous dissemination, which carries significant mortality. Sarcomas predominantly metastasise to the lungs, although subtypes such as myxoid/round cell liposarcomas and visceral sarcomas tend to spread locally or to the retroperitoneum and spine [1]. Advanced, metastatic sarcoma is generally incurable, with studies reporting survival in the range of 12 to 19 months [2–4]. In this setting, the philosophy of treatment is to diminish symptoms and maintain a good quality of life for as long as possible. This is particularly important with advanced disease where the symptom burden at the end of life may be substantial requiring expert multidisciplinary palliative care strategies [5]. As such, careful consideration of treatment modalities and timing of therapy can provide effective disease and symptom control.

Metastatic sarcoma can be recognised at the time of diagnosis, or it may eventuate after treatment of the primary tumour. The incidence of metastatic disease on presentation is approximately 10%, of which 80% is pulmonary metastases [6]. 25% of patients develop distant metastases after successful treatment of the original tumour at 2 years of follow-up, with a higher incidence in tumours with poor prognostic factors as defined by size, grade and histologic subtype [7, 8]. Increased

S. Chander
Bone & Soft Tissue Sarcoma Service, Peter MacCallum Cancer Centre, Melbourne, VIC, Australia

Division of Radiation Oncology, Peter MacCallum Cancer Centre, Melbourne, VIC, Australia

C. Ngan
Department of Orthopaedics, St. Vincent's Hospital, Melbourne, VIC, Australia

P. F. M. Choong (✉)
Department of Orthopaedics, St. Vincent's Hospital, Melbourne, VIC, Australia

Bone & Soft Tissue Sarcoma Service, Peter MacCallum Cancer Centre, Melbourne, VIC, Australia

Department of Surgery, University of Melbourne, Melbourne, VIC, Australia
e-mail: pchoong@unimelb.edu.au

P. F. M. Choong (ed.), *Sarcoma*, https://doi.org/10.1007/978-981-15-9414-4_21

tumour size is associated with metastatic potential; the incidence of metastases is 40% in patients with tumours greater than 5 centimetres [9, 10]. Tumour grade is an independent predictor of distant metastases as well as survival for certain histologic subtypes, including malignant fibrous histiocytoma, leiomyosarcoma and liposarcoma [11–13]. Specific subtypes are also known to be highly metastatic, such as leiomyosarcoma, synovial sarcoma, neurogenic sarcoma, rhabdomyosarcoma and epithelioid sarcoma [8, 14].

The principle of managing metastatic sarcoma is to maintain quality of life while balancing any side effects of palliative treatment. Therapeutic options include watchful waiting, local therapy and systemic therapy. Watchful waiting may be suitable for indolent subtypes and is guided by symptom progression. Local therapies, such as radiotherapy and surgery, can be offered to control symptomatic or rapidly progressive disease. Chemotherapy is a final consideration, as most subtypes tend to be resistant to treatment. It can, however, be effective for certain tumours and contribute to substantial improvement in survival.

21.1 Radiotherapy

Radiotherapy is an effective modality for achieving local disease control and should be considered in symptomatic metastases. It is frequently used to palliate painful bony lesions, haemoptysis from pulmonary metastases and neurologic symptoms and signs from spinal cord compression [15–17]. An Australian patterns-of-care study for advanced soft tissue sarcoma showed that about 37% of patients with advanced sarcoma required radiotherapy for palliation of symptoms [18].

Targeted radiotherapy is a versatile technique that can be applied to patients unfit for surgery and can treat inoperable disease with effective symptomatic response in 80 to 90% of cases [19, 20]. When delivered as stereotactic ablative radiotherapy, it has been shown to be particularly effective in treating pulmonary and spinal metastases [21–24]. Treatment is relatively convenient for the patient, as it is administered as a short course over days to weeks without requiring inpatient hospital stay. Side effects to the skin (redness and irritation) can be minimised with modern radiotherapy regimens, and systemic effects are minimal.

A variety of dose and fractionations are used such as from 8 Gy in 1 fraction, 20 Gy in 5 fractions, to 30 or 36Gy in 10 or 12 fractions. For inoperable primary sarcomas of the soft tissue and bone, a more protracted course maybe used such as 50 to 70Gy in 20 to 35 fractions to maximise chances of durable local control and symptom relief. Local control at critical metastatic sites is an important consideration even in the face of widely spread disease given the relatively longer survival of some patients with metastatic sarcoma, such as those with myxoid liposarcoma and leiomyosarcoma. Stereotactic body radiotherapy (SBRT) may offer an advantage of short course (1–2 treatments) and more durable local control at these critical sites, such as the spine [25].

21.1.1 Treatment of Oligometastasis

Hellman and Weichselbaum in 1995 first introduced the concept of oligometastasis to describe the state in which the number and sites of systemic spread are limited [26]. Two clinical groups characterise oligometastasis, namely, those with subclinical metastatic disease and those with such limited metastatic disease that cure may be contemplated if the disease can be eradicated. The clinical implication of this hypothesis for the latter group is that locally extirpative or ablative treatments may be effective in prolonging survival in these patients with small numbers of metastases and perhaps curing a few. In this regard, ongoing survival in patients with minimal metastatic disease has been reported where the disease was amenable to resection.

21.1.2 Stereotactic Body Radiotherapy

Many subtypes of bone and soft tissue sarcomas are often considered relatively unresponsive to conventional treatment modalities such as chemotherapy and radiation therapy. This has led to surgery being the primary modality of local ablation. However, with the evolution of radiotherapy planning and delivery techniques, stereotactic body radiotherapy (SBRT) using highly conformal image-guided techniques has increased the efficacy of radiation therapy. Bauman et al. in their recent publication propose stereotactic body radiotherapy as an equivalent alternate to surgery for oligometastatic sarcoma [27]. Yu et al. also propose stereotactic radiotherapy could have similar outcomes as surgery for pulmonary metastasis from osteosarcoma [28]. Yamada's group at the Memorial Sloan Kettering Cancer Center in New York [22] have published on their experience of specifically treating spinal metastasis from sarcoma with stereotactic body radiotherapy. Their series which includes 88 patients with 120 sites of spinal metastasis is the largest published series to date. At 12 months local control was 87.9%, and overall survival was 60.6% with a median survival time of 16.9 months. They updated their data recently and found isolated local failure in treated area or adjacent spine extremely rare [29].

21.2 Surgery

Surgery in the setting of metastatic sarcoma can be performed with curative or palliative intent. Curative resection is rare and generally refers to the complete removal of disease in patients with oligometastatic tumours. This may be considered in the setting of isolated lung disease, where pulmonary nodules can be entirely resected with adequate respiratory reserve and the primary disease is controlled or controllable [30–33]. However, the impact of local surgery on survival after metastatic disease outside of the lung remains controversial. Notwithstanding, the limited studies do suggest that good local control does influence survival and this seems to be best seen after resection of oligometastases to lymph nodes [34, 35] and bone [36].

More commonly, surgery is used to achieve local disease control in the palliative setting. In this regard, the surgical intent is focused on improvement of quality of life and symptom control. Removal of resectable disease can rapidly manage local complications from locoregional metastatic spread, such as ulceration, bleeding, pain and malodour [37]. In the setting of bony metastases, fixation of pathological fractures and impending fractures offer symptom relief and preservation of limb function [38–41]. In this circumstance, the predicted survival from multiple bone metastases may be well compensated by the protection afforded by prophylactic fixation which is known to be durable for treating bone metastases in the short to medium term [41, 42]. In exceptional instances, palliative amputation of an extremity with fungating growth, intractable pain and loss of function may be the final option [43, 44]. The caveat to all surgical interventions is that the patient must be medically appropriate for an operation, post-operative recovery is relatively slow, and wound healing can be impaired from prior chemotherapy or radiotherapy [45–47].

21.3 Chemotherapy

While the combination of neoadjuvant chemotherapy and surgery has been highly effective for certain primary bone sarcomas, the effectiveness of systemic therapy for treatment of metastatic sarcomas is low, with a response rate that ranges from 0 to 50% depending on subtype [48, 49]. Moreover, limitations to systemic therapy are its general toxicity (hair loss, mucositis, neurotoxicity, bone marrow toxicity) [50]. Suitable chemotherapy regimens vary based on histologic type, with anthracyclines and alkylating agents (doxorubicin and ifosfamide), gemcitabine with taxanes or dacarbazine and dacarbazine alone being the main therapeutic options.

Notwithstanding, metastatic sarcomas, which often comprise the higher-grade and more aggressive phenotypes, make excellent candidates for novel approaches with newer agents as these tumours manifest some levels of chemosensitivity. Targeted therapy may be considered for certain subtypes such as dermatofibrosarcoma protuberans (DFSP), perivascular epithelioid cell tumours (PEComas) and alveolar soft-part sarcoma (ASPS) [51–53]. Emerging therapies now include small molecule, receptor inhibitors and immune modulators, amongst others, and these may be effective in combination with the above-mentioned local treatment strategies and particularly if the subtype is susceptible to the agent [54].

The combination and timing of the above therapeutic options must be individualised to the patient. Metastatic sarcoma is a largely incurable disease, and treatment must be titrated to the patient's experience. In addition to medical management, it is important to employ a multidisciplinary approach to patient care, including social and psychological support, physiotherapy, specialist palliative care and involvement in cancer support groups and community services.

References

1. Nakamura T, Matsumine A, Matsubara T, Asamuma K, Niimi R, Uchida A, et al. Retrospective analysis of metastatic sarcoma patients. Oncol Lett. 2011;2(2):315–8.
2. Billingsley KG, Burt ME, Jara E, Ginsberg RJ, Woodruff JM, Leung DH, et al. Pulmonary metastases from soft tissue sarcoma: analysis of patterns of diseases and postmetastasis survival. Ann Surg. 1999;229(5):602–10; discussion 10-2
3. Billingsley KG, Lewis JJ, Leung DH, Casper ES, Woodruff JM, Brennan MF. Multifactorial analysis of the survival of patients with distant metastasis arising from primary extremity sarcoma. Cancer. 1999;85(2):389–95.
4. Leahy M, Garcia Del Muro X, Reichardt P, Judson I, Staddon A, Verweij J, et al. Chemotherapy treatment patterns and clinical outcomes in patients with metastatic soft tissue sarcoma. The SArcoma treatment and burden of illness in North America and Europe (SABINE) study. Ann Oncol. 2012;23(10):2763–70.
5. Kawashima H, Ariizumi T, Yamagishi T, Ogose A, Ikoma M, Hotta T, et al. Symptom burden and end-of-life palliative treatments during the last two weeks of life in patients with advanced musculoskeletal sarcoma. J Palliat Med. 2019;22(8):908–14.
6. Christie-Large M, James SL, Tiessen L, Davies AM, Grimer RJ. Imaging strategy for detecting lung metastases at presentation in patients with soft tissue sarcomas. Eur J Cancer. 2008;44(13):1841–5.
7. Lindberg RD, Martin RG, Romsdahl MM, Barkley HT Jr. Conservative surgery and postoperative radiotherapy in 300 adults with soft-tissue sarcomas. Cancer. 1981;47(10):2391–7.
8. Zagars GK, Ballo MT, Pisters PW, Pollock RE, Patel SR, Benjamin RS, et al. Prognostic factors for patients with localized soft-tissue sarcoma treated with conservation surgery and radiation therapy: an analysis of 1225 patients. Cancer. 2003;97(10):2530–43.
9. Amin M, Greene F, Edge S, Compton C, Gershenwald J, Brookland R, et al. The eight edition AJCC cancer staging manual: continuing to build a bridge from a population-based to a more "personalized" approach to cancer staging. CA Cancer J Clin. 2017;67:93–9.
10. Ramanathan RC, A'Hern R, Fisher C, Thomas JM. Modified staging system for extremity soft tissue sarcomas. Ann Surg Oncol. 1999;6(1):57–69.
11. Coindre JM, Terrier P, Guillou L, Le Doussal V, Collin F, Ranchere D, et al. Predictive value of grade for metastasis development in the main histologic types of adult soft tissue sarcomas: a study of 1240 patients from the French Federation of Cancer Centers Sarcoma Group. Cancer. 2001;91(10):1914–26.
12. Hashimoto H, Daimaru Y, Takeshita S, Tsuneyoshi M, Enjoji M. Prognostic significance of histologic parameters of soft tissue sarcomas. Cancer. 1992;70(12):2816–22.
13. Lahat G, Tuvin D, Wei C, Anaya DA, Bekele BN, Lazar AJ, et al. New perspectives for staging and prognosis in soft tissue sarcoma. Ann Surg Oncol. 2008;15(10):2739–48.
14. Pisters PW, Leung DH, Woodruff J, Shi W, Brennan MF. Analysis of prognostic factors in 1,041 patients with localized soft tissue sarcomas of the extremities. J Clin Oncol. 1996;14(5):1679–89.
15. Chang UK, Cho WI, Lee DH, Kim MS, Cho CK, Lee SY, et al. Stereotactic radiosurgery for primary and metastatic sarcomas involving the spine. J Neuro-Oncol. 2012;107(3):551–7.
16. Price P, Hoskin PJ, Easton D, Austin D, Palmer SG, Yarnold JR. Prospective randomised trial of single and multifraction radiotherapy schedules in the treatment of painful bony metastases. Radiother Oncol. 1986;6(4):247–55.
17. Wulf J, Haedinger U, Oppitz U, Thiele W, Mueller G, Flentje M. Stereotactic radiotherapy for primary lung cancer and pulmonary metastases: a noninvasive treatment approach in medically inoperable patients. Int J Radiat Oncol Biol Phys. 2004;60(1):186–96.
18. Bae S, Crowe P, Gowda R, Joubert W, Carey-Smith R, Stalley P, et al. Patterns of care for patients with advanced soft tissue sarcoma: experience from Australian sarcoma services. Clin Sarcoma Res. 2016;6:11.

19. Alektiar KM, Brennan MF, Healey JH, Singer S. Impact of intensity-modulated radiation therapy on local control in primary soft-tissue sarcoma of the extremity. J Clin Oncol. 2008;26(20):3440–4.
20. Wilson AN, Davis A, Bell RS, O'Sullivan B, Catton C, Madadi F, et al. Local control of soft tissue sarcoma of the extremity: the experience of a multidisciplinary sarcoma group with definitive surgery and radiotherapy. Eur J Cancer. 1994;30A(6):746–51.
21. Dhakal S, Corbin KS, Milano MT, Philip A, Sahasrabudhe D, Jones C, et al. Stereotactic body radiotherapy for pulmonary metastases from soft-tissue sarcomas: excellent local lesion control and improved patient survival. Int J Radiat Oncol Biol Phys. 2012;82(2):940–5.
22. Folkert MR, Bilsky MH, Tom AK, Oh JH, Alektiar KM, Laufer I, et al. Outcomes and toxicity for hypofractionated and single-fraction image-guided stereotactic radiosurgery for sarcomas metastasizing to the spine. Int J Radiat Oncol Biol Phys. 2014;88(5):1085–91.
23. Levine AM, Coleman C, Horasek S. Stereotactic radiosurgery for the treatment of primary sarcomas and sarcoma metastases of the spine. Neurosurgery. 2009;64(2 Suppl):A54–9.
24. Navarria P, Ascolese AM, Cozzi L, Tomatis S, D'Agostino GR, De Rose F, et al. Stereotactic body radiation therapy for lung metastases from soft tissue sarcoma. Eur J Cancer. 2015;51(5):668–74.
25. Sprave T, Verma V, Forster R, Schlampp I, Bruckner T, Bostel T, et al. Randomized phase II trial evaluating pain response in patients with spinal metastases following stereotactic body radiotherapy versus three-dimensional conformal radiotherapy. Radiother Oncol. 2018;128(2):274–82.
26. Hellman S, Weichselbaum RR. Oligometastases. J Clin Oncol. 1995;13(1):8–10.
27. Baumann BC, Nagda SN, Kolker JD, Levin WP, Weber KL, Berman AT, et al. Efficacy and safety of stereotactic body radiation therapy for the treatment of pulmonary metastases from sarcoma: a potential alternative to resection. J Surg Oncol. 2016;114(1):65–9.
28. Yu W, Tang L, Lin F, Li D, Wang J, Yang Y, et al. Stereotactic radiosurgery, a potential alternative treatment for pulmonary metastases from osteosarcoma. Int J Oncol. 2014;44(4):1091–8.
29. Leeman JE, Bilsky M, Laufer I, Folkert MR, Taunk NK, Osborne JR, et al. Stereotactic body radiotherapy for metastatic spinal sarcoma: a detailed patterns-of-failure study. J Neurosurg Spine. 2016;25(1):52–8.
30. Chao C, Goldberg M. Surgical treatment of metastatic pulmonary soft-tissue sarcoma. Oncology (Williston Park). 2000;14(6):835–41; discussion 42-4, 47
31. Kim S, Ott HC, Wright CD, Wain JC, Morse C, Gaissert HA, et al. Pulmonary resection of metastatic sarcoma: prognostic factors associated with improved outcomes. Ann Thorac Surg. 2011;92(5):1780–6; discussion 6-7
32. Robinson MH, Sheppard M, Moskovic E, Fischer C. Lung metastasectomy in patients with soft tissue sarcoma. Br J Radiol. 1994;67(794):129–35.
33. Shimizu J, Emori M, Murahashi Y, Sonoda T, Mishina T, Miyajima M, et al. Pulmonary metastasectomy is associated with prolonged survival among patients with bone and soft tissue sarcoma. Mol Clin Oncol. 2020;12(5):429–34.
34. Fong Y, Coit DG, Woodruff JM, Brennan MF. Lymph node metastasis from soft tissue sarcoma in adults. Analysis of data from a prospective database of 1772 sarcoma patients. Ann Surg. 1993;217(1):72–7.
35. Riad S, Griffin AM, Liberman B, Blackstein ME, Catton CN, Kandel RA, et al. Lymph node metastasis in soft tissue sarcoma in an extremity. Clin Orthop Relat Res. 2004;426:129–34.
36. Brandal P, Bjerkehagen B, Bruland OS, Skjeldal S, Bogsrud TV, Hall KS. Synchronous and metachronous skeletal osteosarcomas: the Norwegian radium hospital experience. Acta Oncol. 2009;48(8):1165–72.
37. Blakely AM, McPhillips J, Miner TJ. Surgical palliation for malignant disease requiring locoregional control. Ann Palliat Med. 2015;4(2):48–53.
38. Bauer HC. Controversies in the surgical management of skeletal metastases. J Bone Joint Surg Br. 2005;87(5):608–17.

39. Hansen BH, Keller J, Laitinen M, Berg P, Skjeldal S, Trovik C, et al. The Scandinavian sarcoma group skeletal metastasis register. Survival after surgery for bone metastases in the pelvis and extremities. Acta Orthop Scand Suppl. 2004;75(311):11–5.
40. Healey JH, Brown HK. Complications of bone metastases: surgical management. Cancer. 2000;88(12 Suppl):2940–51.
41. Moon BS, Dunbar DJ, Lin PP, Satcher RL, Bird JE, Lewis VO. Is it appropriate to treat sarcoma metastases with intramedullary nailing? Clin Orthop Relat Res. 2017;475(1):212–7.
42. Tanaka T, Imanishi J, Charoenlap C, Choong PF. Intramedullary nailing has sufficient durability for metastatic femoral fractures. World J Surg Oncol. 2016;14:80.
43. Merimsky O, Kollender Y, Inbar M, Chaitchik S, Meller I. Palliative major amputation and quality of life in cancer patients. Acta Oncol. 1997;36(2):151–7.
44. Parsons CM, Pimiento JM, Cheong D, Marzban SS, Gonzalez RJ, Johnson D, et al. The role of radical amputations for extremity tumors: a single institution experience and review of the literature. J Surg Oncol. 2012;105(2):149–55.
45. Cannon CP, Ballo MT, Zagars GK, Mirza AN, Lin PP, Lewis VO, et al. Complications of combined modality treatment of primary lower extremity soft-tissue sarcomas. Cancer. 2006;107(10):2455–61.
46. O'Sullivan B, Davis AM, Turcotte R, Bell R, Catton C, Chabot P, et al. Preoperative versus postoperative radiotherapy in soft-tissue sarcoma of the limbs: a randomised trial. Lancet. 2002;359(9325):2235–41.
47. Peat BG, Bell RS, Davis A, O'Sullivan B, Mahoney J, Manktelow RT, et al. Wound-healing complications after soft-tissue sarcoma surgery. Plast Reconstr Surg. 1994;93(5):980–7.
48. Pezzi CM, Pollock RE, Evans HL, Lorigan JG, Pezzi TA, Benjamin RS, et al. Preoperative chemotherapy for soft-tissue sarcomas of the extremities. Ann Surg. 1990;211(4):476–81.
49. Van Glabbeke M, van Oosterom AT, Oosterhuis JW, Mouridsen H, Crowther D, Somers R, et al. Prognostic factors for the outcome of chemotherapy in advanced soft tissue sarcoma: an analysis of 2,185 patients treated with anthracycline-containing first-line regimens--a European Organization for Research and Treatment of cancer soft tissue and bone sarcoma group study. J Clin Oncol. 1999;17(1):150–7.
50. Schein PS, Winokur SH. Immunosuppressive and cytotoxic chemotherapy: long-term complications. Ann Intern Med. 1975;82(1):84–95.
51. McArthur GA, Demetri GD, van Oosterom A, Heinrich MC, Debiec-Rychter M, Corless CL, et al. Molecular and clinical analysis of locally advanced dermatofibrosarcoma protuberans treated with imatinib: Imatinib target exploration consortium study B2225. J Clin Oncol. 2005;23(4):866–73.
52. Stacchiotti S, Pantaleo MA, Astolfi A, Dagrada GP, Negri T, Dei Tos AP, et al. Activity of sunitinib in extraskeletal myxoid chondrosarcoma. Eur J Cancer. 2014;50(9):1657–64.
53. Wagner AJ, Malinowska-Kolodziej I, Morgan JA, Qin W, Fletcher CD, Vena N, et al. Clinical activity of mTOR inhibition with sirolimus in malignant perivascular epithelioid cell tumors: targeting the pathogenic activation of mTORC1 in tumors. J Clin Oncol. 2010;28(5):835–40.
54. Amankwah EK, Conley AP, Reed DR. Epidemiology and therapies for metastatic sarcoma. Clin Epidemiol. 2013;5:147–62.

FSC
www.fsc.org
MIX
Papier aus verantwortungsvollen Quellen
Paper from responsible sources
FSC® C105338

If you have any concerns about our products,
you can contact us on
ProductSafety@springernature.com

In case Publisher is established outside the EU,
the EU authorized representative is:
Springer Nature Customer Service Center GmbH
Europaplatz 3, 69115 Heidelberg, Germany

Printed by Libri Plureos GmbH
in Hamburg, Germany